ART THERAPY *in* MUSEUMS AND GALLERIES

of related interest

Art Therapy with Older Adults
Connected and Empowered
Erin Partridge
ISBN 978 1 78592 824 6
eISBN 978 1 78450 940 8

Art Therapy with Adults with Autism Spectrum Disorder
Beth Gonzalez-Dolginko
ISBN 978 1 78592 831 4
eISBN 978 1 78450 972 9

The Handbook of Art Therapy and Digital Technology
Edited by Cathy Malchiodi, PhD
Foreword by Dr Val Huet
ISBN 978 1 78592 792 8
eISBN 978 1 78450 774 9

Portrait Therapy
Resolving Self-Identity Disruption in Clients with Life-Threatening and Chronic Illnesses
Susan M. D. Carr
ISBN 978 1 78592 293 0
eISBN 978 1 78450 605 6

Art Therapy in Private Practice
Theory, Practice and Research in Changing Contexts
Edited by James D. West
Forewords by Joan Woddis and Chris Wood
ISBN 978 1 78592 043 1
eISBN 978 1 78450 297 3

Art Therapy and Substance Abuse
Enabling Recovery from Alcohol and Other Drug Addiction
Libby Schmanke
ISBN 978 1 78592 792 8
eISBN 978 1 78450 774 9

ART THERAPY *in* MUSEUMS AND GALLERIES

Reframing Practice

EDITED BY ALI COLES AND HELEN JURY

FOREWORD BY JORDAN POTASH

Jessica Kingsley Publishers

London and Philadelphia

First published in 2020
by Jessica Kingsley Publishers
73 Collier Street
London N1 9BE, UK
and
400 Market Street, Suite 400
Philadelphia, PA 19106, USA

www.jkp.com

Library of Congress Cataloging in Publication Data
A CIP catalog record for this book is available from the Library of Congress

British Library Cataloguing in Publication Data
A CIP catalogue record for this book is available from the British Library

ISBN 978 1 78592 411 8
eISBN 978 1 78450 775 6

Printed and bound in Great Britain

Contents

About the Front Cover Image 11
Helen Jury

Foreword 13
Jordan Potash

Acknowledgements 15

Introduction 16
Helen Jury and Ali Coles

Part I The Context

Chapter 1 Art Therapy in Museums and Galleries: Evidence and Research 26
Sue Holttum

Chapter 2 What Do Museums Mean?: Public Perceptions of the Purposes of Museums and Implications for their Use in Art Therapy 44
Ali Coles

Chapter 3 *Making Space Safe* at Modern Art Oxford 63
Mary Chamberlain

Part 2 Art Therapists Working with Museums and Galleries

Chapter 4 From Isolation to Relation: Reflections on the Development of Museum-Based Art Therapy in Russia 82
Nana Zhvitiashvili

Chapter 5 *Starting with Art*: Ben Uri Artworks as a Stimulus for Art Psychotherapy in Dementia Care 108
Emma Hollamby, Elaine Homer and Jane Landes

Chapter 6 *Creative Dialogues*: A Journey from Recovery to Discovery for People Using Drug and Alcohol Services 133
Simon Hackett, Ruth McGovern and Fiona Fitzpatrick

Chapter 7 The Caring Museum/Le Musée qui soigne: Art Therapy at the Montreal Museum of Fine Arts 157
Stephen Legari, Marilyn Lajeunesse and Louise Giroux

Chapter 8 Expanding the Frame: Developing and Sustaining a Long-Term NHS Art Museum Partnership Within a Workforce Development Strategy for Enhanced Quality of Care 181
Sheila Grandison

Chapter 9 Art Therapy at the Bilbao Fine Arts Museum: A Gaze Through Emotions, Culture and Social Integration 202
Karen Lund

Chapter 10 BALTIC Art Therapy Project: A Collaboration Between NHS Art Therapists and BALTIC Centre for Contemporary Art Gateshead 223
Michael Fischer and Whittaker Scott

Part 3 Wider Perspectives

Chapter 11 Further Conversations with Rembrandt in Space, Place and Time: How Rembrandt's Self-Portraits and the Gallery Setting Inform the Art Psychotherapy Review 244
Helen Jury

Chapter 12 Temporary, Portable and Virtual: Making Galleries on the France–UK Border at Calais 265
Miriam Usiskin, Bobby Lloyd and Naomi Press

Chapter 13 Art Therapy and Museums in the Colombian Context: Co-leading Collective Transformations 289
Andrée Salom

Biographies 310

Subject Index 313

Author Index 317

Figures

Figure 3.1 *Making Space Safe* shelf within the storage cupboard 71

Figure 3.2 The Project Space (photo credit: Stu Allsop) 73

Figure 3.3 'Our' corner in the Project Space 74

Figure 3.4 The basement space 75

Figure 4.1 Ivan Aivazovsky, 'The Ninth Wave' (1850), oil on canvas, © State Russian Museum, St Petersburg 91

Figure 4.2 Painted sculptures. 'From monologue to dialogue' workshop (1997) 95

Figure 4.3 'The Shadow' by patient A (2017) 103

Figure 5.1 Samuel Hirszenberg, 'Sabbath Rest' (1894), oil on canvas. Ben Uri Collection 119

Figure 5.2 Chana Kowalska, 'Shtetl' (1934), oil on canvas. Ben Uri Collection 119

Figure 5.3 Alfred Wolmark, 'In the Synagogue' (1906), oil on canvas. Ben Uri Collection 120

Figure 5.4 David Breuer-Weil, 'The Edge' (2007), oil on canvas. Ben Uri Collection 122

Figure 5.5 Albert, 'Waiting in Line', pencil and pastel drawing 125

Figure 6.1 Doing an Orozco 143

Figure 6.2 Collective collage workshop 144

Figure 6.3 The flyer invitation 149

Figure 6.4 The exhibition 149

Figure 6.5 The exhibition: detail 150

Figure 7.1 Alberto Martini, 'Self-Portrait' (1929), oil on canvas. The Montreal Museum of Fine Arts, purchase, Horsley and Annie Townsend Bequest. Photo MMFA, Brian Merrett 164

Figure 7.2 'Totem-Muses', collective artwork by participants from Le Cap 165

Figure 7.3 'Expérience de mort imminente' ('Near Death Experience'), part of the *contrasts* project. Participant artwork portraying experience as a patient with traumatic brain injury 169

Figure 7.4 *Sharing the Museum* (*Le Musée en partage*) (Photo: Pierre Arsenault) 176

Figure 8.1 Connecting: Art as a bridge across site and context 184

Left: Entrance to the Newham Centre for Mental Health. Supplied courtesy of East London NHS Foundation Trust. Photo credit: © Sheila Grandison, 2012

Centre: Tate Modern from St Paul's, 2016, Tate Photography. © Tate, London 2019

Right: '4 casb 2 '67', 1967; Barry Flanagan (1941–2009). Purchased 1976; © The estate of Barry Flanagan/ Bridgeman Images; Photo © Tate, London 2019

Figure 8.2 'Babel' 2001; Cildo Meireles (born 1948). Purchased jointly by Tate, London (with the assistance of the Latin American Acquisitions Committee) and the D. Daskalopoulos Collection, 2013, as a promised gift to Tate; © Cildo Meireles; Photo © Tate, London 2019 198

Figure 9.1 Participant artwork after viewing 'The Rape of Europa' 216

Figure 9.2 Participant artwork after visiting the 'Messages from the Wall' exhibition 218

Figure 9.3 Participant artwork after viewing 'Albia' 219

Figure 10.1 BALTIC 225

Figure 12.1 Plasticine installation 272
Figure 12.2 Stage-managing the boat 274
Figure 12.3 Postcard exhibition on the table 276
Figure 12.4 Drawing postcards in the shipping container 278
Figure 12.5 Viewing the map and exhibition 280
Figure 12.6 Viewing the map at night 281
Figure 13.1 'La Lechuga' (drawing by author) 294
Figure 13.2 A personal chiva (drawing by author) 304

About the Front Cover Image

Helen Jury

Cover artwork: © Philippa Beveridge
Photography: © Paul Louis

'Lost and Found'

> 'Lost and Found' is a series of works created during my artist's residency in France and deals with the concept of collective and individual identity through the everyday form of a purse: an object which is often lost, stolen or mislaid, an easily identifiable form which fits into the hand or a pocket and contains hidden memories – a testimony to a stage of their life. To create this body of work, I invited the local residents to visit the studio and show me the contents of their purses. I then photographed the different elements and transferred the imagery onto glass which I then cast into moulds. The images distort as the glass melts, leaving imprints of the objects and clues, or traces of their owners' identities. (Philippa Beveridge)

Philippa Beveridge's work connects to many of the chapters in this book. Her work questions the idea of temporality and how belongings that are lost still retain personal memories, using notions of time, memory and identity. In her artwork, Philippa captures in glass the ephemeral memories connected with the idea of the lost item. This bears relevance to the place of the museum and gallery, where the collections and displays inspire us to engage with our personal responses and histories and to question anew our relationship with objects and artworks, revealing emotions and feelings – sometimes hitherto unexplored. These ideas can be encapsulated in the artwork and museum objects that, as Philippa has discovered with glass, can be both robust and delicate at the same time. Through using memories as source material, she crafts an object that takes on the character of the memories and emotional stimulus that inspired it. We are given the opportunity to view the inner world of the person who might have owned the purse and to glimpse their memories and identity, made visually and materially permanent. Philippa describes the 'parallel between what we want to reveal and what we want to keep private, intimate or secret' (Beveridge in Van Butsele 2010). This is similar to the art therapy practice explored in this book where, through making artwork, clients discover how to balance a sense of self and identity with encountering what memories and emotions reveal to them.

Philippa Beveridge was born in London in 1962. She studied Landscape Architecture at the University of Greenwich, and then Glass at the Massana School of Applied Arts in Barcelona, where she lived until 2018. She received the Jutta Cuny-Franz Memorial Award in 2003, and in 2006 the Barcelona ARTFAD (Association of Art and Design) first prize, alongside gaining a master's degree in Art in Architecture at the University of East London. She has taught in the USA and Europe and directed the Syracuse University Visual Arts Study Abroad programme from 2005 to 2010. Her website is www.philippabeveridge.com.

Reference

Van Butsele, G. (2010) Catalogue: *Philippa Beveridge, Lost and Found/Objets Trouvés*. Conseil Général, Département du Nord, Musée-atelier du verre à Sar-Poteries.

Foreword

Jordan Potash

I am fortunate to live in Washington DC, a city known for politics but which also has a rich arts scene. Out of the range of available history, science and cultural museums, I frequently find myself returning to the National Gallery of Art. Sometimes it is to visit an old favourite artwork, such as Thomas Cole's existential 'Voyage of Life' series or Wayne Thiebaud's inviting 'Cakes'. Other times it is to wander through the collection, perhaps for a fantastical escape into Alexander Calder's mobiles. Still other times, it is to meet something new. Within a two-year period, I was introduced to the work of artists Theaster Gates and Rachel Whiteread (National Gallery of Art 2017, 2018). Gates, an American black man from Chicago, Illinois, seeks out abandoned places, deconstructs them, and reconstructs sculptures that combine original narratives with new ones. Whiteread, a British white woman from London, casts the negative expanse of rooms and around furniture to call our attention to the in-between. Gates invites viewers to repurpose and recontextualise places while honouring their original purpose, whereas Whiteread offers an opportunity to contemplate what is obvious about an area but untouched.

When I reflect on these exhibits, I am enthralled by the intersection of how they alter conceptions of space in thoughtful and intentional ways. Like these two artists, art therapists have always found ways to re-invigorate overlooked settings, such as dark basements, locked wards, converted broom closets and dilapidated store fronts. It only makes sense that art therapists have discovered the potential of high culture forums to transform them from leisurely, art for art's sake, educational, or scholarly purposes, into public opportunities for promoting health and social concerns. Like Gates, art therapists have mined historical artefacts and celebrated artworks to encourage clients, students and workshop participants to further personal insight, strengthen relationships and consider social issues. Like Whiteread, art therapists have discovered the unseen potential to benefit health and mental health goals, as well as to foster cross-cultural engagement.

I have frequently utilised the museums in my work as both an art therapist and educator. The editors and contributors of this volume conceptualise how revisioning spaces, both galleries and studios, can firmly integrate the grand purposes of museums and the noble pursuits of art therapy. Even though these projects take place outside the traditional milieu of clinics, hospitals, schools and community studios, they honour core art therapy tenets. In responding to exhibits, we find that the creative process furthers meaning-making. By considering alternative approaches to viewing collections, we discover that metaphor heightens symbolic communication. In developing a professional relationship, purposeful structure allows for meaningful encounters to occur. Museums and art therapy in partnership unleash vast opportunities for encouraging each of these distinct fields to discover how their overlooked spaces are creative grounds for inspiration, imagination and wellbeing to flourish.

Jordan Potash
Associate Professor, Art Therapy Program,
The George Washington University and Editor in Chief
of *Art Therapy: Journal of the American Art Therapy Association*

References

National Gallery of Art (2017) 'Theaster Gates Presents New Body of Work in Solo Exhibition at National Gallery of Art, Washington.' National Gallery of Art. Accessed on 21/2/19 at www.nga.gov/press/exh/4927.html.

National Gallery of Art (2018) 'Rachel Whiteread.' National Gallery of Art. Accessed on 21/2/19 at www.nga.gov/exhibitions/2018/rachel-whiteread.html.

Acknowledgements

We would like to thank all the art therapists and other professionals who have inspired us to explore the potential of museums and galleries for art therapy, including members of the British Association of Art Therapists' Museums and Galleries Special Interest Group, which was co-founded by Siân Hutchinson and Ali Coles. Thank you also to all our family members; without their support and encouragement this book would not have come to fruition.

Helen Jury and Ali Coles

Introduction

Helen Jury and Ali Coles

Art Therapy in Museums and Galleries is a timely book, exploring emergent and original thinking and practice in international clinical work in these settings. This is an area of increasing interest to those in the art therapy profession, and the past few years have seen an upsurge in cooperation and partnership between museums, galleries and art therapists, evident in the response to our call for chapters for this book. We are grateful to all those who responded and are delighted to showcase some of this work here, as well as theoretical perspectives that can inform this way of working. This book is the first to present an international view of art therapy in museum and gallery settings and is wide-ranging both in its geographical scope and in terms of client groups; the chapters span Canada to Colombia, Euskadi to East London, children using mental health services to adults and minors in refugee camps.

For the purposes of this book, we consider art therapy to be an activity undertaken by trained art therapists or art psychotherapists. In the UK, for example, the titles 'art therapist' and 'art psychotherapist' are legally protected and those entering the profession require training at master's level and registration with the Health and Care Professions Council (HCPC), demonstrating consideration of the unique role they hold in implementing safe and specialised therapeutic work. It is art therapists' specialised skills that are invaluable in partnerships with settings such as museums and galleries, where community engagement involves working with people who are vulnerable and who might have mental health issues or other difficulties. Museum and gallery professionals are increasingly working with art therapists to re-address the function, scope and meaning of their collections and the opportunities they can offer to the public, in novel and creative ways. At the same time, art therapists are recognising the huge potential of museum and gallery collections and environments for therapeutic work, enabling self-exploration, empowerment and social inclusion. *Art Therapy in Museums and Galleries* is the first book to explore this exciting and resourceful practice which makes an important contribution to the ever-evolving field of art therapy, and we are very grateful to the chapter authors for sharing their knowledge, expertise and insight.

The first part of the book deals with the context for art therapy work in museums and galleries. In Chapter 1, Sue Holttum, applied psychologist and part-time research officer for the British Association of Art Therapists, sets the scene by reviewing some of the key published literature relating to art therapy work in museums and galleries from the past 20 years, including placing this within the wider arts and health arena. The projects she describes span a wide range of client groups and geographical areas, and Holttum uses hypotheses about the health benefits of arts activities in cultural settings and therapeutic factors in art therapy as a basis for exploring how museum and gallery settings have contributed to therapeutic efficacy in the art therapy projects she considers. Finally, Holttum identifies the need for more evidence in this area of work, and suggests how art therapists can evaluate and research their practice in order to advance this work.

Chapter 2 considers how commonly held perceptions about museums (including galleries with collections) might affect engagement in, and experiences of, museum-based art therapy. Ali Coles draws on research undertaken in the UK with the general public about the roles and purposes of museums (including galleries with collections) and considers how the key findings relate to art therapy in these settings. She concludes that many of these public perceptions resonate with key therapeutic principles within art therapy, such as those of holding and containing, trust, exploration and learning, play and acceptance, which suggests that museums have great potential as partners for art therapy practice. Coles also explores how museums might be conducive to addressing issues related to knowing and not knowing, care and neglect, fear, abuse of power, and difference and diversity, relating this to current debates in the museum world, and anticipating a time when the therapeutic value of museums is commonly recognised.

In Chapter 3, Mary Chamberlain explores the concept of 'safe spaces' in the context of a gallery setting, through the lens of an art group for refugees and asylum seekers at a museum in Oxford, England. Discussing the influence of the creative and cultural nature of the setting for the group as well as the impact of the particular characteristics of the spaces that are used, Chamberlain focuses on the structures, both internal and external, psychological and physical, which help to make a space feel safe, drawing on therapeutic principles from art therapy. In the gallery setting, she has created a safe space that provides participants with a sense of being seen and cared for, and which encourages agency and control, in distinct contrast to what they may have experienced in the outside world.

Part 2 contains descriptions of, and reflections on, art therapy work with museums and galleries from around the world, in a variety of institutional frameworks and with a range of client groups. Nana Zhvitiashvili reflects on her work as a museum curator in Russia in the 1990s in Chapter 4. Motivated by a desire for integration, equality and respect, she collaborated with a psychologist to bring together museums and art therapy approaches in projects for marginalised people, a process that was influenced by the post-communist political, cultural and social transformations at that time. The chapter focuses particularly on a project for young people with learning difficulties, and Zhvitiashvili, now a qualified art psychotherapist, identifies the key factors for the efficacy of museum-based art therapy based on her experiences. She makes general recommendations that will be of use to others when developing work of this kind and which she has applied in her current museum-based art therapy work with oncology patients (children and adults) at a private hospital in London. Zhvitiashvili also explores the resonances between curatorial and art therapy practice from her dual perspective as curator and art psychotherapist, discussing key ideas which inform both areas of work.

Chapter 5 takes us to recent work in the UK, where a small London art gallery established a partnership with an art therapy training institution and an experienced art therapy supervisor to deliver a project for older adults living with dementia. Emma Hollamby, Elaine Homer and Jane Landes describe how the project was established, and reflect on how the gallery collections were used as the focus for weekly art therapy groups in a National Health Service day centre, as well as how visits to temporary exhibitions and curatorial talks contributed to therapeutic outcomes. In particular, they discuss the influence of the collections' themes of migration and identity on the therapeutic work with this client group, showing how the gallery's collection helped group members to tell their own stories, create artwork, and connect to each other, to the gallery and to wider cultural life.

In Chapter 6, Simon Hackett, Ruth McGovern and Fiona Fitzpatrick present a case study of an arts and museums project in northern England for people using drug and alcohol services, which included visits to museums and galleries and an exhibition of the participants' work. Drawing on theory associated with the concept of recovery capital, the project was devised to span the three overlapping areas of art therapy, visual and fine arts practice, and museums/galleries and health and wellbeing, and was co-led by an art therapist, artists, museum staff and drug and alcohol recovery centre staff. It aimed to stimulate creative dialogues in order to help participants to develop their confidence, social networks and community engagement, and participants had the opportunity to be creators, art critics, curators and exhibitors. The authors conclude that creative engagement with museums and galleries can support people who are in recovery from substance misuse, noting the importance of the role of the art therapist in providing a safe framework for the therapeutic work.

Chapter 7, by Stephen Legari, Marilyn Lajeunesse and Louise Giroux, describes pioneering work in Montreal in a fine arts museum where the first full-time art therapy post in the world in a museum context has been established, and where art therapy is now fully integrated. The post has a mandate to facilitate work with a variety of client groups, to collaborate in research, supervise, and manage a community studio to implement projects for wellbeing. Humanistic principles and art therapy practice guide the foundation of projects, with integration of art therapy trainings that benefit from engaging in clinical opportunities and research in the context of the museum setting. Projects are co-created with organisations and agencies, thereby benefiting from close collaboration with other experts in their field and allowing the authors to conclude that here, art therapy in the museum is thriving.

Similarly, Sheila Grandison's work in Chapter 8 highlights the advantages that can be gained by long-term, phased projects in partnership with museum and NHS (UK National Health Service) professionals, and how each profession's skills set can benefit both the client group and those working with them. Drawing on the varying levels of cultural access available to mental health service users in a deprived part of London, Grandison calls our attention to promoting cultural understanding and working with the community. Over three phases of a project that is ongoing, she and her colleagues have developed a flexible working model to provide gallery-based training with both the client group and staff working with them for reflecting on compassionate care creatively. Their ideas and practice have bridged in-patient and cultural sites, building greater links between an NHS Trust and a major gallery eight miles away.

Chapter 9, by Karen Lund, explores art therapy and social projects with a fine arts museum in northern Spain, outlining the benefits of a participatory meeting space for people at risk of social exclusion. She emphasises the institution's community role and refers to the range of client groups involved, from offenders to unprotected minors in foster homes. The important role of the art therapist to safeguard the emotional frame for participants is outlined. She describes working closely with the museum, which employed her as a member of staff to facilitate the groups. Using artwork in the museum, Lund explores cultural heritage, enabling and empowering group members to express artistic responses and safely communicate feelings and thoughts. Group members are integrated into public life and enjoy improved participation in their community environment, negating a tendency towards isolation. The gallery as a sensory space acts as an instigator for group members' personal responses, and Lund emphasises the positive responses from collaborating staff who view museum users from a new perspective.

Michael Fischer and Whittaker Scott, in Chapter 10, describe another model of collaborative working in a contemporary art gallery in Gateshead, England. They developed a project with the NHS for children and young people, questioning what it was about the gallery encounter that could add to art therapy group experience. They provide evidence of the feasibility of their project and results, so others can use this experience to establish similar projects. A central tenet of the work is the belief that for art therapists and artists, art galleries add something to the therapeutic process through the environment, which is inspirational to young people. The aim of the project was accessing hard-to-reach adolescents to address issues around confidence-building, self-esteem and relationships. Young people had the opportunity to learn new skills from the freelance artist and exhibit their own artwork in response to an exhibition, aiding promotion of positive mental health awareness in the community. This chapter demonstrates intricacies, benefits and challenges in developing a flexible balance between reflective and educational elements, and in overseeing working relationships with gallery staff, resident artists and NHS management.

Part 3 considers wider perspectives on the interaction between art therapy and museums and galleries and here, in Chapter 11, Helen Jury considers how galleries and art collections extend our thinking around the scope of art therapy not only theoretically, but also as practising artists. She details how responses to the two Rembrandt self-portraits in the National Gallery in London, and development of ideas concerning keeping them in mind, informed concepts around time, place, space and the roles of the review and supervision in art therapy. Jury draws on parallels between absence and presence of the image in the therapy space; how we hold in mind individual and collective artworks of the client is considered, along with thoughts and feelings about artwork that are evoked in the review. She refers to the collapse of sense of time and its impact on clients when their artwork is set out collectively, side by side as in a gallery setting, and how the psychological effect of different temporal structures can be considered theoretically, through drawing on our experience of gallery viewing. Supervision is considered in relation to clients' artwork in the absence of the client, with the opportunity to develop explorative approaches.

In Chapter 12, Miriam Usiskin, Bobby Lloyd and Naomi Press discuss a radical approach to working with psychosocial groups, through crisis support for refugees living in transit on the France–UK border at Calais. They refer to the setting becoming multipurpose and multifunctional, interpersonal and improvisational, responding to the necessary humanitarian needs of the population group that is both homeless and highly vulnerable. They describe how, at times, the potential spaces occupied by the art therapists and participants become temporary, virtual and portable galleries, thereby recognising the importance and significance of the art object as a constant in otherwise impermanent and insecure surroundings. They describe the work that has been carried out in this context with partner organisations responding to the needs of the refugees, and how their methods and planning as a team are an essential element of their successful interventions. Mapping, representation of the experience of the refugees, context-specific materials and exploration of refugee experience are all recounted, as well as theoretical underpinnings as rationale for this provision of psychological, virtual – and at times physical – gallery space.

Chapter 13 explores how art therapists can unlock the therapeutic potential of museum exhibitions. In the particular context of the political situation in Colombia and the way in which arts in health and art therapy work has developed in that country, Andrée Salom focuses on four particular exhibitions. She frames them in therapeutic terms and describes art therapy directives which could be used to enhance their therapeutic efficacy for informal museum visitors as well as scheduled groups, considering the possibility of delivering art therapy to large numbers of people or to individual visitors wishing to engage on a personal level with exhibits. She argues that a union between art therapy and museums results in the transformation of both fields, and that it can also be transformational for the individual in terms of how they view and experience the world, thus facilitating reparation and social justice.

These chapters form an exciting and impressive collection of projects and theoretical viewpoints from which to consider an expansion of the already growing work in this field, and the foreword from Jordan Potash in the USA reiterates how, as both artists and art therapists, we bring exceptional and innovative skills to work in conjunction with museum and gallery settings. The chapters demonstrate versatile and original thinking in developing new projects and responding to gallery and museum resources, confirming the huge potential for collaborations between art therapy and museums and galleries. We believe that this book represents only a fraction of the work that is taking place in this area internationally and we hope that it will inspire others to develop, expand and share this area of practice in the future.

Please note: Chapter authors have obtained the necessary consents to include information about clients and service users, and pseudonyms have been used to ensure anonymity.

PART I

The Context

CHAPTER 1

Art Therapy in Museums and Galleries

Evidence and Research

Sue Holttum

Introduction

In this chapter, I describe work by art therapists in museums and galleries, draw out the contribution of the settings, and suggest ways forward for research. I am engaged in art therapy research as an applied psychologist at England's Canterbury Christ Church University, and as part-time research officer for the British Association of Art Therapists. It would be difficult to do justice here to the full range of innovative work by art therapists in museums and galleries, so I focus on just a few projects from the past 20 years. My aim is to discuss work that art therapists are doing in museums and galleries with a range of participant groups and in different countries.

Art therapy in museums and galleries has been seen as one of a number of kinds of arts and health approaches, and was included in the UK's All-Party Parliamentary Group on Arts, Health and Wellbeing (APPGAHW) report (2017). This report suggested two main ways in which arts and health projects may produce benefits for their participants. First, the report suggested that the enriched environment of arts engagement may reverse harmful effects of deprivation and stress. The report drew on a biopsychosocial model and understandings of animal and human biology (e.g. Bygren 2013;

Rasmuson *et al.* 1998). Environmental stresses can affect our genes, determining whether certain genes are switched on or off (Borghol *et al.* 2012). New knowledge has also indicated that the human brain continues to adapt and grow new brain cells throughout life (see Cozolino 2018 for an overview), and one study has reported beneficial brain changes in response to art classes for older people in a museum (Bolwerk *et al.* 2014). If we draw on Bygren (2013), enrichment may be provided not only through cultural venues and their exhibits, but also through the opportunities afforded for social connection, interaction, creativity and play during participation.

The second proposed therapeutic mechanism in the APPGAHW (2017) report was the way that absorption in arts activities may reduce stress hormones through calming, and there is some evidence to support this in relation to drumming (Fancourt *et al.* 2016) and art therapy (Visnola *et al.* 2010). Considered alongside evidence that simply visiting museums and galleries and viewing artworks can be calming (Clow and Fredhoi 2006; Roberts, Camic and Springham 2011), it seems possible that a museum and gallery setting can add to any calming effect of arts activities themselves.

A variety of hypotheses have been put forward regarding the way in which art therapy in its own right may yield therapeutic benefits. The review by Gabel and Robb (2017) is particularly relevant in that it examined group art therapy, the form most often used in museums and galleries. Gabel and Robb (2017) reviewed 119 sources across art therapy teaching material, practice reports and empirical studies, and suggested five main mechanisms of action for group art therapy. Their reviewed literature incorporated clients across the lifespan and in different contexts (medical, psychiatric, wellbeing and re-habilitation). Their five suggested mechanisms were: symbolic expression (the use and sharing of symbols), relational aesthetics (communication and attachment through artworks), embodiment (expressing mental contents through art-related actions), pleasure and play (relaxation and mastery through interacting with and manipulating art materials), and ritual (special places such as the art studio and consistent boundaries and practice). The following section explores how a museum or gallery setting might contribute to these, and other, therapeutic aspects of art therapy practice.

Evidence on art therapy involving museums and galleries

People diagnosed with cancers

Deane, Fitch and Carman (2000) evaluated 16 sessions of art therapy for 21 people with cancer diagnoses in Canada. Participants received a tour of the McMichael Canadian Art Collection, and then made art in a studio with the art therapist. Deane *et al.* (2000) evaluated the programme using a questionnaire and audio-recorded telephone interviews. They reported that both the gallery tour and hearing stories about artworks and artists inspired participants to create their own expressive artwork. Deane *et al.* (2000) also reported that some participants found new ability to discuss their condition with friends and family, thus increasing their ongoing support, which became possible once participants had depicted unspoken emotional material and verbalised it with support from the art therapist.

While this may have been possible without inspiration from the gallery tour, some participants appeared to find learning about the artists and gallery artworks helpful in enabling them to be creative in their own use of art for expression and self-exploration. Many enjoyed learning about art and artists, and some continued to visit art galleries or engaged further in other arts such as theatre.

Young people

Some art therapy projects in museums and galleries have involved young people. Linesch (2004) piloted art therapy in the USA's Museum of Tolerance, which houses exhibits concerning the Holocaust. In a young people's five-day summer camp, where the focus was learning about tolerance, participants toured the museum with a guide and made art in a group with an art therapist in response to the exhibits. At the end of the week they exhibited their artwork. Although Linesch (2004) did not conduct a formal evaluation, she suggested that art therapy facilitated an 'experience of museum viewing that transitions the participant from passive viewer to self-expressive artist and potential exhibitor' (p.57). This suggests that basing art therapy in a museum or gallery might bolster the potential for identity transformation of art therapy participants through an artist status (Thompson 2009; Wood 1997).

Also in the USA, Treadon, Rosal and Thompson Wylder (2006) piloted group art therapy for seven secondary school children with behavioural and emotional problems. Numerous studies have implicated environmental stress in the development of such problems (e.g. McLaughlin 2016; Sandler *et al.* 2015). The children worked partly at school and partly in an art museum. Treadon *et al.* (2006) did not report outcomes formally, but suggested that participants developed new interests in art and gained confidence in school art classes. The children were absorbed in the activities and surprised their teachers by their 'lack of resistance or negative behaviours' (Treadon *et al.* 2006, p.299). They were able to connect with the artworks and produce their own expressive art with technical support from the art therapists.

Family carers of people with severe mental health diagnoses

In the UK, Shaer *et al.* (2008) aimed to enable mental health service users and carers (in separate groups) to create podcasts about their experiences, using artworks in London's Tate Britain gallery to stimulate discussion followed by the opportunity to make art. Shaer *et al.* (2008, p.31) stated, 'Participants greatly increased their understanding and engagement of both gallery paintings and their own images through a relationship negotiated via shared viewing.' As with Linesch (2004) and Deane *et al.* (2000), the art therapist here contained the participants' emotional reactions to difficult themes when viewing exhibits and making art.

Building on Shaer *et al.* (2008), Roberts *et al.* (2011) evaluated a two-session group art-viewing and art-making programme for eight family carers of people with severe mental health problems, again in Tate Britain. Participants appreciated the venue as providing a sense of privilege and as a safe space. In one participant's words, it was 'like being somewhere very grand or something...and just for you' (Roberts *et al.* 2011, p.154). Interest in art increased, and viewing a tranquil seascape reminded some participants of their capacity for coping by being outdoors or by the sea, for relaxation.

Mental health staff

Huet (2011) also built on Shaer *et al.* (2008), again employing art-viewing and art-making in Tate Britain. Huet (2011, p.3) referred to her one-off session as piloting 'art therapy-based organisational consultancy' for staff who cared for residents of a forensic learning disabilities unit. The curator told the artist's story, inviting a human connection to art and artist, and Huet (2011) suggested that this facilitated participants' subsequent artworks that depicted powerful work-stress themes. Two of the viewed artworks portrayed people without homes, and among the themes Huet (2011) identified through using thematic analysis (Braun and Clarke 2006), the pictures prompted staff to voice their feelings about their clients being seen as outsiders and about themselves being marginalised due to their work.

Older people

Salom (2011) piloted museum-based art therapy in Colombia for ten older people resident in a care home, which involved a visit to the Archaeological Museum in Bogotá. The aim was to allow them to connect to their past through the Archaeological Museum and its exhibits, and to open up to new experiences. Salom (2011) proposed therapeutic roles for museums, for example 'museum as group' (p.83) due to containing objects that signify a range of human experience. Thus, participants can have their own experiences validated by museum objects as they can do by other therapy group members, a therapeutic factor that Yalom (1995) termed universality (Salom 2011).

Many publications have reported evaluations of arts and health projects in different countries with older people in museums and art galleries, and I mention these in passing because they tend to involve artists, but not art therapists (e.g. Age and Opportunity 2012; Flatt *et al.* 2015; Harper and Hamblin 2010; McGuigan, Leggett and Horsburgh 2015). The aim of many of these projects is to improve the social inclusion and general wellbeing of older people, often in the context of dementia and with an emphasis on stimulation and enjoyment rather than processing difficult feelings or psychological issues. They use the museum or art gallery to assist in this aim, and benefits may accrue partly through the enriched environment discussed in the APPGAHW (2017) report. As the study by Bolwerk *et al.* (2014) suggested, art-based activities in a museum or gallery may lead to positive brain changes for older people. However, as has been illustrated already, art therapists often work with the expression of difficult feelings and thoughts.

Adults with severe mental health difficulties

In a UK study, Colbert *et al.* (2013) interviewed seven participants with psychosis-related diagnoses after a four-session programme of art-viewing and art-making, at the Dulwich Picture Gallery in London. Consistent with Linesch (2004), Colbert *et al.* (2013, p.255) suggested that there was 'the emergence of a sense of personhood over patienthood or professionalism' in that both mental health professionals and service users began to see themselves and each other as part of the 'socially valued community of gallery-goers and art-makers'. For one mental health service user, seeing strong emotion in a painting ('Samson and Delilah' by Anthony Van Dyck) contributed to his sense of strong emotion becoming seen as normal rather than being a sign of illness. This seems to echo Salom's (2011) description of museum objects as representing human life and providing a sense of universality (Yalom 1995).

Coles and Harrison (2018) describe an 18-session art therapy programme in two museums in Gloucester, England. Seven of their ten participants with severe mental health difficulties completed the programme. Their mixed-methods systematic case study included three short validated measures: the University College London (UCL) Museum Wellbeing Measure for young adults (Thomson and Chatterjee 2013), the Psychological Outcome Profiles (PSYCHLOPS, Ashworth *et al.* 2005), which allows service users to set their own therapy goals and rate their progress on these, and the Rosenberg Self-Esteem Scale (Rosenberg 1989). Five of the seven participants self-reported as improved on PSYCHLOPS. Two who rated themselves as slightly worse had experienced difficult life circumstances during the programme, and this finding highlights the value of gathering additional contextual data. The mean change was positive, with a large effect size, indicating clinically as well as statistically significant change. Self-rated changes on the self-esteem scale were smaller but consistent with PSYCHLOPS. Scores on the UCL Museum Wellbeing Measure after each session suggested positive feelings.

Coles and Harrison (2018) outline the possible contribution of the museum settings and exhibits, which their qualitative data seemed to support. First, participants could make emotional connections with exhibits and express these emotions in their own artworks, which in turn seemed to assist self-understanding. Second, exploring boxes of museum objects or viewing exhibits together fostered playfulness, communication and mutual understanding, as when several people chose the same object and it elicited similar feelings. Some participants began to meet for coffee before sessions and formed friendships, which suggests the enhancement of social connection as in Deane *et al.* (2000) and Delucia (2016). Third, attending the activities in museums helped participants to feel like 'a person not a patient' (Coles and Harrison 2018, p.122). This is reminiscent of Linesch (2004) and Colbert *et al.* (2013). Fourth, the museum settings and exhibits appeared to inspire participants' imagination and creativity. Some participants became motivated to set themselves artistic and other goals, such as getting to the museum on public transport.

It appears that the participants' gains were facilitated by the therapeutic context and approach, beginning with boxes of museum objects within a confidential space for early sessions, and then moving out into the museum and to another museum later on. One could suggest that the therapists gradually increased the terrain for exploration in line with the progress of attachment via the triangular relationship. Gabel and Robb (2017) located the triangular relationship within what they saw as the larger concept of relational aesthetics operating in group art therapy. They defined relational aesthetics as 'the overlapping triangular relationships between group members, artworks and leaders' (Gabel and Robb 2017, p.129), and reported this concept to be present in 64 per cent of the 119 sources reviewed. In museums and galleries, the artworks and surroundings may extend what is possible in clinical settings by significantly expanding the available space for the operation of relational aesthetics (see also Coles, Harrison and Todd 2019).

Military veterans

Delucia (2016) in the USA has described group art therapy with the opportunity to exhibit artwork in a community-based art therapy studio and gallery dedicated to veterans. Delucia (2016) suggested that when participants exhibited their artwork they experienced empathy from viewers, stating that when friends and family visited the gallery and saw veterans' artwork, some veterans were able to discuss distressing experiences with them for the first time.

Experiential avoidance (a feature of persistent post-traumatic stress) was the focus in Lobban and Murphy's (2018) two-week residential programme of art therapy for four veterans with a diagnosis of post-traumatic stress disorder (PTSD) at UK charity Combat Stress. The programme included two art therapy sessions (viewing and making) in galleries as well as group and individual art therapy at the residential facility. Although Lobban and Murphy (2018) reported a mean reduction in self-rated experiential avoidance, there was no statistical test. During the first gallery visit, participants were drawn to an etching ('Map of Nowhere', 2008) by the British artist Grayson Perry (who is well known in the UK) and, the following day, made art in response to it. Participants drew on their knowledge of the artist and his 'alter ego, and reputation for cross-dressing' (Lobban and Murphy 2018, p.104) to discuss the issue of how one is perceived by others, but the authors did not provide further detail of this particular resonance.

Adults with eating disorders

Thaler *et al.* (2017) added a one-day, museum-based, group art therapy session to an existing clinical programme for adults with severe eating disorders, in a rolling programme of art therapy at the Montreal Museum of Fine Arts in Canada for groups of up to 12 participants. Baddeley *et al.* (2017) have described this programme, which included lunch and an art educator-led tour, followed by art-making in an on-site studio. There were 78 participants in total, and, in addition to carrying out thematic analysis on their written answers to a short questionnaire, Thaler *et al.* (2017) used quantitative measures of mood, preoccupation with eating, and body satisfaction. There were no significant therapeutic changes in body satisfaction or preoccupation with eating, but anxiety decreased (Thaler *et al.* 2017). The qualitative data suggested that visiting the museum and learning about artworks served as distractions from hospital routines, stimulated creativity and enabled seeing different perspectives. Thaler *et al.* (2017) suggested that the creative, playful aspect of the art therapy component in this setting challenged rigid thinking.

Adults without identified health difficulties

In Greece, where art therapy is not yet well established, Pantagoutsou, Ioannides and Vaslamatzis (2017) worked with ten members of the public in a 12-session pilot art therapy group in the National Museum of Contemporary Arts, Athens, with the aim of enabling them to explore emotional issues in the context of Greece's economic struggles. No formal evaluation was reported, but the authors suggested that viewing selected artworks and hearing about the artists who had made them helped participants to make connections to their own lives and, similar to Deane *et al.* (2000), inspired them to create their own expressive artworks. The art therapists created an atmosphere of acceptance, assisted by the museum staff welcoming participants and encouraging 'a critical stance towards contemporary art' (Pantagoutsou *et al.* 2017, p.70).

Two studies drawing on art therapy, in the USA and Hong Kong respectively, have used the concept of relational aesthetics to increase citizens' political awareness (Betts *et al.* 2015; Ho *et al.* 2017). Betts *et al.* (2015) reported that self-rated empathy increased more in participants who made response art after viewing exhibits in the USA's Holocaust Memorial Museum, compared with those who only viewed the exhibits without the art-making process. Ho *et al.* (2017) reported a reduction in desire for social distance from people with mental health difficulties after selecting, reflecting on, and making art in response to artworks by mental health service users.

Therapeutic factors in art therapy based in museums and galleries

Almost all the projects discussed here describe how participants made personal and often emotional connections with exhibits in the setting. These personal connections with exhibits could be viewed as either an aspect of relational aesthetics (Gabel and Robb 2017), or Yalom's (1995) universality (Salom 2011). However, the important thing about these connections seems to be that in many reports, they inspired participants' own art-making and self-expression. In some cases (e.g. Huet 2011; Pantagoutsou *et al.* 2017), there was a suggestion that the art curator or museum guide encouraged the forming of personal connections with artworks, prior to therapeutic art-making, rather than positioning the artworks as above such ordinary responses.

Having made a personal connection with an exhibit, participants of most projects were described as expressing their thoughts and feelings in the subsequent art-making sessions, which may be viewed as either embodiment and/or symbolic expression (Gabel and Robb 2017). Although these are concepts applied to group art therapy outside art galleries and museums and mostly in clinical settings, the exhibits in museums and galleries could be said to assist the art therapist in encouraging art-based expression, invoking Salom's (2011) idea of the museum as therapist.

Several authors mentioned an enjoyable or playful aspect of their projects, which is consistent with Gabel and Robb's (2017) idea that pleasure and play lead to relaxation and mastery, and with the APPGAHW (2017) report, which suggests calming as a therapeutic mechanism in arts and health projects. In museums and galleries, this may be enhanced because the cultural setting celebrates creativity and human expression or experience. McNiff (2004) has described the art therapy space within a clinical setting as an asylum (refuge) within an asylum (medically dominated mental health system). By contrast, museums and galleries and their exhibits can be seen as enhancing the already containing space: Jury and Landes (2015, p.27) have suggested that museums and art galleries can be a 'non-clinical, safe and containing setting' for art therapy, and Ioannides (2017, p.104) referred to 'valuable and priceless items that are very well protected', which she suggested may in turn help some people to feel secure.

Coles and Harrison (2018) referred to participants setting themselves new challenges, and although this could have been due to their active involvement in setting and rating their own therapy goals, another possible aspect was the stimulation and enrichment (APPGAHW 2017) provided by museum objects in the early stages, alongside the museum and gallery exhibitions and the buildings themselves. The 'specialness' of a museum or gallery may add a sense of ritual, possibly also enhancing security (Gabel and Robb 2017). Specialness and value conferred by a cultural setting was mentioned in Roberts *et al.* (2011), and also featured in Stevens *et al.* (2018) in their study of arts-based recovery college courses held in cultural venues. This might be an insufficiently acknowledged component of art therapy in museums and galleries.

The long-standing view within art therapy of considering clients as artists (Thompson 2009; Wood 1997) is potentially supported by museums and galleries as cultural venues (Colbert *et al.* 2013; Coles and Harrison 2018; Linesch 2004). Making, and particularly exhibiting, artwork might serve not only to validate participants as artists (Linesch 2004; Thompson 2009) but also to enable friends and family to empathise with their feelings, perhaps for the first time (Delucia 2016). This may arise without exhibiting, as a result of an enhanced ability to communicate personal experiences through viewing and making art (Deane *et al.* 2000), but exhibiting in a culturally valued space may enhance this therapeutic outcome.

Where next for research?

Few of the reports on art therapy in museums and galleries used formal evaluations, and this means that many of the findings and therapeutic processes described here have to remain tentatively stated. The APPGAHW report (2017) recommends the use of rigorous mixed-methods designs for evaluating arts and health projects. One such example is Coles and Harrison's (2018) systematic case study. This approach enables researchers to gauge the degree to which different sources of data converge on the same findings and to understand unexpected outcomes. Systematic case studies involve careful pre-planning of what data to collect, based on hypotheses about processes and outcomes. This data is then collected systematically and represented transparently (see Yin 2018 for an overview of this approach). If art therapists wish to pursue a purely qualitative approach to evaluation, there are some helpful texts for guidance on how to make this rigorous and less open to a common criticism of descriptive case studies: that reported findings are influenced by researcher bias. Willig's (2013) text represents a useful introduction to a range of qualitative methods in that it covers many commonly used approaches, and discusses their comparative strengths and weaknesses.

As a basic start, art therapists could routinely use short questionnaires to audit their work. For example, behaviour problems in young people might be rated by teachers using the Strengths and Difficulties Questionnaire (SDQ) (Goodman and Goodman 2011). Social participation (new friendships or greater arts participation) could be examined in a range of client groups, but may require careful devising and validation of a new questionnaire to incorporate arts participation. The role of the museum or gallery and its exhibits could feature more in qualitative evaluations to test the suggestions of Salom (2011) about their possible inherent therapeutic functions for different participants, and to investigate the prevalence of the idea of 'specialness' and what this might mean. The self-esteem component of a sense of enhanced social identity might be captured in participants who experience societal stigma using the Rosenberg Self-Esteem Scale (Rosenberg 1989), which is a freely available and widely used short questionnaire.

For examining changes in wellbeing, the APPGAHW report (2017) points out that the Warwick-Edinburgh Mental Wellbeing Scale (Stewart-Brown *et al.* 2009) has been used extensively in arts and health studies in different countries. It utilises a seven-item short form, making it especially useful for participants who find long questionnaires daunting. PSYCHLOPS (Ashworth *et al.* 2005) is also short and enables service users in collaboration with their therapist to create their own goals for therapy and rate them pre, post, and in-between. The UCL Museum Wellbeing Measure (Thomson and

Chatterjee 2013) is intended for regularly gauging immediate positive and negative emotions during arts and health projects and could be useful for evaluating art therapy interventions when the data is considered in the light of an understanding of clients' particular difficulties.

Thematic analysis (Braun and Clarke 2006; Clarke and Braun 2018) allows for data from interviews and focus groups to be grouped into researcher-determined themes to illuminate participants' experiences and is widely used in psychotherapy and counselling research studies. It can be a valuable component of mixed-methods evaluations (e.g. Huet and Holttum 2017; Stevens *et al.* 2018; Thaler *et al.* 2017).

Research itself (in addition to art therapy) might contribute to enhancing participants' social positioning if it is conducted in a participatory way, for example by utilising an overall framework of participatory action research (Leavy 2017), or experience-based co-design (Point of Care Foundation n.d.). These approaches view service users as active stakeholders in the research, in an equal partnership with professionals, and able to influence the design and execution of the research. UK research funding bodies generally require some level of consultation or active partnership working with service users and members of the public (INVOLVE 2018), and participatory research or co-design can maximise involvement and influence.

None of these rigorous methods rules out the use of artworks themselves to help convey findings. Reproductions of artworks gained with clients' fully informed consent can convey directly something of participants' engagement with the intervention, and of their communication through the use of art materials (Gabel and Robb 2017). However, images by themselves are open to multiple interpretations and the final interpretation of any artwork created in art therapy sessions always remains with the client. For a more detailed, general discussion of collecting and representing visual material see Pink (2013).

The APPGAHW report (2017) recommends assessing the cost effectiveness of arts-based interventions, for example by recording use of health and social care services before, during and after an intervention, and then ascertaining costs on the basis of actual service costs. The report also highlights a way of establishing the social return on investment (SROI), which ‘allows for the measurement and capture of outcomes that can be intangible and hard to measure’ (Whelan, Holden and Bockler 2016, p.18). The return on investment is expressed in monetary terms, which makes it easier to compare and contrast findings from different studies, and arguably appeals to stakeholders in constrained economic climates. However, estimating these quantities can be problematic and contested, not least because a social return is, in many people’s eyes, not reducible to money.

Conclusion

Research evidence on art therapy in museums and galleries suggests that it is an approach that might enable participants to experience increased understanding of personal identity, to make personalised connections to exhibits and at times be inspired to share their experiences through both art-making and words. In turn, this might enable the processing of personal difficulties. The opportunity of exhibiting one’s own work might enhance participants’ ability to communicate feelings to others, including family and friends, enhancing their social support, as well as amplifying participants’ identity from service user to being considered an artist. There are some commonly used validated measures that have been explored here and that art therapists might make more use of in their work in museums and galleries. It is also likely that thematic analysis as part of a mixed-methods evaluation can illustrate experienced benefits that are hard to capture with standardised scales or are not yet articulated, being qualitative and personal. Following up participants for a time after the intervention is to be recommended, and in order to argue for state funding in current climates, some form of economic analysis is desirable, such as that based on use of other services before and after the art therapy. Through research and evaluation that builds our understanding of the contribution that museums and galleries can make to art therapy practice, and the way in which this happens, the art therapy profession can enhance its offer, and further demonstrate its efficacy to service providers.

References

Age and Opportunity (2012) *Azure: Exploring Greater Inclusion of People with Dementia in Museums and Galleries in Ireland – Pilot Evaluation*. Dublin: Author. Accessed on 9/7/19 at www.lenus.ie/bitstream/handle/10147/325408/AzureEvaluation2012Layoutfinal.pdf?sequence=1&isAllowed=y.

All-Party Parliamentary Group on Arts, Health and Wellbeing (2017) *Creative Health: The Arts for Health and Wellbeing* (second edition). Accessed on 15/7/19 at https://www.culturehealthandwellbeing.org.uk/appg-inquiry/.

Ashworth, M., Robinson, S., Godfrey, E., Shepherd, M. *et al.* (2005) 'Measuring mental health outcomes in primary care: The psychometric properties of a new patient-generated outcome measure, PSYCHLOPS (Psychological Outcome Profiles).' *Primary Care Mental Health 2005,* 3, 261–270.

Baddeley, G., Evans, L., Lajeunesse, M. and Legari, S. (2017) 'Body talk: Examining a collaborative multiple-visit program for visitors with eating disorders.' *Journal of Museum Education 42,* 345–353.

Betts, D.J., Potash, J.S., Luke, J.J. and Kelso, M. (2015) 'An art therapy study of visitor reactions to the United States Holocaust Memorial Museum.' *Museum Management and Curatorship 30,* 21–43.

Bolwerk, A., Mack-Andrick, J., Lang, F.R., Dorfler, A. and Maihofner, C. (2014) 'How art changes your brain: Differential effects of visual art production and cognitive art evaluation on functional brain connectivity.' *PLOS ONE 9,* 7, e101035. Doi: 10.1371/journal.pone.0101035.

Borghol, N., Suderman, M., McArdle, W., Racine, A. *et al.* (2012) 'Associations with early-life socio-economic position in adult DNA methylation.' *International Journal of Epidemiology 41,* 62–74.

Braun, V. and Clarke, V. (2006) 'Using thematic analysis in psychology.' *Qualitative Research in Psychology 3,* 77–101.

Bygren, L.O. (2013) 'Intergenerational health responses to adverse and enriched environments.' *Annual Review of Public Health 34,* 49–60.

Clarke, V. and Braun, V. (2018) 'Using thematic analysis in counselling and psychotherapy research: A critical reflection.' *Counselling and Psychotherapy Research 18,* 107–110.

Clow, A. and Fredhoi, C. (2006) 'Normalisation of salivary cortisol levels and self-report stress by a brief lunchtime visit to an art gallery by London City workers.' *Journal of Holistic Healthcare 3,* 29–32.

Colbert, S., Cooke, A., Camic, P.M. and Springham, N. (2013) 'The art-gallery as a resource for recovery for people who have experienced psychosis.' *The Arts in Psychotherapy 40,* 250–256.

Coles, A. and Harrison, F. (2018) 'Tapping into museums for art psychotherapy: An evaluation of a pilot group for young adults.' *International Journal of Art Therapy 23,* 3, 115–124.

Coles, A., Harrison, F. and Todd, S. (2019) 'Flexing the frame: Therapist experiences of museum-based group art psychotherapy for adults with complex mental health difficulties.' *International Journal of Art Therapy 24,* 2, 56–67.

Cozolino, L. (2018) *Timeless: Nature's Formula for Health and Longevity*. New York, NY: Norton.

Deane, K., Fitch, M. and Carman, M. (2000) 'An innovative art therapy program for cancer patients.' *Canadian Oncology Nursing Journal 10,* 147–151.

Delucia, J.M. (2016) 'Art therapy services to support veterans' transition to civilian life: The studio and the gallery.' *Art Therapy: Journal of the American Art Therapy Association 33,* 4–12.

Fancourt, D., Perkins, R., Ascenso, S., Carvalho, L.A., Steptoe, A. and Williamon, A. (2016) 'Effects of group drumming interventions on anxiety, depression, social resilience and inflammatory immune response among mental health service users.' *PLOS ONE 11,* 3, e0151136, 1–16.

Flatt, J.D., Liptak, A., Oakley, M.A., Gogan, J., Varner, T. and Lingler, J.H. (2015) 'Subjective experiences of an art museum engagement activity for persons with early-stage Alzheimer's disease and their family caregivers.' *American Journal of Alzheimer's Disease and Other Dementias 30,* 380–389.

Gabel, A. and Robb, M. (2017) '(Re)considering psychological constructs: A thematic synthesis defining five therapeutic factors in group art therapy.' *The Arts in Psychotherapy 55,* 126–35.

Goodman, A. and Goodman, R. (2011) 'Population mean scores predict child mental disorder rates: Validating SDQ prevalence estimators in Britain.' *Journal of Child Psychology and Psychiatry* 52, 100–108.

Harper, S. and Hamblin, K. (2010) *'This is Living' – Good Times: Art for Older People at Dulwich Picture Gallery.* Oxford: Oxford Institute of Ageing, Oxford University.

Ho, R.T.H., Potash, J.S., Ho, A.H.Y., Ho, V.F.L. and Chen, E.Y.H. (2017) 'Reducing mental illness stigma and fostering empathic citizenship: Community arts collaborative approach.' *Social Work in Mental Health 15,* 469–485.

Huet, V. (2011) 'Art therapy-based organisational consultancy: A session at Tate Britain.' *International Journal of Art Therapy 16,* 1, 3–13.

Huet, V. and Holttum, S. (2016) 'Art therapy-based groups for work-related stress with staff in health and social care: An exploratory study.' *The Arts in Psychotherapy 50,* 46–57.

INVOLVE (2018) *INVOLVE.* Southampton, UK: Author. Accessed on 12/12/18 at www.invo.org.uk.

Ioannides, E. (2017) 'Museums as therapeutic environments and the contribution of art therapy.' *Museum International 68* (271–272), 98–109.

Jury, H. and Landes, J. (2015) 'Museums and galleries – re-viewing museums: Innovative art therapy practice in museums and art galleries.' *British Association of Art Therapists Newsbriefing,* December 2015, 26–28.

Leavy, P. (2017) *Research Design: Quantitative, Qualitative, Mixed Methods, Arts-Based, and Community-Based Participatory Action Research Approaches.* London: The Guilford Press.

Linesch, D. (2004) 'Art therapy at the Museum of Tolerance: Responses to the life and work of Friedl Dicker-Brandeis.' *The Arts in Psychotherapy 31,* 57–66.

Lobban, J. and Murphy, D. (2018) 'Using art therapy to overcome avoidance in veterans with chronic post-traumatic stress disorder.' *International Journal of Art Therapy 23,* 3, 99–114.

McGuigan, K.A., Leggett, J.A. and Horsburgh, M. (2015) 'Visiting the museum together: Evaluating a programme at Auckland Museum for people living with dementia and their carers.' *Arts and Health 7,* 261–270.

McLaughlin, K.A. (2016) 'Future directions in childhood adversity and youth psychopathology.' *Journal of Clinical Child and Adolescent Psychology 45,* 361–382.

McNiff, S. (2004) *Art Heals: How Creativity Cures the Soul.* London: Shambhala.

Pantagoutsou, A., Ioannides, E. and Vaslamatzis, G. (2017) 'Exploring the museum's images – exploring my image (exploration des images du musée, exploration de mon image).' *Canadian Art Therapy Association Journal 30,* 69–77.

Pink, S. (2013) *Doing Visual Ethnography.* London: SAGE.

Point of Care Foundation (n.d.) *EBCD: Experience-Based Co-Design Toolkit.* London: Author. Accessed on 11/12/18 at www.pointofcarefoundation.org.uk/resource/experience-based-co-design-ebcd-toolkit.

Rasmuson, S., Olsson, T., Henriksson, B.G., Kelly, P.A.T. *et al.* (1998) 'Environmental enrichment selectively increases 5-HT1A receptor mRNA expression and binding in the rat hippocampus.' *Molecular Brain Research 53,* 285–90.

Roberts, S., Camic, P.M. and Springham, N. (2011) 'New roles for art galleries: Art-viewing as a community intervention for family carers of people with mental health problems.' *Arts and Health 3,* 146–159.

Rosenberg, M. (1989) *Society and the Adolescent Self-Image* (revised edition). Middletown, CT: Wesleyan University Press.

Salom, A. (2011) 'Reinventing the setting: Art therapy in museums.' *The Arts in Psychotherapy 38,* 81–85.

Sandler, I., Ingram, A., Wolchik, S., Tein, J.-Y. and Winslow, E. (2015) 'Long-term effects of parenting-focused preventive interventions to promote resilience of children and adolescents.' *Child Development Perspectives 9,* 164–171.

Shaer, D., Beaven, K., Springham, N., Pillinger, S. *et al.* (2008) 'The role of art therapy in a pilot for art-based information prescriptions at Tate Britain.' *International Journal of Art Therapy 13,* 1, 25–33.

Stevens, J., Butterfield, C., Whittington, A. and Holttum, S. (2018) 'Evaluation of arts based courses within a UK recovery college for people with mental health challenges.' *International Journal of Environmental Research and Public Health 15,* 1170.

Stewart-Brown, S., Tennant, A., Tennant, R., Platt, S., Parkinson, J. and Weich, S. (2009) 'Internal construct validity of the Warwick-Edinburgh Mental Well-Being Scale (WEMWBS): A Rasch analysis using data from the Scottish Health Education Population Survey.' *Health and Quality of Life Outcomes 7,* 15.

Thaler, L., Drapeau, C.-E., Leclerc, J., Lajeunesse, M. *et al.* (2017) 'An adjunctive, museum-based art therapy experience in the treatment of women with severe eating disorders.' *The Arts in Psychotherapy 56,* 1–16.

Thompson, G. (2009) 'Artistic sensibility in the studio and gallery model: Revisiting process and product.' *Art Therapy: Journal of the American Art Therapy Association 26,* 159–166.

Thomson, L.J. and Chatterjee, H.J. (2013) *UCL Museum Wellbeing Measures Toolkit.* London: UCL. Accessed on 1/11/18 at www.ucl.ac.uk/culture/sites/culture/files/ucl_museum_wellbeing_measures_toolkit_sept2013.pdf.

Treadon, C.B., Rosal, M. and Thompson Wylder, V.D. (2006) 'Opening the doors of art museums for therapeutic processes.' *The Arts in Psychotherapy 33*, 288–301.

Visnola, D., Sprudza, D., Bake, M.A. and Pike, A. (2010) 'Effects of art therapy on stress and anxiety of employees.' *Proceedings of the Latvian Academy of Sciences*. Section B, 64 (1/2), 85–91.

Whelan, G., Holden, H. and Bockler, J. (2016) 'A social return on investment evaluation of the St Helens Creative Alternatives arts on prescription programme.' Liverpool: Institute of Cultural Capital. Accessed on 26/8/18 at http://iccliverpool.ac.uk/wp-content/uploads/2017/11/Creative-Alternatives-evaluation-report-2016.pdf.

Willig, C. (2013) *Introducing Qualitative Research in Psychology* (third edition). Maidenhead: Open University Press.

Wood, C. (1997) 'The History of Art Therapy and Psychosis 1938–95.' In K. Killick and J. Schaverien (eds) *Art, Psychotherapy and Psychosis*. London: Routledge.

Yalom, I. (1995) *The Theory and Practice of Group Psychotherapy*. New York, NY: Basic Books.

Yin, R. (2018) *Case Study Research and Applications: Design and Methods*. London: SAGE.

CHAPTER 2

What Do Museums Mean?

Public Perceptions of the Purposes of Museums and Implications for their Use in Art Therapy

Ali Coles

Introduction

In this chapter, I explore how commonly held perceptions of museums might affect clients' experiences of art therapy in those settings. These perceptions might impact on someone's decision about whether to engage in museum-based art therapy in the first place. In addition, a client's attitudes towards the setting will be one element in the complex interplay of factors affecting the therapeutic process, particularly if the art therapy includes interaction with museum objects and exhibitions, rather than simply the use of a space within the museum.

A person's attitude to a particular museum is likely to be affected by any direct experience of that institution in the past, or of other museums. However, it will also be influenced by consciously and unconsciously held ideas about the nature and purpose of museums in general. As Bollas (1992) points out, 'If I visit the National Portrait Gallery, this involves me with...a set of notions, feelings, internal relations, and use-potentials evoked by the concept "museum"' (p.34). Trustram (2014) uses the term 'museum in the mind' to refer to the 'conscious and unconscious mental construct that a person holds about a museum' (p.69).

Museums carry different resonances from more traditional settings for art therapy, such as clinical treatment centres. As will be discussed in this chapter, 'museum' can be a highly evocative concept, laden with historical, cultural and personal meaning, and bound up with issues of power, inclusion/exclusion, trust and safety. All these issues are, I suggest, relevant to therapeutic considerations. It is important to remember that clients' ideas about museums may differ from the way art therapists think about museums, particularly art therapists who work with museums, and from the way museum professionals think about their institutions. In addition, clients might find it hard to articulate their responses to the idea of engaging in therapy in a museum environment; indeed, some responses may not be in conscious awareness. Therefore, it could be very helpful for art therapists to reflect on commonly held ideas about museums in order to understand how clients' attitudes towards museums might affect their engagement in museum-based art therapy, and to facilitate positive therapeutic outcomes. A clearer picture of how clients might relate to museums will also further develop art therapists' understanding of why, and how, museums can be valuable partners in therapeutic work.

This chapter draws on the research by BritainThinks (2013), entitled *Public Perceptions of – and Attitudes to – the Purposes of Museums in Society* and carried out with adults in England, Scotland and Wales. It had been recognised that 'little is known about what people think about museums in general and even less about their perceptions of the role of museums and their impacts' (*ibid.*, p.7) and this research sought to explore ideas about the roles and purposes of museums in general, rather than personal experiences of, or attitudes towards, particular museums. It is therefore very valuable for identifying issues which can inform art therapy work in any museum, and the findings have been used as the underpinning structure for the discussion in this chapter.

The research was commissioned by the UK Museums Association, which describes museums as 'institutions that collect, safeguard and make accessible artefacts and specimens, which they hold in trust for society' (Museums Association 2018a), encompassing art galleries with collections of works of art, and this is the definition I use in this chapter. The research involved six day-long workshops with a total of 90 adult participants, carried out in rural and urban areas. The participants were recruited to reflect the overall gender, age, educational profile, occupational grouping and ethnicity of the UK as a whole, and half of them had visited a museum in the last year. The research process included activities designed to encourage participants to adopt a 'citizen perspective' (BritainThinks 2013, p.8), which meant eliciting views about the place of museums within society and what the purpose of museums should be, rather than more personal perspectives. The researchers used a combination of open discussions and hands-on exercises, first facilitating the spontaneous expression of perceptions, and then introducing other potential roles and purposes for consideration. The researchers did not seek to include a representative proportion of participants with mental health or other difficulties which might lead them to receiving psychological therapy; however, this may not have had a significant influence on the findings, particularly given the focus on general perceptions of museums rather than specific experiences. This research was carried out in the UK, and perceptions of museums will differ in other parts of the world due to cultural and historical differences. Additionally, children's perceptions may differ from those of adults. However, I believe that the discussion in this chapter will be useful for art therapists working in other parts of the world, and/or with other client groups, when thinking about the interplay between views about museums and experiences of museum-based art therapy in their particular situations.

Positivity towards museums

The BritainThinks (2013) research found that, overall, there was 'strong, positive emotional attachment to museums' which did not seem to be related to whether, or how often, people visited museums (p.3). Any negativity towards the idea of a museum usually came from people who had not visited a museum for decades, perhaps since being at school, and this view was expressed in terms of museums being 'stuffy, aloof and boring' (*ibid.*, p.11). Most were aware that museums have changed over the years and almost all participants' views became more positive when researchers provided examples of modern museums.

If clients have a generally positive attitude towards museums, this suggests that they might be receptive to the idea of a museum setting for art therapy and to engaging with what they find there. This should be an encouragement to art therapists who are considering using museums in their work. Furthermore, a 'strong, positive emotional attachment' to the idea of a museum (*ibid.*, p.3) has echoes of the concept of secure attachment (Bowlby 1982, first published 1969), the ideal relationship for exploration and growth. It may not be too far-fetched to suggest that positivity towards museums in general might be a helpful emotional framework for museum-based art therapy, facilitating the development of a positive therapeutic relationship between therapist and client, and between clients in a group therapy situation.

At the very least, as Camic and Chatterjee (2013) point out in their discussion of museum-based arts and health activities, museums are 'nearly always non-stigmatising settings in that they are not institutions where diagnosis and treatment of medical and mental problems occur, nor are they settings where one experiences embarrassment, shame or criticism for attending' (pp.66–67). Thus, even if someone did not feel particularly positive towards museums, he or she might be more inclined to feel enthusiastic about a museum setting rather than a clinical setting for therapy, particularly in communities where therapy is 'associated with shame around illness' (Salom 2011, p.81). Coles and Harrison (2018) cite evidence that clients of museum-based art therapy have valued being in a non-clinical environment and, in their own findings, young adults in a museum-based art psychotherapy group appreciated feeling like 'a person not a patient' (p.123). Reflecting on their experiences of delivering museum-based art psychotherapy, Coles, Harrison and Todd (2019) consider that a museum's status as a publicly accessible venue sends a message to people who might have 'withdrawn from society' due to their mental health difficulties that 'you don't have to be excluded because of who you are or what's happened to you' (p.63).

However, some participants in the BritainThinks (2013) research viewed museums as boring or aloof. This could be a result of experiences from many years ago, as the research notes, or could be thought about as an indirect expression of feelings of exclusion. For example, Ander *et al.* (2013) found that some people who took part in museum object handling sessions in hospital and inpatient mental health settings 'regarded museums as "not for the likes of me"' (p.214) as they felt that they did not have the required intellectual ability to interact with museum objects. This potential barrier to engagement in museum-based art therapy could be explored with clients in initial meetings, through describing the setting and how the museum objects and environments will be used within the therapy. For example, it might be important to reassure clients that they are not expected to know anything about the museum's collections, and that the focus is on therapeutic rather than educational outcomes. A client's feeling of the museum being somehow 'above' them in terms of intellectual status might also resonate with any feelings that healthcare professionals are 'superior', perhaps due to having specialist qualifications, and could exacerbate a sense of power inequality between therapists and clients. While there may be value in bringing in museum experts at times during the therapy, it seems important for the therapists not to be seen as museum experts as well as therapy experts. Coles *et al.* (2019) reflected on the value of therapists exploring the collections alongside participants in museum-based group art psychotherapy, with both therapists and clients 'not knowing', rather than the therapists 'having all the answers' (p.64). The idea of a museum being 'aloof' also has connotations of a lack of care and concern, and it is conceivable that this might negatively impact on the development of a positive therapeutic relationship within that setting.

In addition, it is important to recognise that there is likely to be a variation in attitudes towards museums between different sections of the population, at least in part due to the relative relevance of museum collections and how they are presented. For example, a street survey in London in 2004, in which 594 'visible minority ethnic people' were interviewed (Tissier and Nathoo 2004, p.1), found that 63 per cent of participants were either negative or indifferent about museums. Subsequent focus groups of black and minority ethnic (BME) museum non-users identified perceptions that museums are for the 'white middle classes' and that they fail to reflect, acknowledge or engage with BME groups (*ibid.*, p.3). Despite efforts by the museum sector to engage with specific communities, including black, Asian and ethnic minority communities (Museums Association 2018c), 14 years later UK Government figures showed that white people were more likely to visit a museum or gallery than people from other ethnic groups (Department for Digital, Culture, Media and Sport 2018). The issue of relevance is explored later in this chapter.

Museums as custodians of heritage

The BritainThinks (2013) research participants identified three essential roles for museums. The most important role was considered to be 'safeguarding heritage' and preventing museum objects from 'being lost' (*ibid.*, p.12). This was deemed to be important even if museum objects were never seen by the public. It is surely significant for museum-based art therapy that the most important function of museums to emerge from the BritainThinks (2013) research is the care of objects, regardless of whether they are available for public use. As Trustram (2014) notes, it seems that the construct of a museum as a place of 'preservation and permanence' (p.69) has not been significantly affected by the development of new museum functions such as education and economic regeneration. Museums seem to hold a 'consistent meaning for our inner lives' (*ibid.*, p.69) despite the growth of 'blockbuster' crowd-pulling exhibitions, museum shops and cafes, and education and outreach programmes.

This idea of museums as places which take care of objects and prevent them from being 'lost' (BritainThinks 2013, p.12) has powerful resonances with the role of the therapist within art therapy. At one level, the art therapist provides 'consistency of care' for the client (British Association of Art Therapists 2014, p.4) and ensures that the client's artwork is 'safely stored' (*ibid.*, p.7). At a deeper level, there are suggestions of 'holding' (Winnicott 1990, first published 1965) and 'containment' (Bion 1994, first published 1962), which are key to art therapy practice. Just as a museum 'both holds (looks after) objects and contains them (provides a structure that prevents their loss or decay)' (Froggett and Trustram 2014, p.490), the art therapist creates a boundaried arena for the safe expression and exploration of feelings and experiences. Ioannides (2017) talks of the 'museum's ambience of safety and security' and suggests that this allows visitors 'to feel secure such that they can free their minds as they explore' (p.104). Similarly, Silverman (2010) talks about museums providing a sense of 'ontological security' because of the orderliness of exhibitions (p.59) and Carr (2001) considers that 'the museum holds things in place for us, so our minds might move toward, surround, look back at, consider and reconsider them' (p.173); this 'holding in place' has both temporal and spatial aspects when the museum remains relatively unchanged between sessions. There are parallels here with the therapist seeking to provide a consistent, reliable physical environment for therapy and keeping client artworks safe, perhaps for future re-viewing (Case and Dalley 2014, p.90), as well as with the idea of holding a client in mind between sessions. Also, in museum-based art therapy which involves moving between the encounter with objects in the public exhibition spaces and reflective art-making in private spaces, the endurance of the object between sessions is mirrored in the way in which a client holds a chosen object in mind so that it can act as a 'psychological container' even when not physically present (Coles *et al.* 2019, p.60).

Schaverien (1999) discusses how the frames around artworks in a gallery create a boundaried space which 'permits potentially unmanageable images to be contained' (p.71), providing a rigid structure that complements the freedom of the art expression contained within. The display cases and other structural aspects of non-art museum exhibitions could be seen as playing the same role, creating a safe boundary around objects which might evoke powerful feelings. These museum 'frames' echo the 'therapeutic frame', which provides a safe, boundaried physical and mental space for clients to share shameful or distressing thoughts, feelings and experiences (Edwards 2014, p.51). The idea of containment and safety is also echoed in the larger 'frame' of the traditional museum with its grand architecture, managed entrances and exits, security procedures and watchful staff. A further layer of safety is provided by a museum's documentation, which maintains information about the museum objects in accordance with defined procedures and standards, and so helps to facilitate their care (International Council of Museums Documentation Committee 2012). This has similarities with clinical records, which hold data such as personal history and current symptoms in a clear and organised way so that each person can receive safe and appropriate treatment.

However, a museum's physical and procedural strategies for keeping collections safe will not necessarily encourage feelings of safety in clients of museum-based art therapy. For example, exhibition elements such as glass cases and boundary lines on the floor which demarcate zones of exclusion, preventing viewers from getting too close to objects, may resonate with feelings of unworthiness or with internal psychological processes of disconnection from feelings and experiences. They might also evoke memories of locked wards and restricted visiting hours in inpatient settings. The gaze of museum staff may feel intimidating and lead to increased anxiety about being 'under scrutiny' by the therapist, and a museum's grand architecture could feel imposing or overpowering, and even suggestive of 'old style' psychiatric hospitals. In addition, the actual therapeutic frame can be seen as more fluid in museum-based art therapy that involves moving in and out of public exhibition spaces, and this might lead to clients feeling less safe. Coles *et al.* (2019) state that in their experience of using exhibitions within art psychotherapy groups 'it felt as if there was more emphasis on the psychological boundaries of the therapist in holding the therapeutic frame' and note 'the practical steps we put in place to make the work boundaried for the therapist as well as for the participants, for example running the first few weeks of the group solely in the private room using handling objects rather than in the public exhibitions' (p.61). They conclude that the 'fluid museum environment places demands on a therapist's logistical organisation skills as well as their psychological capacity to contain, hold and integrate difficult feelings' (*ibid.*, p.64).

Another aspect of safety in relation to museum purposes is explored by Pearce (1999), who considers that the documenting, organising and storing of objects by museums is in tune with our basic human need to make order out of chaos. This orderliness is in stark contrast to chaotic lives which clients might be experiencing. Pearce (1999) also notes that museum displays are often underpinned by a linear sense of time, while traumatic memories can be 'without temporal narrative organization' (Gantt and Tinnin 2009, p.150); as Van der Kolk (2014) puts it, 'the different sensations that entered the brain at the time of the trauma are not properly assembled into a story' (p.194). Perhaps the way in which a curator works with museum objects, organising, displaying and explaining them, can be linked to the way in which a therapist might help someone give expression to, make sense of and organise traumatic experiences.

It is particularly interesting that the BritainThinks (2013) research suggests that people want museums to look after all the objects within collections, even ones which will never be displayed. This evokes the idea of an acceptance of the hidden, forgotten, unpalatable or dismissed aspects of oneself by the therapist; maybe museums can reassure us that our lives matter and that what has happened has significance and will not be forgotten. The way in which museums notice and value broken or incomplete objects could also resonate with clients. Coles and Harrison (2018) explain that one museum-based art psychotherapy client was encouraged in her attempts to piece her life back together again by encountering a repaired pot on display which had parts missing and visible joins. The broken pot had been considered by the museum as worthy of painstaking care and attention and 'good enough' for display, even with its scars and imperfections. There are clear links here with the therapeutic process, with its emphasis on respect, positive regard, self-acceptance and recovery. Furthermore, Coles *et al.* (2019) consider that in museum-based art psychotherapy the 'ebb and flow between the private and public spaces, and between the intimate and the more social relating, could perhaps help someone to connect vulnerable and more robust parts of themselves and encourage a more embodied, continuous sense of self' (p.64).

Within the BritainThinks (2013) research, participants supported the idea that museums can act as 'society's attic' (p.15). Froggett and Trustram (2014) consider that museums 'enable communities to hold certain objects collectively in mind' (p.490), and this may also apply to cultural concepts and understandings. The idea of a shared heritage has possible implications for museum-based art therapy. Salom (2011) suggests that relating to 'collective imagery that offers information about the human experience' (p.83) might make someone feel less isolated through drawing attention to 'the commonalities among human situations, emotions, difficulties, and achievements' (p.84), linking this to Yalom's (1995) group therapy principle of universality. Thus, within museum-based group art therapy, a sense of collective heritage might encourage interpersonal relating within the group. Coles *et al.* (2019) talk about the museum as 'a repository of marks and traces of people over the centuries' and suggest that through interacting with an object one 'becomes part of its story as well...part of the community of that object', and that this 'might help someone to see that their own narrative is connected to others' narratives' (p.61). However, a particular museum's collection may be more reflective of dominant cultures, with obvious implications for clients who do not identify with those cultures, as noted above in relation to different ethnic groups. It seems important to reflect on this openly, while ensuring that this is done in a way which does not increase any client's feelings of marginalisation.

Museums as places for learning

Another essential role identified in the BritainThinks (2013) research was that of providing information and learning for adults. If we consider that psychological therapies involve learning about the self, then the perception of a museum as a place for learning might make it an appropriate and conducive setting for therapy. The participants in the BritainThinks (2013) research spoke in terms of discovery and exploration rather than education, which has even more resonance with the process of learning about self within psychological therapy; the idea that a visitor to a museum can 'feel she is not being told things so much as discovering them for herself' in a 'non-intrusive' environment (Froggett and Trustram 2014, p.493) has strong echoes of psychotherapeutic approaches. As Carr (2001) puts it, 'The museum offers its users an invitation to guide, connect, and construct their own cognitive or emotional developments' (p.179). In contrast to this idea of a museum as a place for self-directed exploration and learning, a clinical mental health setting might tend to encourage a sense of 'treatment' given by an expert. Indeed, one museum-based art psychotherapy client reflected that the museum setting made her feel that she had been working on her 'own personal goals' rather than just 'going through treatment' (Coles and Harrison 2018, p.123).

The BritainThinks (2013) research also identified a general belief that museums can be highly trusted as 'authoritative, reliable and accurate' repositories of information (p.13), linking with 'the Enlightenment ideal of the museum as a source of rationality' (Trustram 2014, p.69). This perception of museums as reliable and trustworthy may support museum-based art therapy, evoking aspects of the therapeutic alliance which is associated with positive therapy outcomes (Heynen *et al.* 2017). Furthermore, museums were seen as unbiased and as 'presenting all sides of the story' (BritainThinks 2013, p.3), suggesting that they are suitable places for issues to be looked at, thought about and considered. Edson (2015) notes that museums 'represent one of a diminishing number of institutions in which it is acceptable to think, debate, and to disagree' (p.9) and considers that the fundamental attributes of museums include honesty, the promotion of critical thinking and enhancement of open mindedness. According to the Director of the UK Museums Association, reflecting on symbols of discrimination, racism and oppression, 'Museums are exactly the safe and trusted places where difficult histories can be discussed' (Heal 2017), and there is a hint here of the psychological 'environment' which an art therapist seeks to encourage. Bedford (2004) notes that museums offer 'new perspectives and the chance to see the world through others' eyes' (p.5), echoing processes that are at play in art therapy groups. This is encapsulated in Salom's (2011) idea of the 'museum as group', in that museum collections can demonstrate both diversity and commonality, and Ioannides (2017) considers that museums are 'symbols of uniqueness and tolerance towards differences' due to the diversity of their collections (pp.104–105).

However, a view of museums as rational and factual might conflict with an art therapist's attempt to encourage tolerance of 'not knowing', uncertainty, ambiguity and paradox. In fact, as Fleming (2016) points out:

> All museum messages are the creation of the people who work at the museum...every comment they make is an opinion that could be opposed; every object they choose to display is loaded with meaning; every decision to omit something from display could be disputed. (p.74)

The choice of objects and how they are presented and interpreted is a subjective decision, so that 'curatorship is a relational activity' (Froggett and Trustram 2014, p.494). At one extreme, museums have sometimes been deliberately used by those in power as vehicles for strongly partisan views and attitudes. More subtly, museums may have misrepresented or omitted aspects of heritage, such as that relating to black and minority ethic communities. Some are now reinterpreting their collections so that the contribution that marginalised people have made to society is acknowledged; for example, the Victoria and Albert Museum in London has an LGBTQ (lesbian, gay, bisexual, transgender, queer) Working Group which aims to 'unearth previously hidden or unknown LGBTQ histories in the collections' (Victoria and Albert Museum n.d.). It is also true that museums have, historically, appropriated cultural property in exploitative ways. Clients may feel strongly about these aspects of museums, and this will impact on their sense of museums as places that can be trusted or not. Art therapists working in museum settings might choose to actively challenge the 'myth of neutrality' (Janes and Sandell 2019, p.8), using this as a way in to exploring feelings around knowledge, certainty, trust, power (and abuse of power) and difference. For example, the realisation that a museum that presents itself as an objective authority is, in fact, a vehicle for opinion might resonate strongly with people who have experienced certain types of emotional abuse. In this context, therapists' transparency about the subjectivity of their reflections in relation to clients would seem particularly crucial.

Museums as places for play

The third essential role identified by the research participants was providing entertaining education for children as part of a school or family group. The perception of museums as places for children to be entertained is likely to include the notion of play. How might this perception affect adult users' potential for play in the museum setting, and what are the implications for museum-based art therapy with this client group? Coles and Harrison (2018) found that a museum setting which included hands-on exhibits enabled playfulness among young adults in a museum-based art psychotherapy group, and that this aided the formation of relationships within the group. In Winnicott's view, playing facilitates 'growth and therefore health' (2010, first published 1971, p.56). At a more fundamental level, art therapy has drawn heavily on the idea that psychotherapy itself '*has to do with two people playing together*' (*ibid.*, p.51, original italics), and that play can be a form of communication in this context. Coles *et al.* (2019) felt that a museum setting might make it easier for therapists to be playful alongside clients, 'all experiencing something for the first time together' (p.63). Perhaps, therefore, the idea of a museum as a playful place can help the therapist in the essential work of '*bringing the patient from a state of not being able to play into a state of being able to play*' (Winnicott 2010, first published 1971, p.51, original italics) and to play together with clients, in a psychotherapeutic sense. This is in line with the Winnicottian idea of cultural experience as an extension of 'creative living first manifested in play' (*ibid.*, p.135). However, in the context of museums, it is recognised that people 'come with their own values and ideas about how they should behave in public space' and that they 'sometimes need encouragement that "it's ok to play"' (Derry n.d., p.12). A client might feel that it is not acceptable for adults to play in a museum, or that only children benefit from playing, and might need support from the therapist to develop their motivation and ability to be playful in this setting.

Museums as accessible and inclusive

Underpinning the research participants' views about the key role of museums was strong support for accessibility and inclusivity, including towards people seen as vulnerable. Within art therapy, the concepts of accessibility and inclusivity are key. Art therapists seek to ensure that every client has maximum physical, sensory and cognitive access to the therapy, and to adhere to principles of dignity, equality and non-discrimination (Health and Care Professions Council 2013). It is therefore encouraging that the public applies these ideals to museums. Within museums, however, these qualities take on a different aspect as they can contribute to addressing social exclusion (Sandell 2003); as 'places that embrace social inclusion', perhaps museums can offer 'a supporting structure' for challenging discrimination (Ioannides 2017, p.108). By working towards inclusive participation and representation in culture, museums can play a part in helping marginalised people to participate in society more generally. At the same time, integrating social action with art therapy practice (Kaplan 2006) perhaps calls for new types of setting for art therapy. Perhaps, however accessible or inclusive a clinical therapy setting might be, it is intrinsically a place for people set apart by ill-health.

It is interesting to consider the public's view that museums should be accessible and inclusive in the light of Doering's (1999) idea of museum visitors as strangers, guests or clients. Doering (1999) considers that visitors can be conceptualised as strangers (or even intruders) when the museum sees its main responsibility as the collection rather than the public, as guests when a museum wants to 'do good' to visitors from a sense of mission, and as clients when the museum's main focus is on serving the public. The stranger will feel unwelcome, unlike the guest or client. Guests and clients will be welcomed into the museum, but guests might feel that this is a privilege granted by the museum, while the client might see this as an entitlement. Doering (1999) notes that museums were, at that time, moving towards a position of being accountable to the public, in line with the concept of visitors as clients, and this expectation of accountability is now enshrined in the UK Museums Association's ethical guidelines (2018b). In relation to museum-based art therapy, it is likely that a sense of being a client of the museum, with the right to be there, will be most conducive to engagement. There are, of course, clear parallels with the use of the term 'client' within art therapy, referring to someone choosing to make use of services which are available to them. Alternatively, someone might feel like a guest if the therapy involves free admission, visits out of normal opening hours, special access to museums staff or collections, or a designated room which is not normally used by the public, and this could help them to feel valued (Shaer *et al.* 2008; Ander *et al.* 2013; Coles and Harrison 2018).

Although the BritainThinks (2013) research found a public perception that museums should be accessible and inclusive, in practice some museum-based art therapy clients might feel that they do not belong within the museum setting. This could be a result of feeling unwelcome or unworthy when visiting museums in the past, or of a more generalised sense of rejection and low self-worth. Exploring how clients see their relationship to the museum would be helpful in ensuring that they gain maximum therapeutic benefit from the therapy and could also inspire more general reflections on how they see themselves in relation to others and the world at large. This could be done at an initial meeting phase, encouraging the client to reflect on how it might feel to be attending the first museum-based art therapy session, and perhaps explored further during the therapy.

Museums as under threat

Finally, the research found that there was a 'widespread perception that the future of museums is threatened' by decreasing visitor numbers, budget cuts or new technologies (BritainThinks 2013, p.26). Many museums in the UK are under great financial pressure; the Museums Association (2017) reported that 'at least 64 museums in the UK have closed since 2010 – the vast majority due to public funding cuts' (p.4). Clients of museum-based art therapy might be less likely to experience the setting as a place of safe, continuous 'holding' if they know, or believe, that the museum is struggling to make ends meet. Alongside this, a feeling that museums are undervalued, disregarded and vulnerable might resonate with a client's internal world, exacerbating feelings of neglect and potentially feeding into a sense of not getting 'good enough' care from the therapist.

A sense of a museum being 'under threat' could also connect with someone's deep-seated feelings of fear. Clients might, of course, have the same concerns about funding of health services, with similar implications. However, museum closures have the additional factor of the 'loss' of collections (at least in terms of public access to those collections in that particular museum) and if we think about museums as places that contain our collective memory, at a societal level, then fear of collections being 'lost' could be associated with a fear of losing part of our collective sense of who we are. At an even more fundamental level, Trustram (2014) considers that the permanency of museums serves as a 'defense against our anxieties about mortality', assuring us that 'despite death, life will continue' (p.69), so that an anticipated or actual museum closure could resonate with a client's fears around death. Exploring any anxieties around the survival of the museum in which an art therapy intervention is based would seem to be essential in order to maximise the possibility of therapeutic work based on feelings of security and trust.

Conclusion

In this chapter, I have considered the possible implications for museum-based art therapy of various perceptions about museums held by adults in the UK. Many of these perceptions resonate with key therapeutic principles of holding and containing, trust, exploration and learning, play and acceptance, and I feel that this is an encouragement to art therapists who are seeking to utilise museums within their practice. Perhaps a museum is well suited to contributing towards the 'creative and containing environment' which art therapists need to provide for effective therapeutic work (Health and Care Professions Council 2013), and reflecting on these perceptions of museums with clients might help to activate these therapeutic principles within the therapy. I have also identified how views about museums could be harnessed within museum-based art therapy for the exploration of issues such as knowing and not knowing, care and neglect, fear, abuse of power, and difference and diversity.

These resonances between the UK public's 'museum in the mind' (Trustram 2014, p.69) and important aspects of art therapy practice mean that partnerships between museums and art therapy can be 'particularly fruitful' (Silverman 2010, p.45). However, to return to the idea that the concept of a museum evokes a set of 'use-potentials' (Bollas 1992, p.34), the general notion of a museum held by adults in the UK, as explored in the BritainThinks (2013) research, does not yet include a psychological therapy role. For this to become a commonly perceived 'use-potential', there will need to be an increase in museum-based art therapy practice, along with a sharing of information about this work with the wider public. A greater recognition of the therapeutic value of museums would, in turn, further enable engagement by clients and ensure that the partnership of museums and art therapy continues to bear fruit.

References

Ander, E., Thomson, L., Blair, K., Noble, G., Menon, U. and Lanceley, A. (2013) 'Using museum objects to improve wellbeing in mental health service users and neurological rehabilitation clients.' *British Journal of Occupational Therapy 76*, 5, 208–216.

Bedford, L. (2004) 'Working in the subjunctive mood: Imagination and museums.' *Curator 47*, 1, 5–11.

Bion, W. (1994) *Learning from Experience*. Northvale, NJ: Jason Aronson. (Original work published 1962).

Bollas, C. (1992) *Being a Character: Psychoanalysis and Self Experience*. New York, NY: Hill and Wang.

Bowlby, J. (1982) *Attachment* (second edition). New York, NY: Basic Books. (Original work published 1969).

BritainThinks (2013) *Public Perceptions of – and Attitudes to – the Purposes of Museums in Society*. Accessed on 17/9/17 at www.britainthinks.com/pdfs/Museums-Association-The-purposes-of-museums-in-society-Public-report.pdf.

British Association of Art Therapists (2014) *Code of Ethics and Principles of Professional Practice for Art Therapists*. Accessed on 19/1/19 at www.baat.org/Assets/Docs/General/BAAT%20CODE%20OF%20ETHICS%202014.pdf.

Camic, P. and Chatterjee, H. (2013) 'Museums and art galleries as partners for public health interventions.' *Perspectives in Public Health 133*, 1, 66–71.

Carr, D. (2001) 'A museum is an open work.' *International Journal of Heritage Studies 7*, 2, 173–183.

Case, C. and Dalley, T. (2014) *The Handbook of Art Therapy* (third edition). London and New York, NY: Routledge.

Coles, A. and Harrison, F. (2018) 'Tapping into museums for art psychotherapy: An evaluation of a pilot group for young adults.' *International Journal of Art Therapy 23,* 3, 115–124.

Coles, A., Harrison, F. and Todd, S. (2019) 'Flexing the frame: Therapist experiences of museum-based group art psychotherapy for adults with complex mental health difficulties.' *International Journal of Art Therapy 24*, 2 56–67.

Department for Digital, Culture, Media and Sport (2018) *Visits to Museums and Galleries*. Accessed on 13/1/19 at www.ethnicity-facts-figures.service.gov.uk/culture-and-community/culture-and-heritage/adults-visiting-museums-and-galleries/latest.

Derry, C. (n.d.) *Rules for a Playful Museum*. Accessed on 28/1/18 at www.happymuseumproject.org/rules-playful-museum-2.

Doering, Z. (1999) 'Strangers, guests or clients? Visitor experiences in museums.' *Curator 42,* 2, 74–87.

Edson, G. (2015) 'Museums are wonderful places: An introduction.' *Museum International 261–264,* 7–18.

Edwards, D. (2014) *Art Therapy* (second edition). London: SAGE.

Fleming, D. (2016) 'Do museums change lives? Ninth Stephen Weil Memorial Lecture.' *Curator: The Museum Journal 59,* 2, 73–79.

Froggett, L. and Trustram, M. (2014) 'Object relations in the museum: A psychosocial perspective.' *Museum Management and Curatorship 29,* 5, 482–497.

Gantt, L. and Tinnin, L.W. (2009) 'Support for a neurobiological view of trauma with implications for art therapy.' *The Arts in Psychotherapy 36,* 148–153.

Heal, S. (2017) *After Charlottesville*. Accessed on 23/9/17 at www.museumsassociation.org/comment/directors-blog/21082017-after-charlottesville.

Health and Care Professions Council (2013) *The Standards of Proficiency for Arts Therapists*. Accessed on 25/7/18 at www.hcpc-uk.org/standards/standards-of-proficiency/arts-therapists.

Heynen, E., Roest, J., Willemars, G. and van Hooren, S. (2017) 'Therapeutic alliance is a factor of change in arts therapies and psychomotor therapy with adults who have mental health problems.' *The Arts in Psychotherapy 55,* 111–115.

International Council of Museums Documentation Committee (2012) *Statement of Principles of Museum Documentation*. Accessed on 19/1/19 at http://network.icom.museum/cidoc/working-groups/documentation-standards/principles-of-museum-documentation.

Ioannides, E. (2017) 'Museums as therapeutic environments and the contribution of art therapy.' *Museum International 68,* 3–4, 98–109.

Janes, R.R. and Sandell, R. (2019) *Museum Activism*. Abingdon, Oxon and New York, NY: Routledge.

Kaplan, F. (ed.) (2006) *Art Therapy and Social Action*. London and Philadelphia, PA: Jessica Kingsley Publishers.

Museums Association (2017) *Museums in the UK: 2017 Report*. Accessed on 23/9/17 at www.museumsassociation.org/download?id=1219029.

Museums Association (2018a) *FAQs: What is a Museum?* Accessed on 18/1/18 at www.museumsassociation.org/about/frequently-asked-questions.

Museums Association (2018b) *Ethical Guidelines 4 – Access*. Accessed on 3/1/18 at www.museumsassociation.org/download?id=8352.

Museums Association (2018c) *Museums in the UK: 2018 Report*. Accessed on 20/1/19 at www.museumsassociation.org/download?id=1244881.

Pearce, S.M. (1999) *On Collecting: An Investigation into Collecting in the European Tradition*. London and New York, NY: Routledge.

Salom, A. (2011) 'Reinventing the setting: Art Therapy in museums.' *The Arts in Psychotherapy 38,* 81–85.

Sandell, R. (2003) 'Social inclusion, the museum and the dynamics of social change.' *Museum and Society 1,* 1, 45–62.

Schaverien, J. (1999) *The Revealing Image*. London and Philadelphia, PA: Jessica Kingsley Publishers.

Shaer, D., Beaven, K., Springham, N., Pillinger, S. *et al.* (2008) 'The role of art therapy in a pilot for art-based information prescriptions at Tate Britain.' *International Journal of Art Therapy 13,* 1, 25–33.

Silverman, L. (2010) *The Social Work of Museums*. Abingdon, Oxon and New York, NY: Routledge.

Tissier, D. and Nathoo, S.S. (2004) *Black and Minority Ethnic Engagement with London's Museums – Telling It Like It Is: Non-user Research*. London: Strategic Urban Futures. Accessed on 20/1/19 at http://culturehive.co.uk/wp-content/uploads/2013/10/BME-Engagement-with-London-Museums-2.pdf.

Trustram, M. (2014) 'Asylum and the museum.' *American Imago 71,* 1, 67–84.

Van der Kolk, B. (2014) *The Body Keeps the Score: Mind, Brain and Body in the Transformation of Trauma*. London: Penguin Books.

Victoria and Albert Museum (n.d.) *LGBTQ*. Accessed on 20/1/19 at www.vam.ac.uk/info/lgbtq.

Winnicott, D.W. (1990) *The Maturational Processes and the Facilitating Environment: Studies in the Theory of Emotional Development*. London and New York, NY: Karnac. (Original work published 1965).

Winnicott, D. (2010) *Playing and Reality*. Abingdon, Oxon and New York, NY: Routledge Classics. (Original work published 1971).

Yalom, I. (1995) *The Theory and Practice of Group Psychotherapy*. New York, NY: Basic Books.

CHAPTER 3

Making Space Safe at Modern Art Oxford

Mary Chamberlain

Introduction

I am a qualified art therapist and have worked for many years as a creative art practitioner (rather than an art therapist), using some of the therapeutic principles gained during my training. My creative practice involves working with vulnerable people and teaching art in environments that feel relaxing and trustworthy. A huge focus of my work is creating safe spaces (internal and external) for group work. During this chapter, I examine concepts of 'safe spaces' in my work as a creative art practitioner with Modern Art Oxford, a 50-year-old public institution for contemporary art. The name of the group at Modern Art Oxford is *Making Space Safe* and the work is a pilot venture of Modern Art Oxford Associate Artists, set up in response to a perceived need for therapeutic art practice in a public gallery. As well as offering my own perspective, I draw on an evaluation of the project (Radermacher 2019) which explored whether the project had achieved its objectives; how a safe space was created and experienced; and how the project could be improved.

I am interested in exploring themes inherent in the title of the group itself – *Making Space Safe*. I have thought about the name of the group – about each word separately and then joined. Making. Space. Safe. Making Space. Space Safe. Making Safe. These three words and their interactions hold within them the vision and goals of this art group for refugees and asylum seekers. In this chapter, I focus on the physical space that the group meets in. As Papadopoulos (2002) states, 'The most basic form of therapy for individuals who are functioning at a very basic level (at a given period in their life) is the provision of a safe and reliable environment' (p.23). It is this that intrigues me – how to set up and establish a provision with an overt focus on creating a sense of safety within a creative and cultural organisation, and what, if any, difference the setting makes to attendees.

Background to the group

The group was set up in October 2016 and members are referred by external partners: Asylum Welcome, Refugee Resource and Sanctuary Hosting. I am supervised by Dr Michael Korzinski, previously co-founder and clinical director of the Helen Bamber Foundation (HBF), and currently working as an independent psychologist and psychosocial expert. He specialises in work with the victims of complex trauma, including victims of torture and gender-based violence (especially in conflict-affected areas), trafficking and slavery.

Arriving in Oxford in 2014, having previously run a successful weekly art group at HBF in London for six years, I was keen to see if a similar creative art group existed there. My former group at HBF met in the premises of this therapeutic organisation and referrals to the art group were made by HBF clinicians. Occasional creative partnerships and trips to cultural institutions such as the British Museum, Tate Modern and Kew Gardens complemented our programme of work.

I found there was no group of this kind for refugees and asylum seekers in Oxford so decided to establish one. The challenge of setting up a group in a new city almost from scratch seemed to me like having blank canvas, with opportunities of choice about the physical, psychological and theoretical space in which we might meet. Having previously run a group for many years at HBF, I had a successful template in mind that I was keen to draw on and adapt, where needed.

Choice of physical setting for *Making Space Safe*

Options for a physical space where the group could meet included an open space in the foyer of a well-known refugee agency and a private room in another refugee agency. Initial clients were already very familiar with both these spaces and felt in some way 'known' in these settings where clinical, legal and practical work took place. The alternative was to base the group in a cultural and creative venue where the group setting would encourage dialogues around art and the making of artwork and what it is to be an artist, rather than an individual's legal or psychological status as a refugee or asylum seeker. It was this that strongly appealed to me, to work under the aegis of a cultural and creative venue and team, and house the work there, offering clients the experience of belonging to a group in another type of space. Modern Art Oxford, with its strong reputation for engagement and learning activities and location in the city centre, was my home of choice for this group.

As can sometimes be the way, my enquiries to Modern Art Oxford coincided with the gallery wishing to look strategically at how it might become more engaged with different groups and communities within Oxford and the surrounding areas. Work using art with vulnerable people such as refugees and asylum seekers is specialised, requiring the practitioner to have a high degree of sensitivity, understanding and experience of working with therapeutic boundaries. The gallery created a new scheme entitled 'Associate Artists' for this strand of engagement work. My group became the first pilot group to be run under this strand and I became the inaugural Associate Artist at Modern Art Oxford. I stress this, as it highlights two aspects of my involvement with running the group at Modern Art Oxford. First, as a creative art practitioner, having the bespoke role and title of Associate Artist endowed me with a personal sense of safety and being valued, which in turn enabled me to work towards creating a safe space for the group. Second, the kudos of working under such a title helped to enact some of the process I wished my group to experience: the sense that they were being valued and given space at a leading creative cultural organisation in the city centre. There was also a sense of excitement and timeliness about the dialogue for

Modern Art Oxford as this was the first time it had worked with refugees and asylum seekers in this way, offering a regular and fixed place in which to make art within a project that had longevity, and where the group was a closed one with participants referred by external referring agencies.

Associate Artists scheme at Modern Art Oxford

From the gallery's point of view, the project represented a vital and specialised way to engage with a vulnerable population within the city and surrounding countryside, who might not otherwise think to access its building. Modern Art Oxford is renowned for being experimental and bold in its curatorial programming. Its Associate Artists scheme was similarly devised to be bold, working with invited artists who specialise in the development of creative skills for specific groups of vulnerable people and/or with protected characteristics. This strand of work has developed and grown since my initial engagement with Modern Art Oxford. There are currently three Associate Artists working with a range of groups, including vulnerable young people and prisoners and their children, and the groups enable people who may be isolated and vulnerable to engage with art-making and the city's cultural offering. Associate Artists fundraise for their own projects initially and then, ideally, the project becomes embedded into the gallery's core funding streams. Funding for *Making Space Safe* came from private donors, Oxford City Council and the Network for Social Change and the gallery provided the room for free. As well as providing support in kind, the gallery also provided financial support during intermittent periods in the pilot phase when the project was lacking in external funding.

Another vital aspect of *Making Space Safe* that came through strongly in the evaluation is my attitude and manner as Associate Artist, leading the sessions and creating a safe space. Although I am not practising as an art therapist, my training in art therapy underpins my practice as a creative art practitioner and enables me to create a sense of trust that has little to do with the physical space. In my work, I have the opportunity to combine my skills as an artist with my therapeutic training and 'hold' a group of people, some of whom have experienced extreme trauma, enabling them to create artwork of which they are proud. My role involves creating a physical and psychological space where group members can explore and discover their creative voice as well as exercise autonomy over which art materials they will use, or which subjects they will depict. The interplay in my role between creative art practitioner and artist with a training in art therapy is echoed by the external collaboration between a contemporary art gallery and the various therapeutic refugee agencies who refer participants to the project.

Description of the group

About 20 people have participated in the *Making Space Safe* group since it started. Participants are men and women from a range of different countries including Kurdistan, Afghanistan, Syria, Kosovo, Malaysia, China and several African countries, and are mostly aged between 20 and 45 years. Prior to their arrival in the UK, they may have witnessed or experienced displacement, torture, genocide, rape and other human rights abuses. People are referred to the group for many reasons – as a stepping stone to assist their integration into the community, as a place of respite and relief from mental or emotional pressure, to make friends and reduce isolation, or as an impetus to learn new things and gain artistic skills. Among the participants there is often a great range of familiarity with their own art-making process and experiences of being part of a group. To date, an assistant has been present for about half of the sessions. The *Making Space Safe* assistant has a background and training in the visual arts and is experienced in running art groups with refugees and asylum seekers. Their role is to set up the space and ensure safe storage of artwork, help with teas and coffees, support the creative activities, and assist in facilitating a safe and secure environment.

Sessions run for 90 minutes and terms are structured very loosely along the lines of school terms with an autumn, spring and summer term and corresponding holidays and half-term breaks within these. The group aims to be inclusive and welcoming, regardless of artistic skill and experience. Some group members study art in their own time outside the sessions and teach themselves further skills via YouTube, while, for others, it is enough to make it along each week. I have found that if participants return following an initial taster session, they usually attend regularly each week for at least six months or so. One of the group members has been attending for 18 months.

Participants can choose whether to attend each session and when to arrive and leave. I like to think that there is a sense of freedom and care within the whole process. Group members have a sense of being able to come and go as they please, and that is important, but if they choose not to attend, their absence is acknowledged without judgement to ensure they know they are missed when not there. This element of choice and agency of participants was highlighted during an evaluation interview with one of the referring agencies:

> The fact that participants are made aware that they're free to come when they can and feel comfortable doing so and there are no repercussions to missing a class is helpful. As when a participant is unable to come to a session they feel confident that they can come the following week without there being any problems and they will be welcomed and supported. (Radermacher 2019)

Giving traumatised and displaced individuals the opportunity to take part in an art group in a contemporary art gallery, based on principles of a safe space, brings with it possibilities for recovery. While traumatic experiences can lead to a sense of frozenness, I believe that art has a quality of movement inherent within it. Van der Kolk (2014) says that 'trauma robs you of the feeling you are in charge of yourself' (p.203) and 'recovery from trauma involves the restoration of executive functioning and, with it, self-confidence and the capacity for playfulness and creativity' (p.205). The making and exhibiting of art bring variation and choices to participants whose lives might be on hold while in this country, while they may be unable to work and are waiting for resolution of their status. I liken my approach to teaching a language: first the vocabulary of different materials, then devising sentences and paragraphs, before going on to enable group members to discover their own creative process and artistic voice. My work has the sense of the 'present continuous' about it, involving exploring, developing, learning, creating, erasing, undoing, recreating; the process is an ongoing and unfolding one, held within a geographical and psychological safe space. One of the referring agencies touched on this in the evaluation interview:

> It's developing something else, it's being creative, isn't it? It's sort of enabling people to wake up something inside because you know a lot of our clients spend a lot of time trotting in between the different crisis agencies and this is a safe space between all of those. (Radermacher 2019)

Herman (1992) speaks of how 'the first principle of recovery is the empowerment of the survivor. She must be the author and arbiter of her own recovery' (p.133). Within the art group, each participant must make artwork for themselves. No one else will intervene to draw a line for the participant – indeed, it is one of the group rules not to draw or paint on each other's work and to use another piece of paper if you want to demonstrate something. The whole principle of the art group is based on the empowerment of the individual and enabling them to create artwork, and discover and enjoy a quality of agency and control in their lives. As Wertheim-Cahen puts it:

> The activity of the art process itself, involving doing something with your hands and body, offers at least moments in which the asylum seeker regains power over his own life however momentarily, and enables some to have an aesthetic and therefore a positive experience. (Wertheim-Cahen 1998, p.52)

We have 'group rules' or codes of behaviour, from the logistical such as, 'Please clean up your own brushes', to the emotional such as, 'Please treat others with respect even if you don't agree'. In this way, the rules aim to create an internal *locus* of safety both individually and collectively for the group. The group is reminded of these rules at the start of each term and every time a new member joins. These boundaries operate to keep people safely in, and also to keep people safely out; over time, staff at Modern Art Oxford have learned to understand and respect the work and be sure not to enter the space when a session is running.

The referral process

Much of the focus of setting up the group was on developing and liaising with our partners over the referral form for *Making Space Safe*. Conversations mainly revolved around whether there was a need for a form, strengths and weaknesses of running an open or closed group, and organisational logistics of who would fill in the form.

In an initial session with my supervisor, looking at creating the group and getting it off the ground, he used the analogy of building a house. We thought about the vital importance of a robust referral mechanism, operating similarly to the walls of a house and protecting the inhabitants. The referral form is completed by referring organisations, who appreciate its simplicity. It was devised to focus on the individual's relationship with art-making and the best way to contact them. Questions include: whether the participant attends other classes or has attended any classes previously; the participant's familiarity with art materials; what their expectations are for the group and whether they have any goals they would like to achieve; whether they have an interest in art galleries and museums; and the referee's reason for making the referral.

Having referral forms which are filled in by partner organisations helps to ensure that the referral has been thought through by the referee and endows the process with a sense of care. The referral is almost always accompanied by a phone call with the referee in which we briefly discuss the reason for the referral. The process is a relational one, and there is trust and mutual appreciation of skills that have been built up over time. The referral process is not necessarily a mechanism to screen out potential participants, but rather one by which I can find out more information about participants so that I am better able to respond to their needs, as well as a way of building relationships with the referring agencies. I have yet to turn down a referral and would, at the very least, speak with my contact who made the referral to understand their rationale if it seemed unclear. Some referring agencies have taken to this referral process well, whereas others would prefer a more fluid approach where clients can drop in as and when they wish. This is not appropriate with *Making Space Safe* because of the need to create a stable and secure environment for all members of the group.

The setting of Modern Art Oxford

In the evaluation, referring agencies described the gallery as being 'quite a calm and quiet place' in which to run the sessions. This is in contrast to refugee agencies' premises, which can be more chaotic due to the urgent nature of some of the work they undertake. The centrality of the location was also mentioned by all the external referring partners, as the gallery is easy for participants to find and travel to. I feel that having such a prime central Oxford location in which to meet sends out a powerful message to attendees of being valued. This is echoed in the internal space; physical storage space is in great demand within the gallery, but we have been given use of a shelf within a secure cupboard for storing our materials and artworks (Figure 3.1).

I point this out not only to demonstrate how the creation of a safe space operates on many diverse levels, from the micro to the macro, but also for the political nuances that being given dedicated space might carry. There is a political aspect to dialogues of space when working with people who have been dispossessed. A South African artist is quoted as saying, 'It's all about space... Claiming art is reclaiming space' (David Koloane quoted in Deliss 1996, p.265). Although my group is named *Making Space Safe*, it could equally be named 'Reclaiming Space, Safe'. When people have been dispossessed and the land they consider to be their home has been removed from them, the physical backdrop to a therapeutic group becomes of interest and forms part of the landscape of the group.

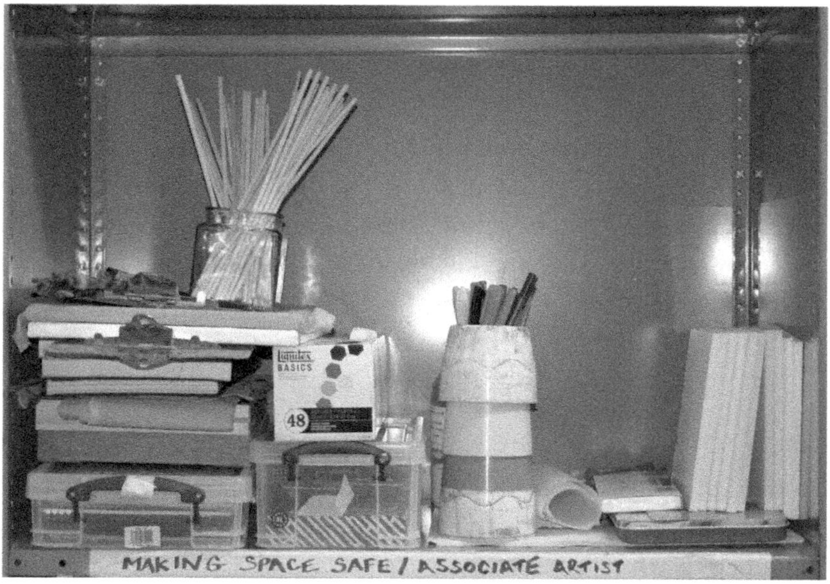

Figure 3.1 Making Space Safe *shelf within the storage cupboard*

The art gallery environment

The art gallery environment points to qualities of beauty and wellbeing. De Botton (2007) writes of how 'we depend on our surroundings obliquely to embody the moods and ideas we respect and then to remind us of them. We look to our buildings to hold us, like a kind of psychological mould, to a helpful vision of ourselves' (p.107). There can be a duality of aesthetics in a modern-day gallery; walls are normally white, artificial lighting bright and natural light often muted or dimmed in order to display artwork to best advantage. A creative, professional and corporate ambience is prioritised in some public spaces in order to appeal to potential funders or for venue hire. On the one hand, from the point of view of a creative art practitioner, credence and authority are given to the work by having a 'cool' space to meet in – a space that conforms to the current received wisdom of a modern art gallery aesthetic with white walls, vinyl black lettering on signage and minimal visual clutter. On the other hand, this aesthetic can have negative associations for the specific client group of refugees and asylum seekers; the bare starkness of the white, the brightness of the artificial light and a lack of 'comfort' might, at worst, be reminiscent of detention centres or suggest a distinctly foreign environment.

Feedback from the group, however, indicates that members like the space where the group is held – they think of it as a studio, and as a place to exhibit work. One member has spoken of how it made her feel important to walk through the gallery doors to attend the group. So, it seems that even if the typical aesthetics of a modern art gallery may verge on the clinical, there is potential for creativity and encouraging the mindset of an artist. In fact, Modern Art Oxford was formerly a brewery and has, to my mind, a sense of external and internal warmth resulting from its original purpose as an industrial space for 'making'.

The Project Space at Modern Art Oxford

Since *Making Space Safe* began in October 2016, we have mostly met in a room called the Project Space (Figure 3.2). This can function as a public space but can also become a private area. It is on the ground floor near to a main entrance, the shop and cafe. Overhead strip lights cast a warm light and create a well-lit space. The art supply cupboard is located in one corner, and the door to the workshop where brushes and art materials can be cleaned at the end of class is situated in the other corner. Although not an ideal art-making space as it is windowless, the space has provided, to my eyes, a warm and secure environment to make work in. The secure nature of the space was picked up on by gallery staff in the evaluation; 'The physical space itself provides a safe space of quiet' and 'The actual physical space, the room, is quiet and removed from other activities, making it a safe space where participants know they won't have to interact with unknown people on the periphery' (Radermacher 2019). Given the aims and objectives of the project – to make space safe – the physical characteristics of the room were significant.

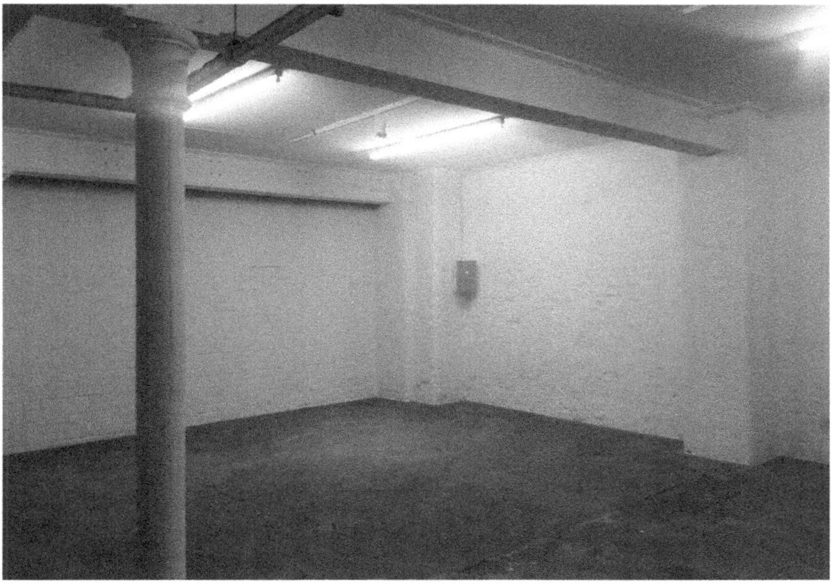

Figure 3.2 The Project Space (photo credit: Stu Allsop)

The room is a good size, with the option of placing the two trestle tables in different positions. Both tables are set up and art materials laid out in advance to create a sense of welcome and an invitation to create within the room. By setting up the room in advance, we make sure that the space is in a state of readiness for the participants' arrival.

However, there is a flexibility on offer with the set-up, and I am keen to understand where group members feel most comfortable in the room to make their artwork. To help encourage familiarity with, and ownership of, the space, I have asked group members where in the space they would like to make their work, encouraging them to walk around the room and examine what it feels like to inhabit different parts of it. So far, the choice has been to place the tables in the far corner, giving the members a little privacy as well as physical space in the room, a space within a space (Figure 3.3). When asked why, a group member said that he liked it because of 'how it feels'.

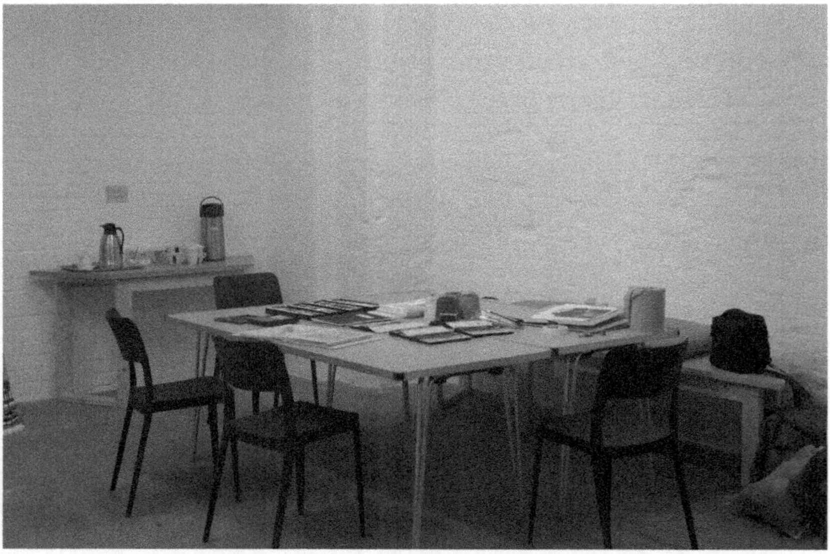

Figure 3.3 'Our' corner in the Project Space

The space is sometimes empty, other than our trestle tables, chairs and art materials, and at other times we have shared the space with a current exhibition. On the occasions we have shared our space with an exhibition, I have yet to see any member of the group go towards, pick up a related item, or engage with the show. We may have conversations about the current exhibitions, all of which are free to enter and easily accessible from the Project Space, but most participants do not choose to visit them. I am unclear about why there is little engagement with the exhibitions during the sessions, and there may be many factors at play. One possible reason is that the focus of the group is very much on participants making their own artwork and being in the present – the 'here and now'.

The basement at Modern Art Oxford

Modern Art Oxford has prioritised the use of the Project Space by the group. However, at times, logistics have demanded we meet in the basement area, a space on the ground floor accessed via steps from the cafe (Figure 3.4). A sign is placed at the head of the stairs when we meet there stating that a session is in progress and that the stairs should only be used for getting to the accessible toilets and baby-changing facilities.

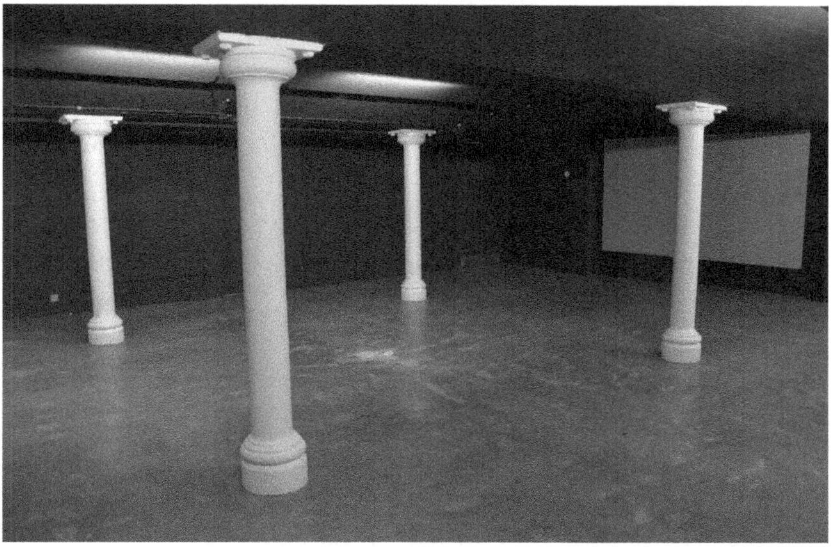

Figure 3.4 The basement space

This space is dimly lit and is an area used for live music and experimental artwork. Bachelard (1964) writes of the cellar as being 'first and foremost the *dark entity* of the house, the one that partakes of subterranean forces' (p.39). This basement area is a public space at a gallery (rather than a house) and thankfully does not quite have that quality, yet I am mindful of the connotations that a basement may have for a group as a place where objects are stored and can become discarded, and even as a place of incarceration.

Since the start of 2018, due to changes to the museum building, we have temporarily moved to this basement space. The table, chairs, art materials and group leader are the same but the spaces are palpably different. The lighting, the placement in the building, the privacy and the size of the two spaces differ enormously. As in the Project Space, I have placed the table and chairs in a corner to make a space within a space and to give some separation from the members of the public who need to come through to access the toilet and baby-changing facilities. To my surprise, the feedback from the group has been entirely positive regarding the move to this space; they told me that this space is 'okay' and 'the same' as or 'similar' to the Project Space upstairs.

The natural and built environments have a profound impact on our health and wellbeing. Within healthcare, access to daylight, fresh air and natural materials aids healing, restoring the integrity between mind, body and soul. Patients and staff alike appreciate health and social care environments that are well designed and animated by the arts (All-Party Parliamentary Group on Arts, Health and Wellbeing 2017, p.11). Perhaps due to past experiences of not getting the help they need, participants may be so grateful for what is provided to them that it is hard to express a negative opinion of a space, facilities or group. It may be that they are seeking to reassure themselves, or me, that the work can continue as before in this new space, or that they might be fearful of losing what they have if they voice objections. Another possible explanation is that the fabric of the group is made up of more than the four surrounding walls, and that the group's perception of itself is based more on relationships and trust and the artwork which is made than the physical setting. Perhaps there is a perception of the venue for the group being the whole space of Modern Art Oxford, the larger building; whether accessing a private room by a main entrance, like the Project Space, or a darker, downstairs space like the basement, the group is still at Modern Art Oxford.

It will be interesting if this basement space becomes the preferred one at the gallery. To my mind, it has fewer associations with the more traditional 'white cube' gallery-type space. According to Brian O'Doherty (1986), 'A gallery is constructed along laws as rigorous as those for building a medieval church. The outside world must not come in, so windows are usually sealed off. Walls are painted white. The ceiling becomes the source of light' (p.15). Continuing with the ecclesiastical theme, Thomas McEvilley (in O'Doherty 1986), speaks of how 'In classical modernist galleries, as in churches, one does not speak in a normal voice' (p.10). Perhaps this spacious basement area, often used for gigs, lends itself to a more relaxed environment that is a little freer. Although access is given to the public for baby-changing and toilet facilities, in a sense this space is more private, tucked away as it is.

There is a need for caution and an awareness of cultural specificity when looking at different areas and rooms. Whereas I perceive the dimness of lighting in the basement as being a negative factor in a space required for making artwork, I must be wary of assuming that group members feel the same. Tanizaki (2001) writes about the value of a certain level of dimmed lighting for accentuating beauty, illustrating the need for the creative art practitioner to try to understand how groups relate to spaces rather than make assumptions:

> And so it has come to be that the beauty of a Japanese room depends on a variation of shadows, heavy shadows against light shadows – it has nothing else. Westerners are amazed at the simplicity of Japanese rooms, perceiving in them no more than ashen walls bereft of ornament. Their reaction is understandable, but it betrays a failure to comprehend the mystery of shadows. (p.29)

The importance of a safe and therapeutic creative space

Van der Kolk (2014) speaks of how 'being able to feel safe with other people is probably the single most important aspect of mental health… For our physiology to calm down, heal, and grow we need a visceral sense of safety' (p.79). Creating that visceral sense of safety for the art group requires a variety of external elements to be put in place. Feedback given in the evaluation by one of the referring agencies highlighted the importance to clients whose lives can be 'so chaotic and unboundaried' of 'having that regular rhythm of being able to go to that place, as part of the structure of their week, and somewhere where they can sort of get lost in their work and get away from their troubles' (Radermacher 2019).

Part of the safety created for the group is a sense of my reliability. Part of this is my weekly contact with group members outside the class, sending reminder texts or emails the day before each session. My intention is also to try to give them a feeling that someone is being mindful of both them and the group between sessions.

As I am the lead artist running the workshops and the key liaison link with our various partners, my own sense of safety and support is fundamental. To this end, I have a variety of important support structures in place. I have regular contact with the Curator of Creative Learning and Creative Learning Assistant at Modern Art Oxford and am assisted each week by an art group assistant who was interviewed and selected for the role. As an external Associate Artist, I value that my work has a psychological home within the organisation, as well as a physical space. I also receive regular supervision from a psychosocial practitioner, which is vital in order to address my own needs and concerns as they arise.

Conclusion

Callaghan (1998) provides a précis of the accumulative effects on body and mind of the experiences of many asylum seekers and refugees, including the sense of exile; the loss of 'home'; the uncertainty and anxiety brought about by the (prolonged) wait to discover the outcome of their asylum process and whether they will be allowed to remain in the UK; separation from families; and financial, physical and emotional stress. *Making Space Safe* provides a regular space within the city centre that is held and supported by a carefully thought-out structure and team of skilled and caring professionals – a space which can provide a sense of attention, of being seen and cared for, and within which the participant can have agency and a sense of control over artistic choices and decisions. This is a group which has been built up over time with mechanisms and procedures in place to allow clients to create, heal and flourish. The project brings together a variety of organisations to create a vital, creative and ultimately safe environment for attendees.

Making. Space. Safe. I conclude by returning to where this chapter started, with a focus on these three words. Within this chapter, I have attempted to look at some of the elements involved in basing the group in a 'making', creative organisation such as Modern Art Oxford, giving a background to the relationship and looking at some of the nuances of holding the group in an art gallery. I have focused on ideas surrounding 'space', concentrating on the physical spaces we have used and how these might affect the group. Finally, I have detailed some of the internal and external structures that make up this work, looking at how they might create a sense of safety for attendees of the group.

In *Making Space Safe* I have the privilege of witnessing people joining the group and experiencing the space, often for the first time. I also witness group members using their autonomy and experiencing a variety of art materials, trying out new things, learning what they like and do not like, and ultimately exploring and seeing if this space might be one in which they want to stay for a while – a safe space.

References

All-Party Parliamentary Group on Arts, Health and Wellbeing (2017) *Creative Health: The Arts for Health and Wellbeing* (second edition). Accessed on 15/7/19 at https://www.culturehealthandwellbeing.org.uk/appg-inquiry/.

Bachelard, G. (1964) *The Poetics of Space*. London: Penguin.

Callaghan, K. (1998) 'In Limbo: Movement Psychotherapy with Refugees and Asylum Seekers.' In D. Dokter (ed.) *Arts Therapists, Refugees and Migrants: Reaching Across Borders*. London and Philadelphia, PA: Jessica Kingsley Publishers.

De Botton, A. (2007) *The Architecture of Happiness*. London: Penguin.

Deliss, C. (1996) *Seven Stories about Modern Art in South Africa*. Paris and New York, NY: Whitechapel/Flammarion.

Herman, J.L. (1992) *Trauma and Recovery*. New York, NY: Basic Books.

O'Doherty, B. (1986) *Inside the White Cube: The Ideology of the Gallery Space*. San Francisco: The Lapis Press.

Papadopoulos, R.K. (2002) 'Refugees, Home and Trauma.' In R.K. Papadopoulos (ed.), *Therapeutic Care for Refugees: No Place Like Home*. The Tavistock Clinic Series. London: Routledge.

Radermacher, H. (2019) *Making Space Safe: An Evaluation*. Melbourne: Radermacher and Associates (unpublished).

Tanizaki, J. (2001) *In Praise of Shadows*. London: Vintage Books.

Van der Kolk, B. (2014) The Body Keeps the Score: *Mind, Brain and Body in the Transformation of Trauma*. London: Penguin

Wertheim-Cahen, T. (1998) 'Art Therapy with Asylum Seekers: Humanitarian Relief.' In D. Dokter (ed.) *Arts Therapists, Refugees and Migrants: Reaching Across Borders*. London and Philadelphia, PA: Jessica Kingsley Publishers.

PART 2

Art Therapists Working with Museums and Galleries

CHAPTER 4

From Isolation to Relation

Reflections on the Development of Museum-Based Art Therapy in Russia

Nana Zhvitiashvili

Introduction

In recent years, the role of museums in wellbeing and healthcare has been redefined. Paradigms have shifted in the last two decades as museums have moved away from a position of 'authority' and adopted more open and integrated approaches to working in dialogue with their audiences (Barrett and Tapia 2003). I have previously worked as a museum curator developing therapeutically minded programmes, and I now work as an art therapist integrating the cultural resources of museums into my clinical practice. What follows is a reflection on my use of museums as therapeutic environments in Russia, an early example of the bringing together of museums and art therapy approaches, and key factors for effective work. I will also review the similarities between my roles as an art therapist and museum curator.

Developing 'museum therapy' in Russia after the collapse of the communist regime

Due to the political and economic turmoil after the collapse of the communist regime in Russia in the early 1990s, The State Russian Museum in St Petersburg, the largest national art museum in the country, significantly reconsidered its mission and began experimenting with new forms of educational work. The museum had to address fast-changing cultural, political and social landscapes in a newly reformed society of freedom of speech. Functioning under the ideological pressure of the government of the Soviet Union for more than 70 years, museums had limited freedom to curate collections and engage the public; as state-funded institutions, they were guided by rigid regulations imposed by the regime. Throughout Soviet museum history, there were attempts to address the relationship between museums and their audiences. For instance, museum experiments from 1932 to 1935, initiated at The State Historical Museum in Moscow, focused on the apperception (the mental process by which a person makes sense of an idea by assimilating it into past knowledge and experience) of diverse young audiences. These experiments were stopped abruptly by the 1936 Decree issued by the Central Committee of the Communist Party, which accused museum curators of 'quasi-scientific and harmful perversions of museum pedagogy' (Yukhnevich 2001, p.23). Almost all innovative programmes were banned for a few decades under Stalin's repressive regime. From the 1950s to the 1960s, the Khrushchev era during which repression and censorship in the Soviet Union were relaxed (the so-called 'Thaw' period), museums remained a conduit of political education. Within this politicised model, the content of educational work was reductionist – museums served as illustrations of political doctrines. The collapse of ideological rule and emergence of new liberties in the early 1990s led cultural institutions to redefine their relationship with the public.

One of the key questions posed was: how can museums operate more as people-focused institutions? Simpson (1996) summarised the position in the 1990s:

> It is time that museums undertook a re-appraisal of the fundamental philosophies upon which they currently operate, to re-evaluate and re-focus their roles in the light of contemporary social thinking, so reflecting in their policies and practices the recognition of other peoples' world views and rights with regard to the ownership, representation and interpretation of material culture. (p.266)

Museum education was the first domain of museum work to respond to societal transformations by offering new opportunities to interpret art in a wider context and connect it to the life experiences of the museum audience. In the light of the political changes in Russia, museum educational and curatorial practice began to deal with new concepts such as representation, power, cooperation and interpretation. Intense distrust of mega-narratives of the Soviet era with its standardisation of knowledge led to a problematisation of the museum as a central tool in regulating cultural politics. Russia's difficult transition from totalitarianism to democracy (the Perestroika phase, 1985–1991) manifested in reforms declaring freedom of speech, political pluralism, modernisation of economics and new relations with the West. However, by 1991 the loss of centralised control and the government's inability to facilitate these changes led to the collapse of the Union of Soviet Socialist Republics (USSR). The consequences of this political event were devastating for the majority of Russian citizens: accelerated impoverishment of the population, high level of unemployment and extreme nationalist conflicts.

In the early 1990s, I belonged to the generation of young professionals who felt empowered by the changes happening in post-Soviet Russia. In 1990, as a curator at The State Russian Museum, I led the team that organised the first exhibition in Russia featuring art by people with disabilities, including those with learning disabilities, visual impairments and cerebral palsy, and people with autism and mental health problems. In the process of collecting artworks for the exhibition, we encountered a hidden reality: most people with 'special needs' (the term we used at the time), young and old, had been living in special care homes away from the public, isolated and forgotten. The exhibition, *Through Different Eyes*, opened in 1991 and provoked heated debates about such 'hidden histories' and the potential for museums to be places where the unrepresented and the misrepresented can have a voice.

Foucault (2009, first published 1961) describes how the creation of disciplinary institutions (such as psychiatric hospitals) was a method of exercising control over 'madness' by power systems. Care homes and psychiatric hospitals in the Soviet Union were used by the regime to restrict and sometimes persecute the 'unwanted' in society. For me as a curator, it was essential to discuss the place of disabled and mentally ill people in Russian society, giving them a chance to demonstrate their creativity, reflect on their experiences and reveal the truth about their marginalisation. Rather than thinking that museums should be neutral and non-biased spaces, we felt strongly that it was our responsibility to initiate a radical shift in the understanding of the need for wider integration of people on the margins of society, and also to encourage museums to address their role in the process. In 1913, Fedorov, one of the key figures of Russian pre-revolutionary philosophy, defined museums as 'supreme institutions of unity', preserving social memory and responding to changes in the world (1995, first published 1913, p.21). This statement is still relevant now, more than one hundred years later; museums as public arenas can articulate the most difficult societal dilemmas and invite the public to discuss them. As Dodd and Jones wrote in 2014: 'Health is increasingly recognised as a societal issue, linked to multiple and complex factors, persistent inequalities such as social and economic deprivation, and lifestyle' (p.3). One of the key questions that emerged from the exhibition was: 'How can we give marginalised people the means to share their experiences in a way which supports their creative development and enhances their social integration?'

Later, having established contact with our museum colleagues (for example, at The Royal Castle in Warsaw and The Slovak National Museum in Bratislava as well as American museums), we realised that our initiatives were part of transformations happening across the museum sector in Eastern Europe, with a particular focus on widening access and dismantling barriers for previously marginalised audiences. Due to all the changes that have happened since the 1990s, we can now see a very different cultural landscape. Treadon, Rosal and Thompson Wylder (2006) refer to two important elements of current museum education discourse: first, 'the power of art objects to elicit feeling and meaning in addition to stimulating appreciation' and second, that 'the profile of a museum attendee must be expanded to include those from various socioeconomic classes, cultures, and ability levels' (p.290).

The experience of the exhibition *Through Different Eyes* led us to create a year-long trial project for people with disabilities, which then developed into a long-term programme. The format of the work was interactive discussions in the museum exhibitions followed by art-making in the studio. Partnerships were formed with two sectors, education for people with special needs and the social care sector; we initially worked with young people with learning disabilities (aged 16–18). The programme started within a framework of educational activities; however, due to the combination of the professional skills of a psychologist who used art as an integral part of her practice and an artist/art historian (curator), it incorporated strong therapeutic elements from the beginning. Art therapy as a profession did not exist in Russia in the early 1990s but during the time of Perestroika, American and European art therapists introduced clinical art therapy practices to Russia and ran various training programmes, enabling us to think about the use of art therapy in the museum framework. We began questioning the outcomes of our practice – growing self-esteem, positive social experience and acquisition of new skills by the participants – and realised that they could be attributed to the therapeutic nature of our sessions.

The numerous challenges we experienced in our work from 1990 until 2000 helped us to formulate some of the fundamental principles which would inform our practice for the next ten years. It became essential to examine the barriers that prevented progression of the programme on a regular basis, both within the museum (understanding the needs of each audience group, establishing reflective practice procedures, articulating outcomes, educating museum staff), as well as outside (funding, forming partnerships, defining and disseminating good practice). The barriers that we were trying to overcome were of a physical, intellectual, cultural, attitudinal and financial nature. From a conceptual point of view, it was important for us to establish a clear distinction between museum education and museum-based therapy. It was equally important to advocate new ideas of museum art therapy as an evidence-based practice within the museum community.

Museum-based art therapy work with young people with learning difficulties – a brief case study

I will focus on a case study of work with a group of young people with learning disabilities, undertaken in the 1990s. Despite a convincing body of publications on art therapy with children and adults with learning difficulties (Rees 1998; Bull and O'Farrell 2012; Critchley 2016), there remains a lack of rigorous research on museum art therapy with this client group. I (as a museum curator) ran the groups with the psychologist Olga Platonova, who was employed by the museum specifically for this project. We had received brief art therapy training provided in Russia by American and British art therapists. Due to the emergence of a new museum paradigm with no precedents of therapeutically minded work to rely on, our ethos and theoretical understanding were based on an eclectic model which incorporated ideas from museum education, psychology of art, art therapy and the concept of disability adopted in Russia at the time.

In 1991, we formed a partnership with one of the orphanages for children and young people with learning difficulties in St Petersburg. We worked with a group of 12 young people, boys and girls aged 17 and 18. In the process of collaborative work with the staff we established that our group of young people experienced difficulties with social interactions and emotional regulation and had high levels of anxiety due to insecure attachments and deprivation in early childhood, and that their use of language was limited. We created a year-long programme in partnership with their carers and other specialists, within which young people contributed their own ideas to planning and delivering the activities. The project aimed to encourage social adaptation and creative rehabilitation: due to changing socio-economic conditions, young people with learning difficulties were able to interact more actively with the wider social context. The young people were preparing to move into an adult care home, a significant forthcoming change in their lives, and we focused on the idea of transition and how we could cope with that individually and as a group.

After a series of preliminary discussions with the carers, we concluded that the museum environment could help the young people to adapt to a wider social context and break the cycle of social isolation. Special attention was given to the process of preparing young people for their museum visits: meeting with them at the orphanage, discussing their expectations, giving them a detailed step-by-step plan of their museum journey in a visual format. They visited the museum fortnightly with their two carers and engaged in group discussions in the museum exhibitions followed by studio-based art-making. Due to their previous isolation in the orphanage, the group found the introduction to the new environment both overwhelming and exciting. At different stages of our work we addressed the concept of 'transition', drawing on the young people's ability to gradually adapt to the museum and studio space and to internalise this experience.

We tried to involve carers as much as possible in order to model interactions with the group for them. As the level of control and restrictions from carers created inhibitions for young people in their verbal and emotional expression, it was important for us to shift negative anticipation to constructive, positive expectations, which supported young people's ideas and made them feel valued. This 'triangular' relationship between young people, their carers and the museum team triggered essential discussions about autonomy and dependence, fears and risks, and continuity and disruptions. It also provoked useful debates with the orphanage staff about conventional models of teaching for young people with learning difficulties, which were often directed towards cognition, thinking function and practical skills, overlooking the role of emotional literacy, creativity and imagination. The relations between museum and care system played an instrumental role in reaffirming for the carers the importance of creative elements in education, and to a certain degree challenged the established hierarchical structures of power between young people and their carers.

We drew on a model of engaging with art collections that reflects the progression from 'associations to appropriations' (Rasanen 2003, p.184). Rasanen's model is based on a triangle:

1. Expression and skills – bridging personal and social knowledge of the viewer with the cultural knowledge mediated by the artwork (reflections).
2. Facts and ideas – a stage of enquiry when an artefact is approached using art historical and critical methods, understanding the meaning of the work in its historical context (conceptualisation).
3. Perceptions and emotions – a stage when the viewer is moving into making his or her own artistic response to museum work (production) (Rasanen 2003, p.184).

This incorporated a diversity of forms of activity, from a multisensory approach (touching, smelling, looking, listening) which would assist with associations, to role play, movement and storytelling. This combination of different approaches helped us to work with young people with varying linguistic skills and to develop the relational aspect of the group. Looking together at museum artworks and sharing feelings was an important part of the entire process; this joint attention can be characterised by a set of behaviours, including sharing of attentional focus and affect around a common object (Isserow 2008). Isserow (2008) refers to early proto-communication between a mother and a child, stating that 'the external behaviour of joint attention can be seen to be determined by the infant's internal capacity to see himself as separate from a whole object as well as able to think triadically about the inter-relationship between objects' (p.37). From our observations, it seemed that for young people who had been deprived of maternal care from birth, joint looking was a phase of re-creating some of the essential processes which they had never experienced in their infancy.

In our sessions, we also utilised a narrative approach, which assisted the young people in keeping the focus on the artefacts and maintaining a sense of personal continuity. As their personal history was fragmentary – they rarely had their life story in photos, or memories of their family members – we used gradual exposure to artefacts which revealed stories and preserved memories to enable them to talk about themselves and validate their experiences. Our sessions were accurately documented (photo and video documentation with consent) and young people were able to create visual diaries of their museum journey. Narrative work can contribute to continuous development for children and help to 'mend the things that are broken' (Bausch cited in Gunaratnam and Olivier 2009). Thus, the use of museum spaces with rich cultural content that lends itself to different types of storytelling and interpretation can have a restorative power.

Initially, the young people did not listen to one another, were inhibited in their choices of art materials and lacked confidence to find their voice in the discussions. When we talked about feelings, most members of the group found it extremely difficult and descended into a 'freeze' mode. This resembled a human response to a stimulus perceived as an imminent threat, and made us aware of the survival-oriented reactions of these young people in the new environment. Their level of concentration did not allow them to stay focused on the artwork for more than five to ten minutes.

After a few months of working with the group, we held a museum session which seemed to be pivotal for the dynamics of our interactions. The group focused on a well-known painting by Russian marine artist Ivan Aivazovsky called 'The Ninth Wave' (1850) (Figure 4.1), which depicts a sea after a night storm and a small group of people attempting to save themselves by clinging to the debris of a wrecked ship. The colour palette and the composition do not give the viewer a definitive answer about the outcome of this drama; the painting is open to interpretations, and the viewer may use the visual and verbal, analytical and intuitive modes (Barrett 1994). In Russian art history, this is an iconic image and it encapsulates the dramatic tensions of human struggle against the enormity of nature's force. The title refers to an old sailing expression meaning a single and decisive wave, larger than the others, which threatens to engulf people. The ambivalence of this painting inspired the group to speculate about possible scenarios of either death or survival, and to use their imagination to identify with the characters on their journey. We incorporated sensory, drama and artistic forms of expression within the boundaries of the therapeutic process, and the use of different modalities channelled communication in the group and enabled members to talk about their strong feelings. The fear, anger, hope and sadness that emerged in the group resonated with the overwhelming life changes the young people were facing at the time, in moving into adult care. This intense experience of engaging with the museum artwork played a transformative role in the dynamics of the therapy and served as a catalyst for establishing a more cohesive group.

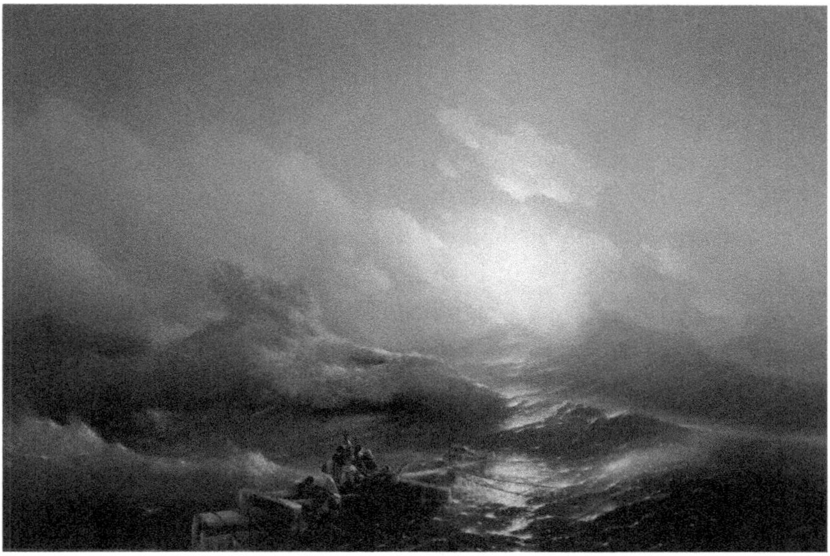

Figure 4.1 Ivan Aivazovsky, 'The Ninth Wave' (1850), oil on canvas, © State Russian Museum, St Petersburg

Gradually, the young people felt safe enough to experiment with new types of behaviour, balancing between being autonomous of and dependent on the group, articulating their thoughts and feelings and experimenting with art-making. Their concentration and attention spans increased and their communication skills improved. The social aspect of the group, which occurred outside their usual environment, proved to be beneficial for the teenagers, increasing their adaptability to new situations. The group format allowed young people to be seen and heard by their peers. The role of peers becomes important for adolescents and often replaces the family as the primary support group, especially in the context of an orphanage. For young people with learning difficulties, the question of negotiating their autonomy and finding their voice in light of moving on to the new adult care home became of existential importance.

In the course of our work with this group, and subsequent engagement with other client groups over the next ten years (1991–2001), we established some of the key factors which determined, in our opinion, the efficacy of museum-based art therapy (Zhvitiashvili and Platonova 2000). These are outlined below.

1. Establishing partnerships

We now perceive museums as places that contribute to social cohesion and that can act as catalysts for cultural and social change. However, working in partnerships with other sectors requires the constant negotiations of shared goals and expectations. It was vital to acknowledge the role of partners as it is unrealistic to think that the museum can have any significant impact on social inclusion on its own. The nature of our collaboration with a number of non-governmental organisations as well as hospitals, orphanages and educational institutions was consultative, focusing on specific aspects of each project. We realised the benefits of employing the skills, experiences and contributions of people from different professional backgrounds. Prolonged marginalisation and institutionalisation of the target groups created a degree of resistance among professionals towards engaging with museums, and so establishing trusting, long-term relationships and continuity of work were the key factors in the formation of working partnerships.

2. Interpreting museum collections from multiple perspectives

Using museum resources in a more integrated way and creating new ways of establishing the dialogue between people and art collections was central to our work. When working with an artefact, one cannot reduce it to a simple summary of its technical or historical elements – it triggers a complex process of projections and responses (Osorina and Nekrasova-Karateeva 1998). Collaborative 'curator-psychologist' work facilitated the process of experimentation, which led us to the use of a museum art therapy model: it unified physical, emotive and cognitive elements. This model can be described as gradually moving through different stages of visual thinking: the 'contact' stage – the first encounter with an artefact, collecting and processing observations, which may include kinaesthetic and multisensory aspects (for instance, people can use their body to express responses to the artwork); the 'orientation' stage, which entails in-depth examination of different aspects of the artefacts (colour, forms, composition, themes), viewers testing ideas contextualised by art historical knowledge and articulating emotional responses with reference to their life experiences; and finally the 'meaning-making' stage, when the therapeutic format encourages participants to trust their own process in formulating thoughts, insights and ideas. At this final stage, the process may culminate in art-making, through which people can internalise their experience and achieve a degree of symbolisation. The enhanced capacity to think symbolically suggests a gradual transformation from experiencing the world as concrete and two-dimensional to seeing it as a psychologically animated and extended space (Isserow 2013).

3. Introducing reflective practice

Our museum team devised two modes of reflective practice: a small working group that met on a fortnightly basis (including our colleagues from the education department), serving an almost supervisory function; and termly seminars with larger groups, involving museum educators, artists, psychologists, and representatives from hospitals, social care, education and parents' associations. The latter groups debated a wider range of issues related to the social integration of disabled people, which resulted in a series of publications. These ongoing discussions were instrumental in reshaping the established approach of the museum towards people with disabilities, such as the museum imposing its values and knowledge on the audiences rather than giving them a chance to select suitable modes of interaction. We learned the importance of moving from a 'museum-centric' to an 'audience-centric' model, integrating the voices of the people we worked with right from the planning phase of each project. Collaborating with different disciplines was not always easy, but by taking this opportunity for reflection, definition and growth, we broadened our perspectives and kept our new audiences' needs in focus.

4. Identifying evaluation tools

Finding meaningful evaluation tools was a challenging task. There was pressure from the museum to find qualitative and quantitative evidence to demonstrate that museum-based art therapy programmes were effective. One of the methods, alongside more traditional ones (such as observations, questionnaires and facilitated discussions) was video and audio recording of our interactions during the sessions. We developed a list of seven behaviours by participants (including us) that we thought would indicate active engagement, interaction and a level of change (some of them are: making comments about art, creating connections with prior experiences, engaging in group interactions, demonstrating new levels of understanding and engagement, exercising creativity). It could be a time-consuming exercise; however, this type of evaluation was beneficial in assessing the quality of changes for the groups we worked with as well as for the museum staff. The carers were also involved in observing changes in the young people at their orphanages or care homes, which helped us to understand what was going on outside the museum.

5. Fostering integration

At one point in our programme development we focused our efforts on integration, aiming to bring young people with disabilities and young people from mainstream education together. We started organising week-long workshops twice a year, 'From monologue to dialogue', where young people (with and without disabilities) were able to meet and engage in a creative process. For five days, a multidisciplinary team of professionals (museum educators, artists, art and music therapists, musicians and actors) worked with young people, using different art forms (movement, drama, art, music) and taking inspiration from the museum's collection (Figure 4.2). The end product was an exhibition or a performance. With consent from all the participants, these events were presented to the local community and contributed to establishing a wider acceptance of integrative practices, confronting the segregation of certain groups. It was important to address issues related to group dynamics, such as setting boundaries, conflict resolution, and accepting differences. The psychodynamic framework of these groups served as a holding environment and provided safety and support as well as enhanced social contact, which members could take at their own pace.

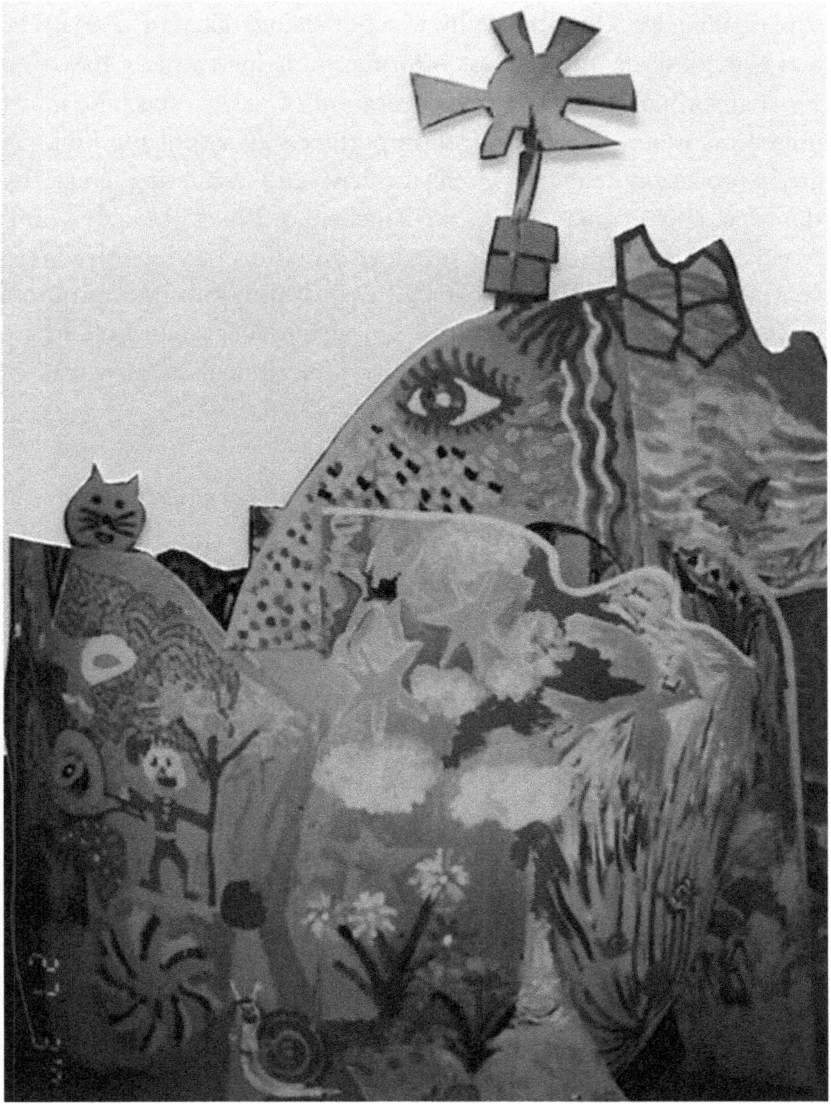

Figure 4.2 Painted sculptures. 'From monologue to dialogue' workshop (1997)

6. Focusing on the visual in the art museum and linking it to art therapy

In the art museum, we encounter a pictorial, rather than textual, model of the world. The visual format of representation played a significant role in assisting the young people in 'activating and re-experiencing emotions through the act of seeing' (Chaney 2001). The way we consume and process information is increasingly based on a visual format, and visual representation of ideas, especially in art museums, is now gaining more importance as a tool for building group cohesion, enhancing engagement and triggering creativity (Housen 2007; Yenawine 1999; Zinchenko 2006). This museum-based art therapy programme provided a platform for creative interventions, which led to better integration of the skills and resources of both cultural and social sectors. For instance, carers started to use drawings with young people with learning difficulties as a way of reflecting emotional states.

7. Educating museum staff and sharing skills

Initially, we encountered resistance and criticism from our museum colleagues in the professional community. This response could have been attributed to a number of factors, including anxiety related to their lack of understanding of this audience group, negative attitudes towards people with disabilities and disbelief that there could be effective outcomes. These tensions prompted us to think about education for museum professionals and we introduced experiential training programmes for those who intended to start museum-based art therapy programmes. Some of the museum initiatives ended up being 'inclusion and access' programmes, which led to debates on how to distinguish between museum-based art therapy programmes and those which provide wider access to marginalised audiences. One might ask: 'What is the difference/similarity between educational and therapeutic practice?' Waller (1993) has debated the similarities and differences between art teaching and art therapy, referring to the historical links of the two disciplines. She points to the fact that they overlap when teachers use therapeutic insights to teach children, and art therapists facilitate artistic experimentation. Our museum team strongly believed that through both processes we participate in creating spaces (both physical and intellectual) that support dialogue and integration. In the next section, I will draw on my own dual experience as a curator and as an art therapist to discuss the similarities and differences between the two professional positions.

Dual perspective – as an art therapist and as a museum curator

Since the 18th century, the definition of a curator, who assembled, maintained and interpreted museum objects, has been transformed. Now the role of the curator is to revitalise the dialogical potential of the museum and to comment critically on the relationship between reality and representation (Schubert 2000). As a museum curator in the 1990s, I collaborated with a psychologist who practised art therapy as a primary mode of work but did not have any museum work experience. By bringing our diverse skills together we were trying to establish common ground and negotiate the differences in our approaches. Hawley Reagan (2017) points out that there is a lack of research which considers the different attempts 'to translate principles from the field of art curating into art therapy practice' (p.1). A number of art therapists have written about the subject: Gilroy (2008), for example, suggests a view that art therapists can enrich their practice by incorporating their implicit knowledge of art history and art-making in their work. She reflects on the role of the curator as an 'interpretative bridge' (Gilroy 2008, p.260) between an artist and their audience, and focuses on the importance of the social context of production for art and art therapy. Marxen (2009) parallels concepts from contemporary art with art therapy practice, referring to relational aesthetics, the concept formulated by cultural theorist Bourriaud (1998) when artistic forms are given to social intervention and relation.

Hawley Reagan (2017) made a systematic attempt to address the connectivity between the two disciplines, using grounded theory to establish the link between art therapy and art curating. As an art therapist, she analysed the changes in the museum field which led to the emergence of participatory, process-based and audience-focused approaches in the last 20 years. She outlined principles which would be equally applicable to art therapy practice and a curator's practice, including creation of multiple points of access, an emphasis on experiences of the objects in the museum context, and a focus on trust in the non-linear process of art. She wrote:

> Similar to curating art exhibitions by beginning with a familiar piece, art therapists have also used familiar images as a starting point. Art therapists often employ images from art history or techniques inspired by famous artists as a point of access to engage clients and enrich their experience with art therapy. (Hawley Reagan 2017, p.44)

Some of her findings resonate with my experience and I will briefly discuss the ideas which, in my opinion, would equally inform both an art therapist's and a curator's practice.

1. Engaging people

Current curatorial practice dismantles the 'authoritative' model of museum communication with the audience and replaces it with another model, which can be characterised as 'process-oriented', that is, based on collaboration of all the participants of museum interactions. A growing body of research supports the link between cultural attendance and public mental health. Bygren *et al.* (2009) conducted a large-scale study to 'ascertain the possible influence of attending various kinds of cultural events or visiting cultural institutions as a determinant of survival' (p.65). They established that cultural attendance contributes to a higher quality of life and recommended that it should be an integral part of any public health policy. For instance, they found 'a higher mortality risk for those people who rarely visited the cinema, concerts, museums, or art exhibitions compared with those visiting them most often', leading to the conclusion that attendance of cultural events 'may have a beneficial effect on longevity' (Bygren *et al.* 2009, p.70).

O'Neill (2010) comments on the outcomes of this study in the UK context: 'Social prescribing, art therapy and community art projects should have providing inductions to mainstream cultural services as a core aim, so that people's capacity to use these on their own is enhanced' (p.26). He gives all-encompassing practical recommendations, including 'an efficient and easily accessible method by which public health and voluntary organisations could refer people to cultural institutions' (O'Neill 2010, p.27). Empirical and evidence-based examples in literature (Huet 2011; Peacock 2012; Ioannides 2014; Coles and Harrison 2018) suggest that museum-based art therapy projects can frame the entry experience in a way that enables participants to feel valued and connected and gives people confidence to encounter unfamiliar opportunities, as well as deepen their pre-existing interests and experiences.

2. Creating narratives and communicating ideas through objects

There are similarities between the symbolic, historical and cultural value of museum objects and the use of objects in a psychotherapeutic context. Greenblatt (1991) describes a museum as a 'memorial complex' (p.46), a cultural machine 'that generates an uncontrollable oscillation between homage and desecration, longing and hopelessness, the voices of the dead and silence' (p.48). This relates to Freud's idea of suppressed memory (1958, first published 1914). The museum presents not only objects, but also ideas, emotions, stories and interpretations related to the objects. Uncovering and presenting the hidden meanings of an artefact through curatorial practice resembles the therapeutic process of bringing unconscious material into consciousness and familiarity. The evolution of the perception of an object from the phase of the 'transitional object' (Winnicott 1971) to complex symbolic interpretations not only signifies the formation of personal cultural experience, but serves as a prerequisite to the development of the self. Froggett and Trustram (2014) apply object relations theory to museum practice and illustrate how the capacity for reflection and symbolisation can be enhanced by engaging with artefacts: 'Museum objects have been described as functioning as symbols of identity, relationships and social group... By internalising a relation to objects we become subjects with distinctive capacities for relatedness in which we can accept a world of other people' (p.5).

In a systematic review of material objects in the context of psychological theory, Solway *et al.* (2015) refer to the use of transitional objects 'in the service of projects originating in the inner world' (p.5), dwelling on Winnicott's work *Playing and Reality*. Winnicott (1971) describes the location of cultural experience in the 'potential space between the individual and environment' (p.100). In the context of museum practice, Jordanova (1989) concludes that 'The "knowledge" that museums facilitate has the quality of fantasy because it is only possible via the imaginative process...objects are the stepping-stones towards fantasies, which can have aesthetic, historical, macabre or a thousand other attributes' (p.23).

3. Belief that generating meaning is a collaborative effort

In recent museum developments, the experience of the viewer/visitor has been placed at the centre: the viewer who is making their own meanings, controlling the extent of their engagement and creating connections with their own life experiences. Contemporary museums invite the public to speak for themselves in order to 'maintain their legitimacy as public institutions' (Thumim 2010, p.293), and curators and educators facilitate this process through various means. Thumim (2010) talks about the 'valorisation of emotional experience' in the museum context, concluding on the basis of case studies that the discourse of self-representation invokes a therapeutic discourse as much as a democratic one (p.302). Message and Healy (cited in Thumim 2010) advocate for the centrality of emotion in the museum experience, explaining that visitors' experiential accounts are offered as trustworthy because they do not claim to be objective. Shaer *et al.* (2008), writing about an art therapy-based intervention at the Tate Britain gallery for people with long-term mental health conditions, reflect that the project promoted the gallery 'as a place that welcomes the individual's personal thoughts on any of the works' and signalled that insight that 'does not only come from experts and personal experience can be as illuminating as historical knowledge when it comes to interpreting art' (p.26).

In art therapy, meaning emerges through the therapeutic relationship, enhancing the client's sense of agency. The provocative question posed by art critic and writer John Berger (1972, p.32), 'To whom does the meaning of art of the past properly belong? To those who can apply it to their own lives, or to a cultural hierarchy of relic specialists?' is now being answered by the museum community through inviting visitors to make sense of their museum experiences, and offering visitors physical and digital platforms to share their views, to complement art historical knowledge.

4. Containing: a multiplicity of different levels of interactions

If we consider the cultural space as a 'container' of material and non-material values, we can see how within its framework the perception of such fundamental values as tolerance, personal dignity, self-actualisation and the development of creative activities are taking shape. It seems that there are certain similarities between the containing function of the museum and the therapy space. The containing function of the museum is not only of a physical nature (preserving objects and presenting them to the public), but also of a symbolic nature, enabling viewers to share culture in a safe environment and hold it in their minds. 'Holding' (Winnicott 1971) or 'containing' (Bion 1984, first published 1962) is central to the process of therapeutic work as it resembles the early pre-verbal relationship between mother and infant, which later forms a child's ability to symbolise psychic events. Froggett and Trustram (2014) talk about a containing museum as a place where cultural experience is located, enabling visitors 'to discover for themselves objects that symbolise personal experience' (p.12).

Both museum and art therapy spaces can facilitate visualising, processing and even reconciling conflicting thoughts and narratives. However, it is debatable whether museum curators can hold emotional responses from the most vulnerable clients as effectively as art therapists, who are professionally equipped to accommodate different levels of interactions with a client. Killick (2000) considers that 'the core anxieties evoked in this journey towards relatedness require experiences of containment before change is possible' (p.113). I want to emphasise the importance of the containing function at the institutional level as well as in the wider community; structure and support become essential factors for the work to be effective. In the current political and economic climate, changes in healthcare seem to have partially eroded the containing ability of the wider community and systems in which we work, therefore museums emerge as invaluable resources for therapeutic work in the community.

5. Making links which lead to meaningful interpretations

In therapy, making links between external and internal, between what is known and unknown, is important. A similar process happens when curators 'contribute to cross-referential understandings of art between different artistic, ethnic, cultural, sexual, gender and class locations and works' (Hawley Reagan 2017, p.23). There are almost unlimited ways of seeing the image, and some of them involve our own projections and depend on our ability to symbolise. This transformative experience may eventually lead to the increased capacity to integrate insights:

> Personal vital value of perception and interpretation of a work of art may be determined by a limitless number of factors, but is fixed (and therefore checked) by one integral sign: whether the interpretation became, in the end, an event of the inner personal life of the interpreter. (Boyko 2006, p.200)

Conclusion

In this chapter, I have attempted to review my experience of developing museum-based art therapy programmes in Russia, a process that was influenced by political, cultural and social transformations in post-communist Russia. The model we used might not be fully transferable, but essential elements will be applicable to different cultural contexts. I have presented a set of recommendations that can potentially be utilised in various institutional scenarios; my work at The State

Russian Museum has informed a museum-based art therapy project with oncology patients (children and adults) which started in 2014 at the private hospital in London where I currently work, and which appears to be effective in addressing the needs of people with long-term life-threatening conditions (Figure 4.3). As museums bridge conceptual and practical aspects of work, I conclude that they offer therapeutic resources which can be employed to benefit vulnerable client groups, although this new field of art therapy practice requires more rigorous research in terms of understanding the specificity of conditions, processes and outcomes.

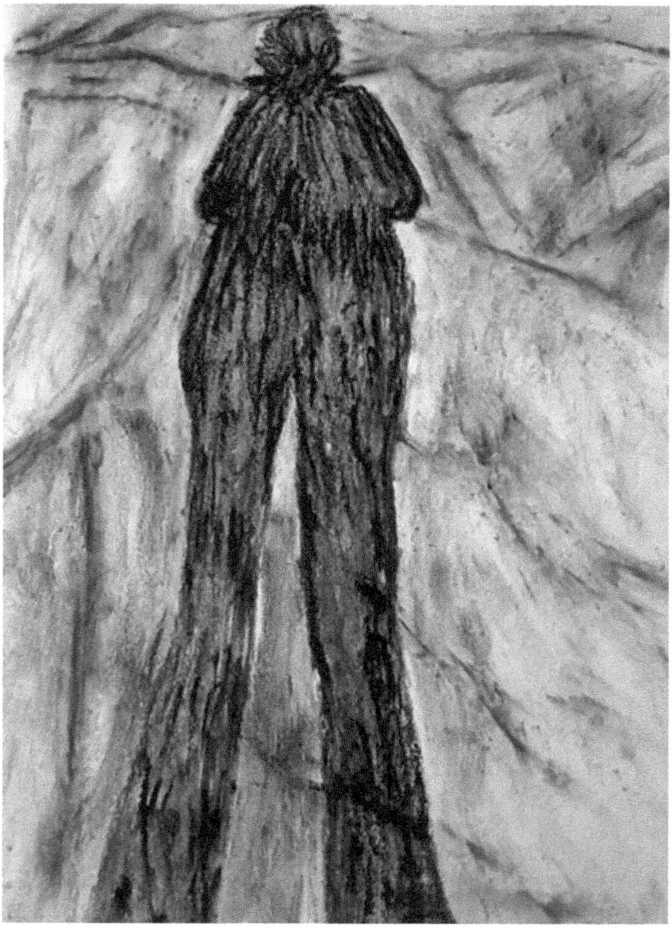

Figure 4.3 'The Shadow' by patient A (2017)

The similarities of the two positions of art therapist and museum curator suggest that the art therapy–museum alliance can be productive, but this entails the constant revision of roles and professional boundaries. It might be useful to explore further how these professional stances can complement each other in therapeutic situations. In the light of changes happening in the museum curatorial field, Schaverien's (1989) statement becomes debatable:

> the agreed task of looking deeply into and behind the apparent in the images distinguishes the role of the art therapist from that of the art critic. The therapist, unlike the art critic, sees the visual relationships in the context of the personal relationship. (p.154)

On a personal note, I want to stress that by engaging with an artwork in the museum, we engage with the elements of our own experience. In an attempt to connect with and understand artworks, we become aware of our changing self and the need for continuous reinterpretation of our experience. As art therapists, we need to advocate for the efficacy of this approach and instigate further research and discussions about the ever-changing state of our professional practice.

References

(Russian texts translated by author)

Barrett, S.H. and Tapia, J.M. (2003) 'Postmodernism and art museum education: The case for a new paradigm.' In M. Xanthoudaki, L. Tickle and V. Sekules (eds) *Researching Visual Art Education in Museums and Galleries*. Dordecht, The Netherlands: Kluwer Academic Publishers.

Barrett, T. (1994) 'Principles for interpreting art.' *Art Education 47*, 5, 8–13.

Berger, J. (1972) *Ways of Seeing*. London: British Broadcasting Corporation and Penguin Books.

Bion, W. (1984) *Learning from Experience*. London: Routledge. (Original work published 1962).

Bourriaud, N. (1998) *Relational Aesthetics*. Paris: Les Presses du réel.

Boyko, A. (2006) 'Ecological approach to interpreting works of visual art in conditions of museum educational communication.' In *Fine Arts and Ecology of Visual Aspects. Collection of Methodological Articles*. Scientific Research Project 'Ecological Role of Fine Arts in Conditions of an Intensive Visual Stream'. St Petersburg: The State Russian Museum Publishing.

Bull, S. and O'Farrell, K. (eds) (2012) *Art Therapy and Learning Disabilities: Don't Guess My Happiness*. London: Routledge.

Bygren, L.O., Johansson, S.-E., Konlaan, B.B., Grjibovski, A.M., Wilkinson, A.V. and Sjöström, M. (2009) 'Attending cultural events and cancer mortality: A Swedish cohort study.' *Arts and Health 1*, 1, 64–73.

Chaney D. (2001) 'Contemporary socioscapes.' *Theory, Culture and Society 17*, 112–117.

Coles, A. and Harrison, F. (2018) 'Tapping into museums for art psychotherapy: An evaluation of a pilot group for young adults.' *International Journal of Art Therapy 23*, 3, 115–124.

Critchley, S. (2016) 'Art Therapy for Adults with Learning Difficulties at Baltic Centre for Contemporary Art.' Accessed on 21/1/19 at www.baat.org/About-BAAT/Blog/76/Art-Therapy-for-Adults-with-Learning-Difficulties-at-BALTIC-Centre-for-Contemporary-Art.

Dodd, J. and Jones, C. (2014) *Mind, Body, Spirit: How Museums Impact Health and Wellbeing*. Research Centre for Museums and Galleries, School of Museum Studies, University of Leicester.

Fedorov, N. (1995) 'Museum, its Meaning and Function.' In *Philosophy of the Common Goal: Articles, Letters and Works of Nikolay Fedorov. Volume 2.* Moscow. (Reprint of the original 1913 work).

Foucault, M. (2009) *History of Madness*. London: Routledge. (Original work published 1961).

Freud, S. (1958) 'Remembering, Repeating and Working Through (Further Recommendations on the Technique of Psychoanalysis).' In J. Strachey (ed. and trans.) *The Standard Edition of the Complete Psychological Works of Sigmund Freud Volume 12*. London: Hogarth Press. (Original work published 1914).

Froggett, L. and Trustram, M. (2014) 'Object-relations in the museum: A psychosocial perspective.' *Museum Management and Curatorship 29*, 5, 482–497.

Gilroy, A. (2008) 'Taking a long look at art: Reflections on the production and consumption of art in art therapy and allied organisational settings.' *International Journal of Art and Design Education 27*, 3, 251–263.

Greenblatt, S. (1991) 'Resonance and Wonder.' In I. Karp and S. Lavine (eds) *Exhibiting Cultures: The Poetics and Politics of Museum Display.* Washington, DC: Smithsonian Institute Press.

Gunaratnam, Y. and Olivier, D. (2009) *Narrative and Stories in Health Care: Illness, Dying and Bereavement*. Oxford: Oxford University Press.

Hawley Reagan, L. (2017) *Translating Principles from Art Curating to Art Therapy Practice: A Grounded Theory Research Study*. PhD essay, Mount Mary University, Milwaukee, Wisconsin. Accessed on 21/1/19 at https://lesleyreagan.files.wordpress.com/2017/03/lhr-contextual-essay-2017-lesley-reagan1.pdf.

Housen, A. (2007) 'Art viewing and aesthetic development: Designing for the viewer.' In P. Villeneuve (ed.) *From Periphery to Center: Art Museum Education in the 21st Century*. Reston, VA: National Art Education Association.

Huet, V. (2011) 'Art-based organisational consultancy: A session at Tate Britain.' *International Journal of Art Therapy 16*, 1, 3–13.

Ioannides, E. (2014) 'New forms of interactions: National Museum of Contemporary Art, Athens.' *British Association of Art Therapists Newsbriefing, June 2014.*

Isserow, J. (2008) 'Looking together: Joint attention in art therapy.' *International Journal of Art Therapy 13,* 1, 34–42.

Isserow, J. (2013) 'Between water and words: Reflective self-awareness and symbol formation in art therapy.' *International Journal of Art Therapy 18,* 3, 122–131.

Jordanova, L. (1989) 'Objects of Knowledge: A Historical Perspective on Museums.' In P. Vergo (ed.) *The New Museology*. London: Reaktion Books.

Killick, K. (2000) 'The Art Room as Container in Analytical Art Psychotherapy with Patients in Psychotic States.' In A. Gilroy and G. McNeilly (eds) *The Changing Shape of Art Therapy.* London and Philadelphia, PA: Jessica Kingsley Publishers.

Marxen, E. (2009) 'Therapeutic thinking in contemporary art: Or psychotherapy in the arts.' *The Arts in Psychotherapy 36,* 3, 131–139.

O'Neill, M. (2010) 'Cultural attendance and public mental health – from research to practice.' *Journal of Public Mental Health 9,* 4, 22–29.

Osorina, M. and Nekrasova-Karateeva, O. (1998) 'Psychological aspects of art perception in museums.' In B. Stolyarov (ed.) *Art Museum and Learning Process.* St Petersburg: The State Russian Museum Publishing.

Peacock, K. (2012) 'Museum education and art therapy: Exploring an innovative partnership.' *Art Therapy: Journal of the American Art Therapy Association 29,* 3, 133–137.

Rasanen, M. (2003) 'Interpreting Art Through Visual Narratives.' In M. Xanthoudaki, L. Ticke and V. Sekules (eds) *Researching Visual Arts Education in Museums and Galleries.* Dordecht, The Netherlands: Kluwer Academic Publishers.

Rees, M. (ed.) (1998) *Drawing on Difference: Art Therapy with People Who Have Learning Difficulties.* London: Routledge.

Schaverien, J. (1989) 'The Picture Within the Frame.' In A. Gilroy and T. Dalley (eds) *Pictures at the Exhibition: Selected Essays on Art and Art Therapy.* London: Routledge.

Schubert, K. (2000) *The Curator's Egg.* London: One-Off Press, Christie's Books.

Shaer, D., Beaven, K., Springham, N., Pillinger, S. *et al.* (2008) 'The role of art therapy in a pilot for art-based information prescriptions at Tate Britain.' *International Journal of Art Therapy 13,* 1, 25–33.

Simpson, M.G. (1996) *Making Representations: Museums in the Post-Colonial Era.* London: Routledge.

Solway, R., Thompson, L., Camic, P. and Chatterjee, H.J. (2015) 'Museum object handling groups in older adult mental health inpatient care.' *International Journal of Mental Health Promotion 17,* 4, 201–214.

Thumim, N. (2010) 'Self-representation in museums: Therapy or democracy?' *Critical Discourse Studies 7,* 4, 291–304.

Treadon, C.B., Rosal, M. and Thompson Wylder, V.D. (2006) 'Opening the doors of art museums for therapeutic processes.' *The Arts in Psychotherapy 33,* 288–301.

Waller, D. (1993) *Group Interactive Art Therapy: Its Use in Training and Treatment.* London: Routledge.

Winnicott, D. (1971) *Playing and Reality*. London: Routledge
Yenawine, P. (1999) 'Theory into Practice: The Visual Thinking Strategies.' Paper presented at the conference Aesthetic and Art Education: A Transdisciplinary Approach. Lisbon, Portugal.
Yukhnevich, M. (2001) *I Will Take You to a Museum*. Moscow: Russian Institute of Cultural Studies.
Zhvitiashvili, N. and Platonova, O. (2000) *Art Therapy Programme at The State Russian Museum*. St Petersburg: The State Russian Museum Publishing.
Zinchenko, V. (2006) 'Psychological aspects of art's impact.' In *Fine Arts and Ecology of Visual Aspects. Collection of Methodological Articles*. Scientific Research Project 'Ecological Role of Fine Arts in Conditions of an intensive visual stream'. St Petersburg: The State Russian Museum Publishing.

CHAPTER 5

Starting with Art

Ben Uri Artworks as a Stimulus for Art Psychotherapy in Dementia Care

Emma Hollamby, Elaine Homer and Jane Landes

Introduction

Starting with Art began as a small-scale, qualitative art therapy pilot project exploring the potential for a gallery and museum to promote wellbeing for a group of older people living with dementia (PLWD). It sits within the context of wellbeing work delivered by the Ben Uri Gallery and Museum, as well as a broader trend for art therapy/museum collaborations. Ben Uri is based in North London and centres its work around a strong collection of émigré art from the 20th century to today, exploring themes of identity and migration.

The gallery collection provided the focus for weekly art therapy groups in a UK National Health Service day centre. A trainee art therapist facilitated the groups over two academic years while on clinical placement with the gallery. The project involved establishing a role for art therapy in the gallery setting and a strong gallery presence in the day centre. As well as the core collection from which replica artworks were produced and used in therapeutic sessions, the broader experience of the gallery, including temporary exhibitions and curatorial talks, was integral to the project. In this chapter, we reflect on our collaboration over the first two years of *Starting with Art*, focusing on one of the groups.

Dementia and the arts

Dementia is an umbrella term which describes a wide set of symptoms (Alzheimer's Society 2017) and includes a range of incurable progressive brain diseases. These can lead to a severe decline in mental abilities – most markedly in language, judgement, reasoning and memory (Waller 2002, p.122). Each person's experience of dementia is different and can be made harder to deal with by concurrent depression, anxiety and personality changes. Difficulty in finding the right words can decrease social confidence and increase feelings of isolation. Consequences for family members are also far-reaching as they adapt to change, and they may experience frustration and despair alongside their loved ones (Waller 2002).

It is predicted that by 2025 numbers of people living with dementia will reach one million (Alzheimer's Society 2014a). The National Institute for Health and Care Excellence recommends that 'People with dementia are enabled, with the involvement of their carer, to maintain and develop their involvement in and contribution to their community' (National Institute for Health and Care Excellence 2015). Consequently, there is a demand for appropriate services for the two-thirds of people with dementia who live in the community (Alzheimer's Society 2014b). The arts are increasingly being employed to fill some of this need, reflecting growing awareness of the positive impact of arts engagement on health and wellbeing. The Taylor Review (Taylor *et al.* 2015) emphasises the social and therapeutic benefits of such participation for PLWD and the potential role for galleries and museums in offering accessible person-centred arts initiatives (London Arts in Health Forum 2015). Personal growth through art activity is possible at any stage of life (Ehresman 2014), an ethos that fundamentally underpins this project.

Ben Uri Gallery and Museum

Ben Uri Gallery and Museum is a public art gallery founded in 1915 by Russian-Jewish émigré artist Lazar Berson in Whitechapel in the East End of London. Its name was taken from biblical craftsman Bezalel Ben Uri, creator of the tabernacle in the Temple of Jerusalem.

It began as an art society providing support for Yiddish-speaking, Jewish immigrant artists and craftsmen who were working outside the cultural mainstream. By the 1920s, it had moved to London's Bloomsbury, then on to Soho and the West End, before settling in its current North London home.

Today, Ben Uri has a core collection of more than 1300 works with an ambitious temporary exhibitions programme addressing the gallery's core themes of identity and migration. The collection comprises predominantly British and European art reflecting the work, lives and contributions of émigré artists and their journeys to London. It features major works by David Bomberg, Mark Gertler, Frank Auerbach and Leon Kossoff, and regularly lends to other institutions, reflecting its importance in the narrative of early 20th-century British art. The collection holds work from some 380 artists from 35 countries and continues to grow. Ben Uri's focus today is to celebrate the impact of these émigré artists and their work on British art and culture.

Ben Uri receives no core government funding and operates as a registered charity. Part of its charm lies in the sense of intimate connection and ownership engendered in Jewish and other minority community visitors (Glasser 2015). It runs an ambitious range of projects with the aim of meaningfully and sustainably connecting to new audiences; using art differently.

How the project began

In 2000, David Glasser was elected as Ben Uri Executive Chair, bringing a focus on 'creating a new style of visitor-engaging museum addressing contemporary issues and social integration through the visual and creative arts' (Ben Uri 2018a). In 2013, co-author and art therapist Jane met David. This was a fortuitous meeting, at a time when the gallery was considering how best to develop a wellbeing strand alongside its education programme and Jane was interested in creative innovation within art therapy, having recently left an NHS art therapy post. In their meeting, they discussed the gallery space and its suitability for on-site group visits, nascent ideas for taking reproductions to outside partners as a way of reaching people who would not otherwise be able to access the collection, how this might differ from the main education programme and what working safely and effectively with vulnerable client groups might entail. Working with PLWD was first mooted. There was an air of excitement about the possibilities and a loose collaboration was envisaged whereby the gallery could use Jane's expertise to help set up and advise on what were ostensibly arts and health projects.

Shortly thereafter, Aimée Taylor joined the gallery as Learning Manager. Aimée was interested in a growing consensus that museums and galleries can have a therapeutic function for visitors (Ioannides 2016) and that the diversity of their contents (held safely within their walls) can enable people to find commonalities with others while affirming their own unique identity (Salom 2008). Aimée was particularly interested in the potential of a gallery/art therapy collaboration and she, together with Jane, spearheaded the project. They decided to offer a placement to an art therapy trainee who, under supervision from Jane, would use the collection to work safely and in some depth with clients. Jane's role was Consultant to Ben Uri and University Trainee Supervisor. Initially, her work was conducted on a pro bono basis until project funding was secured by the gallery to cover supervision and other meetings. Emma Hollamby was then appointed as a learning intern, establishing the project partners and acting as the main administrator of the project – responsibilities that led to the establishment of the Learning and Wellbeing Officer role to which Emma was appointed.

At this stage, the aims of the project were to:

- increase access to the gallery and art collection
- stimulate participants' meaningful engagement with art images
- work therapeutically with people living with dementia using the Ben Uri Collection and temporary exhibitions
- improve quality of life for participants
- form partnerships with other agencies (for example, dementia day centres)
- find a suitable trainee to work clinically
- provide that trainee with a good training and learning experience

- measure and record outcomes
- consider the project's potential as a template for working with other groups
- secure future funding.

Why art therapy?

Within the art therapy/dementia literature, a crucial distinction is made between whether project objectives focus on the process of art as a wellbeing/enrichment activity or on treatment outcomes, such as reduction of symptoms and/or behavioural improvements (Beard 2012). Ben Uri's wellbeing programmes with older adults fall into two distinct strands which illustrate this dichotomy. Emma brings art to older audiences and those with dementia through practical art workshops and discussion sessions. *Starting with Art* (as described in this chapter) was facilitated by a trainee art therapist, Elaine, and fits into the second category. Both aim to use the gallery collection to improve the quality of life for participants. In art therapy, however, benefits primarily come from using the arts to communicate inner experience (Ehresman 2014). Connection with others (and concomitant benefits) are arrived at predominantly via this route. Elaine was being trained to work with great sensitivity, paying close attention to non-verbal communication that comes about through image-making and what might be conveyed symbolically. Clients' artwork could reveal painful subjects such as loss that art therapy is able to contain safely (Jensen 1997). Elaine worked alongside other healthcare professionals at the day centre, integrating art therapy into participants' care plan objectives and sharing her professional knowledge where applicable, while being mindful of confidentiality. She had access to personal biographies put together when service users first joined the centre and was able to set therapeutic goals in line with individual needs.

Offering a clinical placement

Art therapists practising in the UK must first complete a mandatory training at postgraduate level, including clinical placements. Two universities were approached for a suitable candidate and following an informal interview, Elaine, from the University of Roehampton, secured the placement. By offering a placement contract to a student, Ben Uri agreed to provide the necessary opportunity for clinical practice, enabling the student to fulfil their course requirements. This included finding a suitable project partner within the local community. The student, in turn, agreed to introduce gallery artworks into their clinical work. A partnership agreement was signed by the student, clinical supervisor, manager of the partner organisation and a representative of the gallery. Once the partnership was established, the gallery maintained an ongoing relationship with the university and the community partner, ensuring that all parties were happy as the project progressed. This clarified aspects of the collaboration, such as provision of art materials and appropriate space to conduct art therapy. Elaine completed an induction period at Ben Uri and attended curatorial talks and regular project team meetings held at the gallery. Similarly, Emma and Jane attended celebration events at the day centre.

Offering such a placement was treading new ground and to our knowledge no other gallery or museum had done so before (British Association of Art Therapists – Museums and Galleries Special Interest Group 2018; Peacock 2012; Peacock, Hamil and Dumison 2014). Working with a trainee enabled the gallery to explore a wider range of responses to the collection, while the student gained a training experience at the cutting edge of art therapy practice (Jury, Landes and MagSIG 2015). The placement ran from October 2014 until June 2015 and was subsequently extended for a second academic year.

Jane and Elaine met regularly throughout the placement for clinical supervision. Elaine also attended a reflective practice group at Roehampton. It is important to note that Elaine came to the placement in her first year of training and stayed for two academic years. The model of supervision therefore needed to be flexible in line with her developing learning needs and skills (Ronnestad and Skovholt 1993). Initially, supervision focused on practical issues such as how to set up groups and how to measure outcomes in a meaningful way. As the first year progressed, exploring visual material began to be crucial. This included consideration of how the gallery images were used as well as processing the content of artwork made by clients in response.

The day centre

From the beginning, developing a relationship with the right project partner was essential. The gallery looked for an organisation that did not have a steady stream of funding, did not offer many activities, was overstretched, or would not otherwise have engaged an art therapist or indeed organised visits to a gallery. For Ben Uri, this represented an ethical obligation to support those services that would most benefit from collaboration. Eight local day centres and residential homes for PLWD were contacted. Three expressed interest and one enthusiastic day centre manager took up the opportunity to work with Ben Uri. Others felt they did not have the capacity to take on a new initiative.

At this time, the day centre offered specialist care for up to 25 people with moderate to severe dementia. The staff team brought energy and verve to their daily programme of activities, which was varied, stimulating and often fun, with good use made of the facilities for group activities and the locality for external visits. Groups came together for quizzes, physical exercise and cooking workshops as well as weekly music and pet therapy. Nevertheless, the centre could be a chaotic and emotionally volatile environment. For PLWD, behaviours that challenge (James 2011) are often a response to an unmet need, or unexpressed emotions such as boredom, frustration and anxiety. Staff working in the centre often used humour as a coping mechanism, and this can disguise a 'hidden culture of despair' (Waller 2002, p.123). Providing art therapy in the centre using the gallery artworks was an attempt to meet some of those needs.

When Emma and Elaine first visited, they found rooms that were comfortable and visually stimulating, with creative wall displays celebrating people's artwork and photographs of centre users in their younger days. People approached Emma and Elaine to ask about the gallery and discuss their own pictures on the walls, giving a feel for the close engagement and vitality that was to come. This initial visit generated excitement, curiosity, optimism and enthusiasm from service users and staff about the project and partnership with the gallery.

The art therapy group

Up to five people attended the art therapy group each session, which was timetabled in six-week blocks over two academic years. Referrals were made through the centre's clinical team and participants were aged between 76 and 97, with a diagnosis of subtypes of moderate to severe dementia and other secondary illnesses. Most were female and the group's range of ethnicities reflected the demographic of the locality. Group membership was stable, and attendance was consistently high from a core group of regular attendees. When three people eventually left to access different services, new members were recruited. The others, Albert and Sheila (names have been changed to ensure anonymity), attended almost all 40 group sessions over the two years.

The group quickly became a focal point of the centre's activities programme. It met each week at the same time in the training kitchen. This was a light and airy room with running water and a view of the garden. The art therapy approach was shaped by the principles of the NHS Trust responsible for governance of the centre and by the gallery's ethos, so as to utilise the unique characteristics of the collection to support wellbeing. Self-directed therapy models can be anxiety provoking and therefore problematic for people already experiencing anxiety due to their condition. Introducing the gallery artworks into the group aimed to reduce this and offer social benefits to the group. The Trust's expectations were for staff to be kind, welcoming, respectful, professional and positive, to work as a team and to make decisions collaboratively with service users.

The group, facilitated by Elaine, offered a safe and confidential space for members to explore reproductions of gallery artworks and experiment with art materials. The same member of centre staff was allocated to support the group each week. The choice of artworks was influenced by the current exhibitions and sometimes by limitations of copyright licensing. In addition, the Mental Capacity Act (HMSO 2005) points to the importance of people being involved in the decisions about them, and a sharing of power. This ethos, along with British Association of Art Therapists best practice guidelines for dementia care (British Association of Art Therapists 2015a, 2015b), was drawn on when thinking about how the artworks were selected, introduced into the sessions and discussed. Members were vocal about what they wanted to see and clear about what they did not like, and in this way helped to determine which paintings were displayed. During sessions, Ben Uri catalogues were also on hand for people to refer to, enabling group members to select and discuss images they were interested in at their own pace. Reproductions and art materials were high quality in order to convey dignity and respect (British Association of Art Therapists 2015a, 2015b). After the group sessions, selected artworks were left on display throughout the week, providing an ongoing connection to the gallery for those who had taken part. Other artworks were displayed in the dining hall for all centre users to enjoy during lunch. Careful consideration was given to how the images might be received and the themes they might bring up for the group and other people in the centre.

Elaine became familiar with the gallery collection and exhibitions, including the history of the artists and their artworks, by attending curatorial talks. She used this information to enrich discussions. Artworks were viewed together in a spirit of shared curiosity and exploration, keeping interpretation open. In this way, the group became as self-directed as possible, with members interacting with each other by talking about the art.

Visiting the gallery

When they could, the group visited each new gallery exhibition, with centre staff organising transport and additional staffing and making changes to the daily schedule. Ben Uri provided a welcoming and intimate space, with adequate time for participants to tour exhibitions and view the artworks they were most interested in, in their own time. Group members overcame physical challenges to get to the gallery, so that they could engage up close with the original artworks. Over time, the group developed a special relationship with the gallery built from regular visits and familiarity with the gallery staff, including the Director. People got to know the artworks intimately, identified deeply with the characters and were delighted to recognise works in the gallery that they had seen before in the catalogues. The importance of this cannot be underestimated for people with dementia. The artworks themselves seemed like familiar friends.

Visits were memorable occasions that generated excitement in the gallery and lively discussion back at the centre as group members shared their experiences on return. Sheila expressed admiration for the works she enjoyed most and asked questions about the artists. Albert recounted being warmly welcomed by the gallery Director, who had given everyone exhibition catalogues.

The groups visited five exhibitions held at Ben Uri Gallery and Museum, as well as an exhibition to celebrate the gallery's centenary, which was held at Somerset House in Central London. Each exhibition had a different theme and a different subsequent influence on art therapy practice within the group. *Refiguring the 50s: Joan Eardley, Sheila Fell, Eva Frankfurther, Josef Herman & L S Lowry (2014)* explored the work of five figurative artists and their strong identification with a place and the people they lived and worked with. This exhibition resonated with the members' life experiences of post-war Britain. By comparison, *No Set Rules (2015)*, an exhibition of works on paper from the Schlee collection in Southampton and Ben Uri's own collection, inspired experimentation with art materials and led to an increase in art-making. The group was fascinated by Ben Uri curator Sarah MacDougall's account of Roger Hilton's life (1911–1975), an artist incapacitated yet still driven to paint from his bed. *Rothenstein's Relevance – Sir William Rothenstein and his Circle (2016)* included Jewish subjects, portraiture and figure studies (in Paris, London and Gloucestershire) and the First and Second World Wars. The exhibition coincided with a deepening of the therapeutic work, and group members depicted characters in their own artwork based on the gallery originals. *Out of Chaos; Ben Uri: 100 Years in London (2015)* was Ben Uri's centenary exhibition held at Somerset House and prompted a wider exploration of the history of the gallery. *Unexpected: Continuing Narratives of Identity and Migration* had explicit themes of journeys, displacement, loss, memory and identity (MacDougall 2016b) and particularly resonated with the group's experiences of living with dementia.

Using the gallery artworks

One of the strengths of group psychotherapy is that people often identify their own difficulties through relating to another group member (Yalom 1986). In the art therapy group, people articulated their difficulties via the narratives they encountered in the gallery reproductions. The images themselves were a conduit to communicate feeling and explore this from a distance. For example, someone might describe the emotional state of a character they viewed when it was perhaps a projection of their own feelings. In this instance, the artworks acted as a container for feelings (Schaverien 2009). This sometimes carried on over several sessions. It was felt that the artworks acted as a spur to art-making or, in some instances, allowed participants to be actively involved in the group without making art.

Having gallery replicas in the therapy room stimulated much animated discussion and interest. Looking together (Isserow 2008) at the artworks offered an opportunity for people to connect empathically as well as to acknowledge their differences, as they expressed varying perspectives and feelings in relation to the works. Pictures affect viewers (Schaverien 2009, p.82) and Elaine noticed that the artworks seemed to directly impact how people were feeling and relating to each other in the sessions. In response, she started to bring in paintings that might specifically evoke calm or reverie to counter people's agitation and anxiety. At one point, it seemed as if an image from the gallery was illustrating for clients how to be in relation to each other; the group, Elaine imagined, began to resemble the family grouping depicted in 'Sabbath Rest' by Samuel Hirszenberg (1894, Ben Uri Collection – Figure 5.1). Gallery artworks, such as Chana Kowalska's 'Shtetl' (1934, Ben Uri Collection – Figure 5.2), firmly grounded the group in the present while also providing a bridge to connect with memories. Group members shared their own happy memories, feelings of excitement and, at times, elation evoked by this painting.

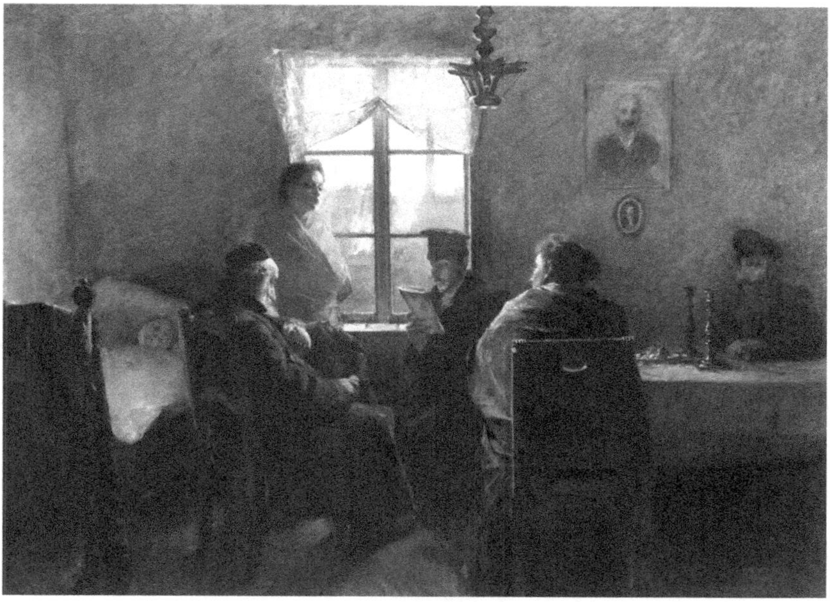

Figure 5.1 Samuel Hirszenberg, 'Sabbath Rest' (1894), oil on canvas. Ben Uri Collection

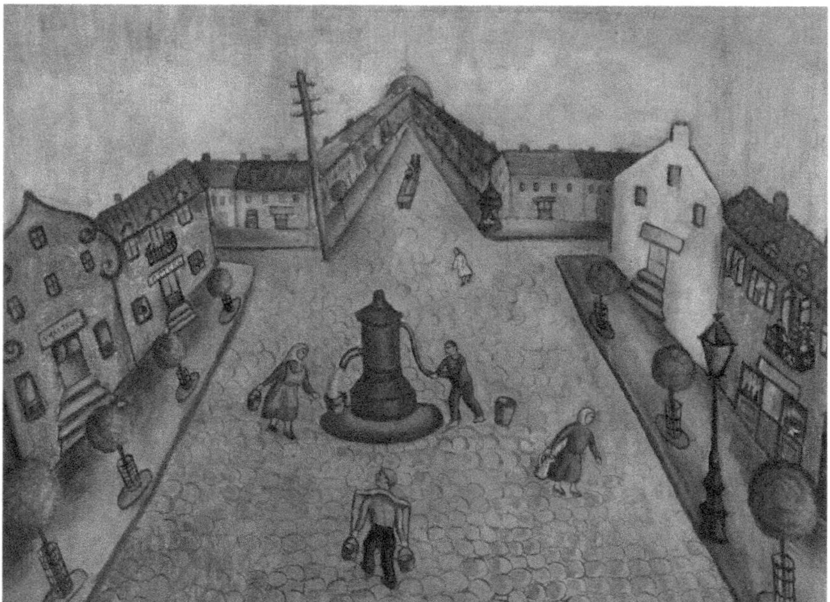

Figure 5.2 Chana Kowalska, 'Shtetl' (1934), oil on canvas. Ben Uri Collection

There were debates around the relative merits of different artworks and their styles, with some preferring the Old Masters and others intrigued by more contemporary art. 'In the Synagogue' by Alfred Wolmark (1906, Ben Uri Collection – Figure 5.3) was much admired by the group, with members recognising the influence of Dutch painter Rembrandt (Smith, Edlin and Goldschmidt 2018) in the tonal values of the painting, the composition and indeed the subject matter.

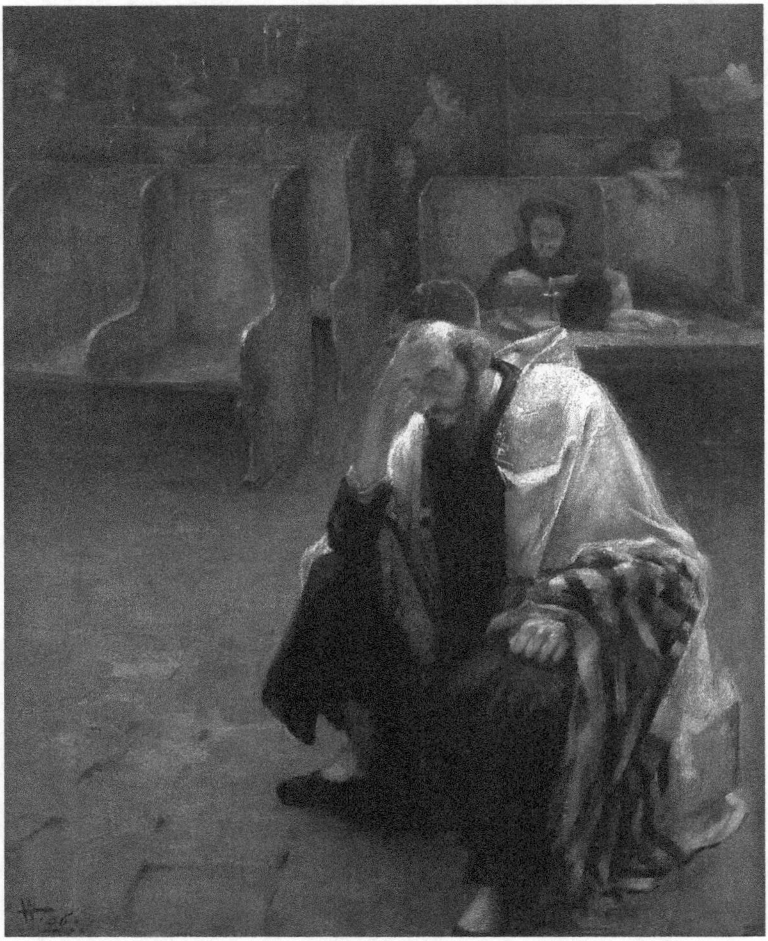

Figure 5.3 Alfred Wolmark, 'In the Synagogue' (1906), oil on canvas. Ben Uri Collection

The gallery artworks facilitated a 'holding in mind' of the clinical work because they evoked, for Elaine, memories of the sessions and how the group had responded. She thought of them as she would the client's own artworks in terms of carrying emotional content for the group members. The gallery itself provided containment for Elaine who referred to it as 'a kind of mothership' – a secure base to return to.

The Ben Uri Collection includes images exploring the lives of Jewish artists and their experience of persecution. While these might not be appropriate to have on general display in the session or at the centre, the catalogues enabled people to choose such content and share it more privately with Elaine if they wanted. One member chose a George Grosz illustration titled 'Interrogation' (1938, Ben Uri Collection) depicting the torture of a man by three Nazi soldiers. Rather than relating to a personal narrative of the past this seemed an expression of experience in 'the here and now' of living with dementia. Although this harrowing image evoked uncomfortable feelings in Elaine, she sat with what she understood to be her client's emotional discomfort, being 'alongside' them in their distress. For the client, this was a way to have an unbearable feeling acknowledged without expressing it in words or sharing it more widely in the group.

Theme: migration

Migration is a key theme in the Ben Uri Collection, which prompted Jane and Elaine to explore within supervision the idea that dementia may be considered as 'a kind of migration of the self'. Certainly, images such as Josef Herman's 'Refugees' (c.1941, Ben Uri Collection) with its expressionistic style and symbolic significance was of great interest to the group, although sometimes difficult to look at; on one occasion, a group member covered this up. In another session, Albert drew attention to 'The Edge' by David Breuer-Weil (2007, Ben Uri Collection – Figure 5.4), in a catalogue. The painting is a direct response to the Holocaust and wider universal themes about humanity, with the broom becoming a symbol of persecution (The Times of Israel 2013). Elaine saw a metaphor here for how PLWD are regarded in society, as having outlived their usefulness. 'The Shoe Shop III' by Julie Held (2004, Ben Uri Collection) depicts a migrant woman as an outsider looking in. This echoed experiences in the group as they looked out into the garden at a different group from the centre, as well as possibly linking to their experience of living with dementia in general.

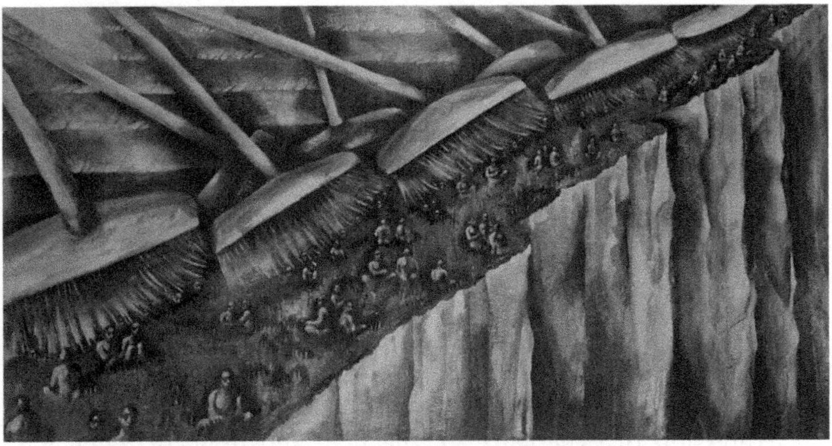

Figure 5.4 David Breuer-Weil, 'The Edge' (2007), oil on canvas. Ben Uri Collection

Exploring narratives of painful separation in the gallery artworks appeared to help the group members accommodate their own feelings about loss and the proximity of death. Intimate relationships forged in the centre over the years end as people move on to residential care or die. PLWD may not remember why their loved one is no longer there but continue to carry the grief and sense of loss. 'Brother and Sister' by Joan Eardley (1955, Aberdeen Art Gallery and Museums, featured in the Ben Uri exhibition *Refiguring the 50s*) seemed pertinent to processing those feelings with the heartrending, tender depiction of the separation of close siblings. When Emma shared the story behind this work with the group during a gallery visit they were captivated to hear that the brother and sister were reunited 27 years later. The gallery artworks often fostered hope, and stories of migrant artists using art in the face of overwhelming adversity uplifted the participants and all involved.

Working with a gallery collection of migrant artwork was an opportunity for Elaine to acknowledge and incorporate cultural differences in visual symbols and imagery (British Association of Art Therapists 2014) and respond to the cultural diversity of the clients in the centre. Members of the group who were from the Caribbean and South America picked out images such as 'West Indian Waitress' by Eva Frankfurther (c.1955, Ben Uri Collection). These Lyons Cornerhouse workers, known affectionately as 'Nippies' and observed with empathy by the artist, not only represent an archetypal migrant but also celebrate the stoicism and dignity of working people in post-war Britain (MacDougall 2014). The painting opened up opportunities for cultural differences in the group and personal stories of migration to be explored and shared.

Theme: identity

The theme of identity, which underpins the gallery collection, reverberates throughout work with PLWD as they struggle with a shifting sense of identity and self (Falk 2002) due to the progression of the illness. Artworks became a trigger for remembering those who had been important in their lives, such as family members and friends, celebrating the good times and acknowledging losses.

Sometimes the focus was on art appreciation as members offered personal opinions, shared their likes and dislikes, commented on techniques and debated what makes good art. They recounted experiences of visiting museums and galleries, and Albert remembered missing lessons at school in order to visit Tate Britain. Sheila took on an authoritative role reminiscent of her career as an English teacher. She enlivened the group with her keen intellectual curiosity and by reading biographical information about the artists aloud from the gallery catalogues. She identified with them and this reconnected her with her own background as an artist, an identity she expressed in the group with her bohemian vivacity and style of dressing. During gallery visits she often exclaimed, 'I am an artist myself you know!'

The group expressed political views inspired by stories of migrant artists overcoming adversity. When women's rights were discussed in response to Lily Delissa Joseph's 'Self Portrait with Candles' (1906, Ben Uri Collection), Sheila's fist thumped the air, emphatically evoking a sense of being on a 'Votes for Women' rally. Lily Delissa Joseph was involved in the women's suffrage movement, as Sheila's grandmother had been. The group was greatly affected by viewing John Allin's 'Protest at Whitechapel Road and Commercial Street' (1975, Ben Uri Collection), which represents the Battle of Cable Street, a 1936 anti-fascist protest. Sheila expressed strong disapproval of fascism and fondly remembered a Jewish school friend. Identification with the artist's experiences connected the group on an emotional level and with ideals that they felt strongly.

Albert adapted portraits to represent himself at earlier life stages as well as members of his family. He was fond of paintings that depicted older people such as 'The Professor' by L.S. Lowry (1960, private collection, displayed in *Refiguring the 50s*) and Alfred Wolmark's 'Men of Old' (1922, Ben Uri Collection) and which conveyed an empathic understanding of what it is to be old. His comments suggested he felt implicitly understood.

Art-making

Alongside looking at gallery artworks, the group provided a containing space to connect with feelings and other group members through creating art. Art-making was prolific; members made work in response to the gallery collection and often drew inspiration directly from the images in terms of their themes and visual style. Sometimes, Elaine modelled physical tasks and subtly intervened in processes to maintain the flow, such as dribbling water on a watercolour palette if the person had forgotten how to dip the brush. Sessions involved using materials in a sensory way based on the gallery artist's methods (Byers 2011) or at other times emulating narrative and symbolic elements. The members' creative processes included direct copying, drawing on aesthetics such as colour scheme or composition, or using materials in a similar way to the gallery artist. Written accounts of art therapy with PLWD describe incomplete works which are often fragmented, partially completed or confused in composition, with fused symbols and boundaries (Wald 1986). Elaine believed that the artwork produced in the group seemed more coherent and complete compared with Wald's descriptions. Group participants' difficulties depended on the type of dementia and concurrent illness, but overall their creativity and technical competencies were remarkable given their cognitive, motor and visual impairments. To ascertain the role of the gallery artworks in facilitating image-making is an area for further investigation.

Albert was inspired by 'The Old Gardener' by William Rothenstein (MacDougall 2016a) to produce an acrylic painting that he reworked over six sessions, adding and removing elements. Acrylic paints gave him a sense of control over the image, allowing him to overpaint layers and make significant changes or repairs. For him, making art seemed to offer a sense of mastery, of being in charge of something again. He regularly drew inspiration from a Lowry street scene which featured in the exhibition *Refiguring the 50s*, creating a series of drawings of people standing in a line or at a bus stop (Figure 5.5). These images are perhaps symbolic of the experience of being in a day centre, following a daily schedule and waiting around. It is possible that they also allude to the existential anxiety of living with a terminal illness, waiting and wondering (Rayner 1986).

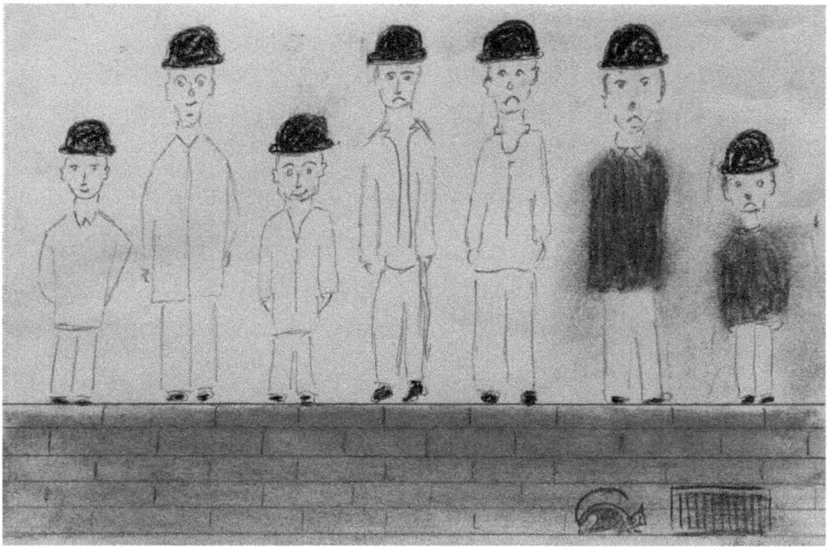

Figure 5.5 Albert, 'Waiting in Line', pencil and pastel drawing

Evaluation

The evaluation process had four main strands arising from the initial project aims:

1. Evaluating the quality of the clinical practice, placement and learning experience for the trainee using the HCPC *Standards of Proficiency for Arts Therapists* (2013) and the university placement assessment process.

2. Measuring and recording improvements in quality of life for participants using criteria adapted from the UCL Museum Wellbeing Measures Toolkit and direct feedback from participants and carers.
3. Exploring the link between meaningful engagement with art images and the outcomes for the group using the supervisory dialogue.
4. Considering the project's potential as a template for future work within the wellbeing team using: records of group attendance; verbal feedback from participants and their carers to Elaine; subjective accounts of what Elaine observed in sessions which were recorded in weekly evaluations and reflections from supervision with Jane.

The four strands of the evaluation process were assessed as detailed below.

1. Quality of the training experience

The placement met the requirements for years one and two of Elaine's art therapy training course at Roehampton University to a high standard, because of the innovative and pioneering nature of the work.

2. Improvements in quality of life for participants

Beard (2012, p.644) states that there are important gaps in the evidence base to support the use of art therapy for PLWD and, according to Waller (2002, p.125), there are considerable problems in trying to measure the effectiveness of such a group. The impact of this group on participants' psychological wellbeing was evaluated using criteria from the University College London (UCL) Museum Wellbeing Measures Toolkit for older adults (Thomson and Chatterjee 2013). The measure was specifically designed for participants in museum activities and piloted with older people with dementia. Its focus on measuring changes in mood and emotion within sessions matched, to some extent, the therapeutic aim of this project, which was to improve quality of life for participants. A limitation was that social wellbeing and communication and creative capacities are not included in the measure. Using a colour-coded 'umbrella' on which to rate mood and emotion, on a 1–5 scale, the measure distinguishes between feeling states which are considered positive and negative. This did not entirely resonate with the potentially cathartic experience of sitting with difficult feelings in a therapy group; rather, it was important to consider the expression of a range of feeling states as potentially beneficial for the group (Coles and Harrison 2018). Additionally, the scales were overly complex for the client group in vocabulary and visual style. Therefore, Elaine evaluated changes in participants' mental state during the sessions based on her observations and verbal responses from group members using criteria mainly selected from the UCL toolkit. These measures of wellbeing and key indicators were:

- *Engagement* – active/interested/alert/entertained/inspired/absorbed/creative
- *Social interaction* – friendly/talkative/interested/lively/listening/observing
- *Feeling safe and secure* – comfortable/relaxed/confident/encouraged
- *Mood* – visible enjoyment/being able to express affect/reduction in distress/feelings contained.

3. The link between meaningful engagement with art images and group outcomes

The gallery artworks were used in tandem with the wellbeing criteria to explore changes. For example, frequently Sheila's mood would improve significantly by the end of the session and this seemed to correlate with changes in how she described the subjects of the paintings. How group members used the gallery artworks was based on qualitative observations of the sessions that were written up and sent to the gallery. Client confidentiality was ensured (HCPC 2016, Guideline 5, p.7) by not identifying individuals by name when sharing data for secondary purposes in line with NHS information governance protocols. Session records were compliant with the legal requirements for data protection, record keeping and information sharing (National Health Service 2018).

4. The project's potential

Group members had a choice whether to attend the group or not and yet consistency of attendance was remarkable given the severity of illness. Albert's and Sheila's carers gave helpful feedback on their perception of the impact attending the group had made. Sheila's carer said that Sheila found attending exhibitions at other galleries difficult because of the noise and crowds. Although Sheila no longer painted, she was maintaining her identity as an artist through being in the group and was able to enjoy exhibitions again; this was important since the visual arts and music had been her main interests all her life. Albert's carer confided that she believed 'he wouldn't be the same without his art'. His interest in making art gave him relief from worry in the early evening and, in turn, respite for her. He established his own art table at home which he used to contain his anxiety; his drawings provided an interest and connection with friends and relations.

Elaine received consistent positive verbal feedback from the group about their experiences, observed their fondness and support for each other and felt their sadness before breaks and the ending. William Rothenstein's 'Blasted Trees' (1917–1919, Cartwright Hall Art Gallery) seemed to capture Albert and Sheila's feelings preceding a break. Albert drew L.S. Lowry's 'Man Lying on a Wall' (1957, The Lowry) in the final session and this seemed to symbolise the ending.

Conclusion

Recent research from Age UK affirms the importance of creative and cultural participation for wellbeing (Age UK Policy and Research Department 2018). This project enabled people to have access to a gallery collection as well as therapeutic support. Being part of a gallery project made participants feel as if they belonged and gave them a personal sense of purpose and agency. In this context, true to Ben Uri's mission statement, they were able to explore their own identity and creativity (Ben Uri 2018b).

In the art therapy group, people responded sensitively to the visual aesthetics and emotional feeling and tone of the gallery artworks. When talking about the paintings, it seemed that members were able to access and articulate their feelings more easily than at other times and share their rich and interesting life histories with one another within the group. The symbolic content of the Ben Uri Collection with its themes of migration and identity was particularly pertinent for this work. The impact of dementia on people's lives is far reaching. PLWD often lose their home as they progressively require more care, family relationships are irreparably disrupted and with cognitive decline come personality changes. All of these vicissitudes contribute to a major shift in identity (Rusted, Sheppard and Waller 2006, p.518). The gallery artists expressed their feelings and experiences of persecution, displacement and loss of their home and loved ones through their art. This undoubtedly resonated very deeply with the group.

Developing the project in the gallery's centenary year was an exciting and auspicious time for Ben Uri to become involved with art therapy. This celebration also fortuitously coincided with the day centre's 25th year. Some of the group's artwork was exhibited to coincide with celebration events at the centre, enabling carers to share in achievements and instilling a sense of pride, purpose and accomplishment in participants. Visiting the gallery became an important feature of the project, connecting the gallery to the community partner and ensuring that the relationship to Ben Uri would continue and be upheld on conclusion of the placement.

The considerable success of the initial two years of the project can be attributed to the hard work and enthusiasm of the whole team and went a long way to achieving aims to increase gallery access and stimulate meaningful engagement with art. Cultural access must be seen as a right for all and this project provided the opportunity for participants to engage in a particularly intimate way with a gallery. The Ben Uri Collection provided the impetus for the group to tell their own stories and create their own artwork, and to feel connected to each other, the gallery and wider cultural life. They embraced the opportunity to engage, responding with boundless humanity and creativity, and warmly appreciated being so intimately involved with Ben Uri Gallery and Museum and its collection.

Starting with Art has since partnered with new organisations working with a range of different client groups, including people living with brain injury, refugees and asylum seekers and young people in schools. This work has been facilitated by new art therapy trainees and, as the project grows, new ways are found to use the universal themes of this unique collection to connect meaningfully with people.

References

Age UK Policy and Research Department (2018) *Creative and Cultural Activities and Wellbeing in Later Life*. Oxfordshire: Age UK. Accessed on 25/6/18 at www.ageuk.org.uk/globalassets/age-uk/documents/reports-and-publications/reports-and-briefings/health--wellbeing/rb_apr18_creative_and_cultural_activities_wellbeing.pdf.

Alzheimer's Society (2014a) *Dementia UK Report*. London: Alzheimer's Society. Accessed on 27/6/18 at www.alzheimers.org.uk/about-us/policy-and-influencing/dementia-uk-report.

Alzheimer's Society (2014b) *Dementia 2014: Opportunity for Change*. London: Alzheimer's Society. Accessed on 27/6/18 at www.alzheimers.org.uk/sites/default/files/migrate/downloads/dementia_2014_opportunity_for_change.pdf.

Alzheimer's Society (2017) *What is Dementia? Factsheet 400LP*. London: Alzheimer's Society. Accessed on 25/5/18 at www.alzheimers.org.uk/sites/default/files/migrate/downloads/what_is_dementia.pdf.

Beard, R.I. (2012) 'Art therapies and dementia care: A systematic review.' *The Royal Society of Medicine 11*, 5, 633–656.

Ben Uri (2018a) *Governance Document*. London: Ben Uri. Accessed on 25/6/18 at benuri.org.uk/about-us/ben-uri-governance.

Ben Uri (2018b) *Mission Statement*. London: Ben Uri. Accessed 26/10/18 at www.benuri.org.uk/about-us.

British Association of Art Therapists (2014) *BAAT Code of Ethics and Principles of Professional Practice for Art Therapists*. London: BAAT. Accessed on 25/6/18 at www.baat.org.

British Association of Art Therapists (2015a) *Art Therapy & Outlook on Later Life (ATOLL) Special Interest Group Guidelines on Art Therapy with Mild to Moderate Dementia*. London: BAAT. Accessed on 25/6/18 at www.baat.org.

British Association of Art Therapists (2015b) *Art Therapy & Outlook on Later Life (ATOLL) BAAT Special Interest Group Full Practice Guidelines for Mild to Moderate Dementia*. London: BAAT. Accessed on 25/6/18 at www.baat.org.

British Association of Art Therapists – Museums and Galleries Special Interest Group (2018) *Art Therapy in Museums and Galleries: Case Studies*. Accessed on 31/10/18 at www.atmag.org/?page_id=46.

Byers, A. (2011) 'Visual aesthetics in dementia.' *International Journal of Art Therapy 16*, 2, 81–89.

Coles, A. and Harrison, F. (2018) 'Tapping into museums for psychotherapy: An evaluation of a pilot group for young adults.' *International Journal of Art Therapy 23*, 3, 115–124.

Ehresman, C. (2014), 'From rendering to remembering: Art therapy for people with Alzheimer's disease.' *International Journal of Art Therapy 19,* 1, 43–51.

Falk, A. (2002) 'A Narrowed Sense of Space; An Art Therapy with Young Alzheimer's Sufferers.' In D. Waller (ed.) *Arts Therapies and Progressive Illness: Nameless Dread.* London and New York, NY: Routledge.

Glasser, D. (2015) *Out of Chaos, Chairman's Essay.* London: Ben Uri. Accessed on 25/6/18 at www.benuri.org.uk/out-of-chaos-chairmans-essay.

Health and Care Professions Council (HCPC) (2013) *Standards of Proficiency for Arts Therapists.* London: HCPC. Accessed on 31/10/18 at www.hcpc-uk.org/standards/standards-of-proficiency/arts-therapists.

Health and Care Professions Council (HCPC) (2016) *Standards of Conduct, Performance and Ethics.* London: HCPC. Accessed on 28/6/18 at www.hcpc-uk.org/aboutregistration/standards.

HMSO (2005) *Mental Capacity Act.* London: HMSO. Accessed on 28/6/18 at www.legislation.gov.uk/ukpga/2005/9/pdfs/ukpga_20050009_en.pdf.

Ioannides, E. (2016) 'Museums as therapeutic environments and the contribution of art therapy.' *Museum International 68,* 3–4, 98–109.

Isserow, J. (2008) 'Looking together: Joint attention in art therapy.' *International Journal of Art Therapy 13,* 1, 34–42.

James, I. (2011) *Understanding Behaviour in Dementia that Challenges: A Guide to Assessment and Treatment.* Bradford Dementia Group Good Practice Guide. Kindle edition. London and Philadelphia, PA: Jessica Kingsley Publishers.

Jensen, S.M. (1997) 'Multiple pathways to self: A multisensory art experience.' *Art Therapy 14,* 178–186.

Jury, H., Landes, J. and MagSIG (2015) 'Re-viewing museums: Innovative art therapy practice in museums and art galleries.' *British Association of Art Therapy Newsbriefing December 2015,* 26–28.

London Arts in Health Forum (2015) *Significant Government Review of Arts Impacts on Health.* Accessed on 29/6/18 at www.lahf.org.uk/significant-government-review-arts-impacts-health.

MacDougall, S. (2014) *Refiguring the 50s.* London: Ben Uri.

MacDougall, S. (2016a) *William Rothenstein and his Circle.* London: Ben Uri.

MacDougall, S. (2016b) *Press Release. Unexpected: Continuing Narratives of Identity and Migration.* London: Ben Uri. Accessed on 25/6/18 at www.benuri.org.uk/exhibitions/unexpected.

National Health Service (2018) *About Information Governance.* England: NHS. Accessed on 29/5/18 at www.england.nhs.uk/ig/about.

National Institute for Health and Care Excellence (2015) *NICE Guidelines. Dementia Resource for Carers and Care Providers: Quality Statement 10.* Accessed on 29/6/18 at www.nice.org.uk/about/nice-communities/social-care/tailored-resources/dementia/statement-10.

Peacock, K. (2012) 'Museum education and art therapy: Exploring an innovative partnership.' *Art Therapy 29,* 3, 133–137.

Peacock, K., Hamil, K. and Dumison, K. (2014) *Project Report: Art Therapy Access Programs.* Memphis, TN: Memphis Brooks Museum of Art. Accessed 8/7/19 at www.speakcdn.com/assets/2259/art-therapy-in-museums-memphis.pdf.

Rayner, E. (1986) *Human Development: An Introduction to the Psychodynamics of Growth, Maturity and Aging* (third edition). London: Unwin Hyman.

Ronnestad, M.H. and Skovholt, T.M. (1993) 'Supervision of beginning and advanced graduate students of counselling and psychotherapy.' *Journal of Counselling and Development 71*, 396–405.

Rusted, L. Sheppard, L. and Waller, D. (2006) 'A multi-centre randomized control group trial on the use of art therapy for older people with dementia in group analysis.' *The Group-Analytic Society (London) 39*, 4, 517–536. doi: 10.1177/0533316406071447.

Salom, A. (2008) 'The therapeutic potentials of a museum visit.' *International Journal of Transpersonal Studies 27*, 98–103.

Schaverien, J. (2009) *The Revealing Image: Analytical Art Psychotherapy in Theory and Practice*. London and Philadelphia, PA: Jessica Kingsley Publishers.

Smith, A., Edlin G. and Goldschmidt M. (2018) *Alfred Wolmark and Judaism Learning Resources*. London: Ben Uri. Accessed on 25/6/18 at www.benuri.org.uk/learning/alfred-wolmark-and-judaism-learning-resources.

Taylor, P., Davies, L., Wells, P., Gilbertson, J. and Tayleur, W. (2015) *A Review of the Social Impacts of Culture and Sport*. CASE. The Culture and Sport Evidence Programme. Accessed on 29/6/18 at www.gov.uk/government/uploads/system/uploads/attachment_data/file/416279/A_review_of_the_Social_Impacts_of_Culture_and_Sport.pdf.

Thomson, L. and Chatterjee, H.J. (2013) *UCL Museum Wellbeing Measures Toolkit*. London: UCL Museums & Public Engagement. Accessed on 9/5/16 at www.ucl.ac.uk/culture/sites/culture/files/ucl_museum_wellbeing_measures_toolkit_sept2013.pdf.

The Times of Israel (2013) 'Rising UK art star gets the go-ahead from his rabbi.' Accessed on 29/6/18 at www.timesofisrael.com/rising-uk-art-star-gets-the-go-ahead-from-his-rabbi.

Wald, J. (1986) 'Fusion of symbols, confusion of boundaries: Percept contamination in the artwork of Alzheimer's disease patients.' *Art Therapy 3*, 2, 74–80.

Waller, D. (ed.) (2002) *Arts Therapies and Progressive Illness: Nameless Dread*. London and New York, NY: Routledge.

Yalom, I. (1986) *The Theory and Practice of Group Psychotherapy* (third edition). New York, NY: Basic Books. (Original work published 1970).

CHAPTER 6

Creative Dialogues

A Journey from Recovery to Discovery for People Using Drug and Alcohol Services

Simon Hackett, Ruth McGovern and Fiona Fitzpatrick

Background

> I was invited to join the *Creative Dialogues* art group at a point where my life was feeling particularly chaotic. I was therefore anxious that I would be unable to engage fully, and that I might feel even more stressed by going and putting myself in a setting of social vulnerability. I am happy to say that my experience has been the total opposite of my fear. I left my first art session feeling so much more grounded than when I arrived and this has been my experience each time since. (Creative Dialogues 2016)

Creative Dialogues was an arts and museums project for people in recovery from substance misuse, including drugs and alcohol. Some people attending the project also had multiple social and health needs, including mental ill-health, instability in their accommodation or homelessness, and contact with the criminal justice system. The aim of the project was to stimulate 'creative dialogues' that might lead people to develop their confidence, social networks and engagement in a wider community. Participants were offered the chance to experience being creators, art critics, curators and exhibitors through a series of workshops, museum and gallery visits, and an exhibition. The project was facilitated by an art therapist, artists from the Newcastle Institute for Creative Arts Practice, staff of the Tyne and Wear Archives and Museums (TWAM) outreach team, and drug and alcohol recovery centre staff.

It all started from a conversation between two art therapists. A newly qualified art therapist, Fiona Fitzpatrick, approached Simon Hackett with the idea of running an 'arts in health' project in a recovery centre where she had been working. Fiona had seen the need for longer-term arts in health projects that could provide people with a wider experience during their recovery. Fiona and Simon discussed partnering with local museums and galleries to develop a project that would aim to build the participants' confidence in the arts to a point where they could exhibit their own work. It was agreed that the project would have an art therapist involved from inception to delivery to help support the participants' recovery journey within a therapeutic and person-centred framework. Simon agreed to be Fiona's supervisor and mentor throughout the project. The recovery centre staff were keen to support the project as it fitted with their aim of helping people to develop a healthy engagement in the community during their recovery. The project proposal was submitted to Newcastle University's 'EngageFMS' fund, which supports collaborative projects between the Faculty of Medical Sciences (FMS) and the Newcastle Institute for Creative Arts Practice (NICAP), and the project received a grant of £5000 for a 12-month period to cover staff fees and art materials, and to fund Ruth McGovern's time as a researcher.

We started with some questions:

- Does engaging in a 'creative dialogue' add something to people's recovery from drug and alcohol problems?
- How do we engage people meaningfully in arts and cultural practice when they are in recovery, through using museum and gallery spaces and artefacts?

The recovery centre staff referred potential participants to Fiona, the art therapist who was leading the project. The art therapist facilitated several introductory meetings for the potential participants alongside artists in order to explain the project, establish relationships and alleviate any anxieties before the project commenced. During the project, a group of 16 people from the recovery centre took part in 20 visual art workshops and eight museum and gallery visits, with time for reflection and art-making in-between visits. The museum and gallery visits were as follows:

1. Segedunum Roman Fort and Museum (guided tour of building)
2. Segedunum Museum (found object activity outside museum, drawing exercise inside)
3. Holy Biscuit Gallery, Shieldfield, Newcastle upon Tyne (visit to see an annual exhibition by Chilli Studio members, entitled 'Curiosity and Grit' – Chilli Studios is a charitable organisation in Newcastle upon Tyne running a user-led creative studio service)
4. Hatton Gallery, Newcastle University (walking outside drawing activity)
5. Hatton Gallery (visit to see Collections exhibition)
6. XL Gallery (site visit)
7. Laing Art Gallery (visit to see exhibition 'The Arts and Crafts House: Then and Now')
8. Segedunum Museum (final visit of exhibition 'Roman Empire: Power and People').

Finally, there was an exhibition of participants' artworks in an art gallery for a week, which then toured to the participants' local museum, Segedunum, situated very close to the recovery centre.

The *Creative Dialogues* participants completed a blog during the project, which is referred to in this chapter, and a focus group was held following the exhibition as an opportunity for participants to feed back about their experience of the project. The art therapist, artists and museum staff planned the museum and gallery programme, reflecting on exhibition content and therapeutic considerations, and anticipating potential anxieties around visiting museums. All agreed that it was important to give enough time within each museum and gallery, take part in guided exhibition and venue tours led by artists and museum staff, and plan visits on quieter days to enable reflection on the content of exhibitions.

The recovery centre where the workshops were based was a few hundred yards from Segedunum Roman Museum and both the centre and the museum were local to most of the participants. The group was given free access to this museum throughout the project and the participants were encouraged to visit independently.

Creative Dialogues themes

The project used *Creative Dialogues* themes drawn from theory associated with recovery capital (Hennessy 2017), including 'choice', 'connecting', 'collective commitment', 'community', and participants becoming 'champions' as artists and exhibition curators of their own work. *Creative Dialogues* drew from three distinct but overlapping areas of practice that can be supportive and engaging for people who are facing challenging circumstances: art therapy, visual and fine arts practice, and museums/galleries and health and wellbeing.

Art therapy has long been used in clinical settings with a wide range of people accessing social and healthcare services, including those with substance dependency (Aletraris *et al.* 2014), people with learning and communication difficulties (Hackett *et al.* 2017a; Hackett *et al.* 2017b), and those within the criminal justice system (Rothwell and Hackett 2018). Although art therapy can take a number of forms, its aims are broadly to support personal wellbeing and growth. An idea that 'the art therapist is like the viewer who visits the artist in her studio' (Schaverien 1999, p.75) is a helpful illustration of the overlapping areas of the art therapist's place within the *Creative Dialogues* team. The art therapist's role was to weave between the participant, the artwork, the artist/art students and the museum and gallery. This role holds the theoretical and practical frame established by art therapists Lloyd and Kalmanowitz (2005) within their 'portable studio', the drawing shed, for working in non-clinical settings: 'central is a belief in people as possessing internal resources rooted in experience, resilience and culture, with the therapist actively holding the potentiality of multi-meanings, and the possibility for sustained immersion in image-making even in the most challenging of circumstances' (paragraph 3).

The concept of recovery capital is the combined sum of internal and external resources available to individuals in recovery from substance misuse (White and Cloud 2008). It focuses on people's ability to access key social, physical, human and cultural resources. Cloud and Granfield's concept of 'recovery capital' (2008) has been used as a theoretical framework to understand the range of benefits that *Creative Dialogues* participants reported. Social capital is perceived as the resources held by people through their membership of a social group (Bourdieu and Wacquant 1992). Herein, reciprocity and trustworthiness develop through the connection between group members (also known as bonding capital) and with external networks and the community (also known as bridging capital) (Putnam 2000). Human capital includes a variety of individual attributes that enable effective functioning within society such as knowledge, skills, education, health and mental health (Cloud and Granfield 2008). Cultural capital is linked to human capital and encompasses values, beliefs, perceptions and appreciations that come from belonging to a particular cultural group (Cloud and Granfield 2008). One of the project's aims was to encourage participants to engage with their local museums and galleries in a confident and independent way. We hoped that by connecting with their local community via museums and galleries they would feel a sense of belonging in a new way that could support their recovery journey after the project had finished. We hoped that a legacy of the project would be for the participants to be able to experience museums and galleries positively, as a safe space, associated with a sense of personal growth and wellbeing.

The museum next door!

At the start of the project, the art therapist guided the group and helped people to think and speak about agreements that were important for the workshops and their hopes and fears (Table 6.1). Both artists were present for this exercise in a listening capacity. All the workshops included space at the beginning and end to reflect on learning and personal experiences, and time to do a relaxation exercise. Schaverien (1999) discusses the 'sacred space' within art therapy: '...the setting aside of space wherein the individual, as a member of a community, can be silent, meditative and self-reflective. Such a place needs to be separated from everyday life and needs of material existence. It must be inviolable; a sacred space' (p.63). A fine arts student volunteer in the group described her own personal experience of this 'sacred space' and how the art therapist facilitated the sessions:

> The art therapist always started and ended the workshops with a meditation breathing exercise to put everyone in a much more open and relaxed frame of mind. I valued the fact she asked what the participants had thought about the previous session at the beginning and how they thought it went at the end. This constant yet non-invasive evaluation enabled *Creative Dialogues* to always be adaptable to the needs of those involved. (London 2016)

The project began with visits to Segedunum Museum, a ten-minute walk down the road from the recovery centre and the site of the most excavated fort along the Hadrian's Wall, built by the Romans by order of Emperor Hadrian in AD 122. Today the site has reconstructions of a bath house and an interactive museum housing an exhibition of Roman artefacts. Alongside this, TWAM staff brought in a collection of artefacts to some of the workshop sessions. We felt that this would encourage a more personal connection to the museums and break down any potential barriers that participants may have about interacting with the collections. Bringing objects out of the museum gives direct access to cultural assets:

> Object handling is the ultimate asset-based approach for museums and helps to create thematic activities based on collections, so that the museum becomes more than just a service providing a space for an activity, rather it actively links audiences and activities with the history of the museum. (Lackoi *et al.* 2016, p.28)

Table 6.1 Group agreement

Group agreement	Hopes and fears
Everyone to arrive on time. Call to give advance notice of lateness or absence. Use clear communication. Show mutual respect: towards other people's ideas and opinions and artwork. Use respectful language to self and others. Know that all contributions are welcome. Let everyone speak and listen to the views of others. Create and maintain a supportive environment. Ensure a drink/drug free zone prior to and during the session. Keep mobile phones on silent during workshop *(unless prior arrangement made due to emergency)*. (Mobile phones for taking photos are fine.) Have an organised break. Keep food and drink in the kitchen when artwork and materials are out. Treat everything disclosed within the session as confidential. Keep an open mind. HAVE FUN!!	**Hopes** Improve myself. Learn something new. Make new friendships. Share ideas and experiences. Feel proud of own artwork. Open new doors and new opportunities. Have involvement with project in future. Make a difference to other people's lives across the globe. Have the arts more integrated in people's recovery. For the exhibition to be brilliant. For project to grow, be sustainable. For project to have a legacy and impact on others. **Fears** Not believing in personal abilities and achievements. People not engaging. Running out of time. Not getting materials I want. Not being able to fulfil ambitions.

At one session, the group explored a museum box which had been created during a project for people with dementia, with objects from the 1940s to stimulate memories. The objects elicited many personal stories from participants and generated associations to the 'everyday'

Roman objects which were present in the Segedunum exhibition, such as shoes, ornaments and clothes. It felt significant that the objects were relatable to the participants and that they offered a sense of connection. Through these museum artefacts, interest and curiosity was sparked about the importance of their own lives, stories and everyday objects. Following on from this, the art therapist observed how the participants were interested in collecting and presenting their own found objects during the workshop. They all gained more confidence within discussions and spoke about their own interests and stories, being able to share about their own 'everyday' objects with each other. The objects were mainly small and held with affection in the participants' hands as they described the personal importance and reason for sharing them. Objects included beer bottle tops, a necklace, sculptures and photographs. Julie Brooker (2010) has explored the benefits of using found objects in art therapy to help improve emotional and mental wellbeing, suggesting that they allow thoughts, feelings and memories to be connected to, recognised and processed.

The following week, the group was brought back to Segedunum Museum and engaged in a workshop outside the museum which was described as an activity in 'seeing deeply' and an experience of 'being' with an object. This creative exercise started outside the museum. The group stood in the Roman fort ruins and were asked to look on the ground and find an object of interest. Rocks, stones and plants were brought back to the circle. The whole group had a minute of silence looking at their objects and then each person was able to share their feelings with the group as they stood in a circle. The group were encouraged to have a further few minutes alone in silence with their chosen objects. The group then moved inside the museum to the 'Roman Empire: Power and People' exhibition. This exhibition brought together over 160 pieces from the British Museum to explore the story of one of the most powerful empires in history. Exhibits included sculpture from the villas of the Emperors Tiberius and Hadrian, coins from the Hoxne treasure, jewellery, and almost perfectly preserved children's clothing from Roman Egypt.

Art materials were given out and shared among the *Creative Dialogues* participants within the space, including watercolours, pencils, pens, oil pastels, chalk pastels and charcoal. The participants were asked to hold in mind how certain objects have 'power' over others and how each person's chosen object could be thought of as sacred for the day. They were then invited to draw in the museum, either drawing their own found object or another object within the exhibition.

One participant had engaged in the 'seeing deeply' and 'being' with an object by sharing with the group personal feelings, past experiences and current family attachment issues that this exercise brought up. This participant chose one of the messier materials, charcoal, when creating her image and she later gave a first-hand account of her museum visit:

> The session today began with a grounding exercise, which involved breathing exercises and feeling grounded within yourself. We then walked down to Segedunum to do a looking and drawing exercise/activity. We did this outside, with each of us picking up an object that took our fancy, and seeing what feelings and emotions it created. I picked a large slate rock. Other members of the group picked flowers and pebbles. To me, my piece evoked feelings of family with the rock being layered with cracked and crumbling sections, much like my family! We next went inside to the exhibition 'Roman Empire: Power and People'. Indoors we continued with the exercise, putting our emotions and feelings onto paper. We had brought paper, pens, paints and charcoals and the group got down to work. This was really interesting for me as I chose to work with charcoal, which I've never used before. After 40 minutes, we packed up and headed back. We then spent 15 minutes eating and discussing the task we had done. I learnt a lot today. I still can't draw, charcoal is really messy and art is very relaxing and therapeutic. Roll on next week. (Creative Dialogues 2016)

Frances O'Brien (2004) has reflected on the use of messy materials in art therapy, stating that 'the chaotic use of materials might express the trauma caused by chaotic relationships of abuse, neglect and fragile attachments' (p.4). Much of the art-making in the workshops was led by professional artists using structured activities to explore techniques and ideas. The art therapist was consistent throughout the project and was present every week. The artists and art therapist jointly planned the project and the art therapist gave guidance to the artists about the therapeutic element of art materials and advised when messier materials such as clay or plaster of Paris could be introduced.

Entering the workshop space the week after visiting the Segedunum museum, the participants found that the tables surrounding the circle of seats were covered in A3 photocopied images taken from the book of the 'Power and People' exhibition. It was as if the museum space had merged with the workshop space. Group participants were given information about collage. The artist facilitators explained that many artists have used collage as a way of making images and showed work made by Gabriel Orozco. Orozco's work fitted well with the activity looking at the exhibit of Roman 'everyday objects' during the museum visit, as 'Playing with ideas of accessibility, Orozco's work revolves around various repeating themes, exploring materials in a way allows the viewer's imagination to discover creative associations between aspects of everyday life that are often overlooked or ignored' (Kurimanzutto 2018, paragraph 1).

The group were invited to choose, cut and merge images together, creating something new. Everyone was encouraged to have a go at 'doing an Orozco' with images from the 'Power and People' exhibition (Figure 6.1), and collective collages also featured as a group activity in other workshops (Figure 6.2).

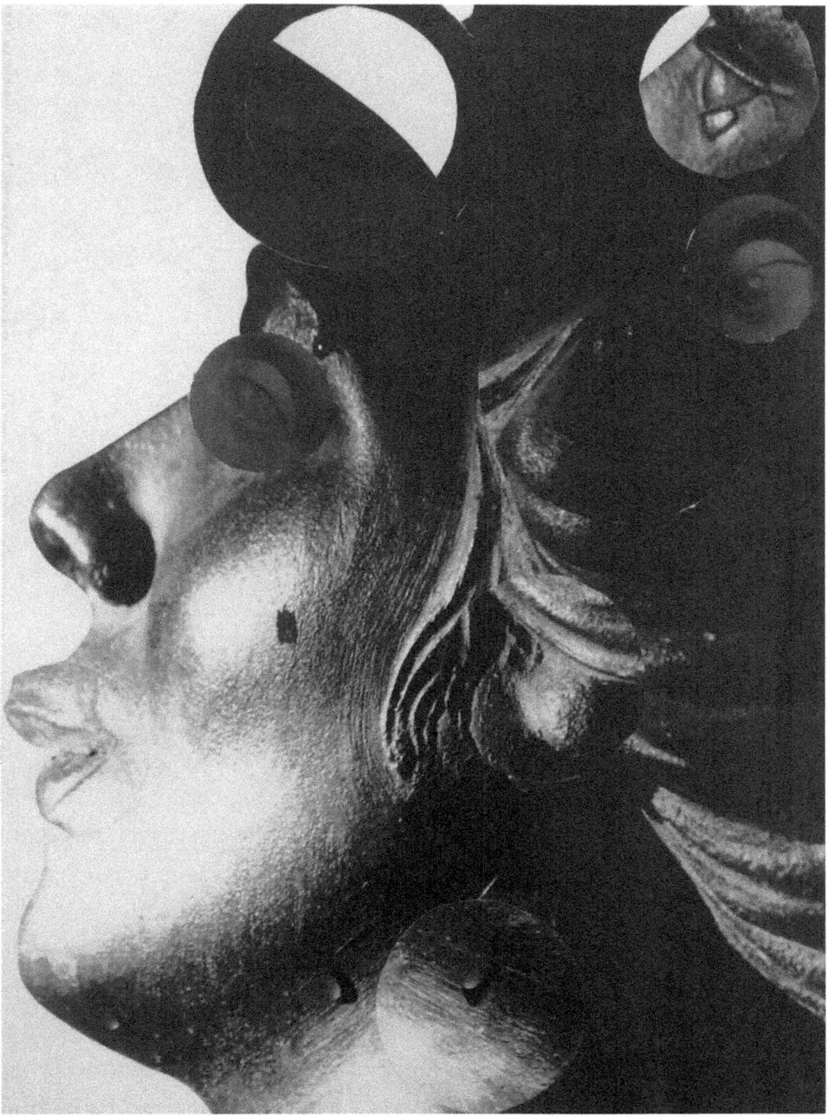

Figure 6.1 Doing an Orozco

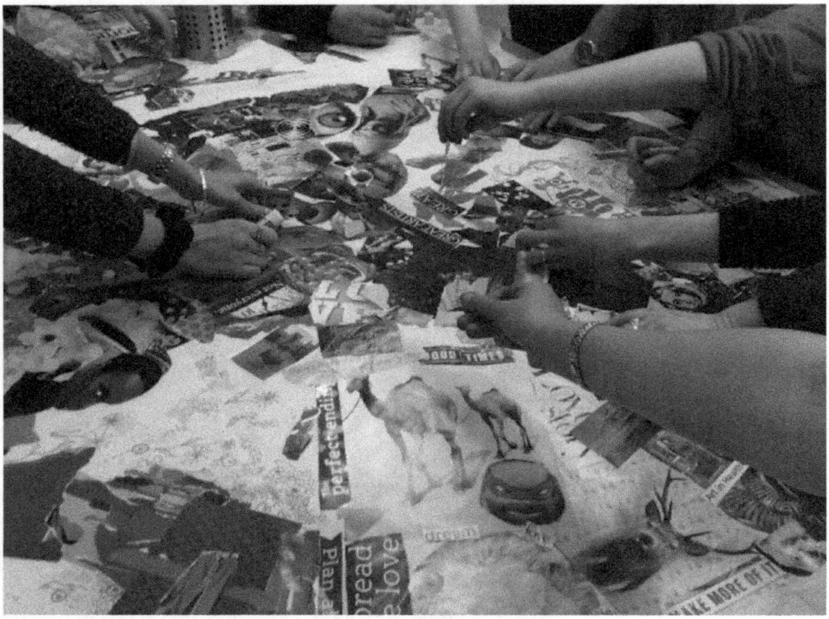

Figure 6.2 Collective collage workshop

The role of the art therapist

The art therapist involvement in the planning stage focused on holding in mind the boundaries which would be necessary to create a therapeutic experience within a project that was mobile and had multiple venues. Safe boundaries are often considered to be important in art therapy and the art therapist will seek to provide a framework, or 'therapeutic frame', to help people differentiate between the literal and the symbolic or between internal and external reality (Edwards 2004); 'The essence of the therapeutic frame is that it provides a physical and mental space where feelings can be held in order to facilitate creativity and emotional growth' (Edwards 2004, p.51). In this project, the art therapist attempted to create a safe therapeutic frame throughout its conception, planning and delivery. Consideration needed to be given to the group's needs within the frame of the workshop space, the museum space (internally and externally) and the various other parts of the project. The art therapist attempted to create a 'safe space', whether in the workshop space or the museums and galleries, where participants could feel free to explore the art media and their own abilities, something that group members had felt apprehensive about prior to commencing the group. Although it was not the primary focus or intention of *Creative Dialogues*, some people in the group found that making art did inevitably communicate something about themselves. In the end-of-project focus group, people spoke about using their art to resolve painful experiences.

Group members spoke about disabling anxieties in their daily lives prior to attendance at the group. These anxieties were sometimes mirrored when visiting museum and galleries, and their initial worries about creating artwork within these spaces was alleviated with the support and reassurance of the art therapist. By the end of the project, the group accomplished a 'walking and sketching' activity outside the Hatton Gallery, surrounded by the general public.

A frequent expression used within the focus group was the 'shared experience' in the art group. It was acceptable to make mistakes, take risks and 'expose' oneself through art because the individual group members were all 'in it together'. Engagement was promoted by a social obligation, enhanced by the enjoyment members experienced from attending the sessions. One group member reported, 'It's the one group I really don't want to miss.'

Reciprocal obligations within the group also encouraged members to complete 'homework' tasks of sketching, drawing and painting at home. In effect, the combined personal enjoyment and responsibility to one another to complete such tasks extended the therapeutic benefit of the art sessions beyond the parameters of the group and into the group members' individual, personal space. Moreover, group members felt that this had also benefited social relationships with others outside the group, through conversations about the project with friends and family members. Two focus group members reported that their families were happy when they painted due to the positive emotional impact it had on them. One of the focus group members also felt that her art had enabled her to communicate more effectively with her husband, allowing her to share difficult things from the past that she had not spoken about to him before. The art she created was about past traumas and through her art she found the language to talk about this with her husband.

'Wow! What a night': the exhibition

> Wow! What a night. How proud I felt. Never before felt like this. The *Creative Dialogues* Team have been wonderful. No judgement, just encouragement to do what I never thought I could do. Thank you all from the bottom of my heart. (Creative Dialogues 2016)

The exhibition was set up to demonstrate and communicate the efforts and value of the group's work (Figures 6.3, 6.4 and 6.5). The museum and gallery visits, and reflecting and responding to them, gave the participants the experience of being the viewer and the viewed, the audience and the artist. The group had five museum and gallery experiences before visiting the XL Gallery where they would showcase their own work. The XL Gallery was situated inside the Fine Art Department of Newcastle University, alongside the Hatton Gallery.

To introduce the participants to the exhibition space gradually, the visit started by the group exploring the outside of the Hatton Gallery and XL Gallery at Newcastle University Fine Art Department, before going inside. The artists distributed cameras to the participants and the task was to observe the interior of the galleries and photograph anything that captured their interest, whether it was the curve of the stairwell, the tiled floor, or an object in their bag. To help the participants to engage with the space, the gallery building was explored like a museum artefact: 'Like the temple and the theatre, the art gallery is a place designed for a particular purpose. Set apart from everyday life by its physical boundary, the building and the rooms within are laid out according to accepted code for exhibiting of pictures' (McNiff 1998, p.69). The space surrounding the building, as well as the building's physical form and structure were studied and explored via art-making. The group physically touched the building and walked through the grounds. The participants were able to look at the space and current exhibitions without feeling too intimidated. A gallery staff member took a group photo within XL Gallery exhibition space, instilling a sense that the participants were valued as prospective exhibitors. Reflecting on the session, each participant was asked to speak a word aloud to describe their experience of being a viewer in a gallery and artists preparing for an exhibition. The words were spoken in a circle within the gallery space and included 'inspired', 'creative', 'jealous' (that they were not a student at the university studying fine art), 'content', 'relaxed', 'curious', 'calm', 'excited', 'energetic' and 'influenced'.

After visiting the XL Gallery the group had an idea of the number of pieces each person was able to exhibit. During the following two group sessions, each person was given one-to-one time with the art therapist and artist to look through their work and decide which pieces they would like to exhibit. This three-way view, from the creator/participant, artist and therapist was important and helped participants to feel confident about the choices they made about showing their work. The art therapist also gave consideration to the content of the work and asked about any vulnerable feelings group members might have about their artwork and themselves. This was also an important private opportunity for participants to identify any work they did not want to display to the public or to talk about anything about the exhibition that might be worrying them.

In planning the exhibition, the group decided to aim to display as many different art forms as possible to show the breadth of work that had been completed during the group's life. There were several discussions within the group over the weeks leading up to the exhibition, such as whether to display group members' names alongside their artwork. The group decided not to do this. There was a collective view that they wanted to be represented as the *Creative Dialogues* group as they felt that this was a group experience and not just about individual artists.

A planning document was created jointly by the art therapist, artists, museum staff and students leading up to the exhibition, which included the installation, marketing and invitation mail-out list that was shared with the participants for their input. The team of staff also created a timeline and distributed this to the participants and partners so that everyone was aware of deadlines. The group discussed the practical and physical elements involved in the installation of the exhibition under the guidance of the artists, art therapist and fine art students.

The group explored different types of interpretation that can accompany a museum or gallery exhibition to explain the work to the audience. It was agreed that the voice of the participants had been important throughout the project and that the information given should reflect the value of the art-making within the museum and galleries and workshop environment for the participants. Therefore, the group agreed that having their own voices within the gallery space as quotes would assist the audience to think about the therapeutic value of the project experience for the participants. A set of quotes from the participants was agreed and sent to a printer to enlarge and laminate so they could be displayed alongside the artwork.

Ideas about how the group could engage the public once inside the exhibition were also discussed, such as a comments book, a board with metallic alphabet letters to write comments on and a projector to display a slideshow of photographic work. The letter board became a safe and playful place within the exhibition where the participants could stand together and communicate through posting up fun phrases. This corner of the exhibition space was filled with laughter and brought its own value to people's experience of the gallery: 'It is play that is universal, and that belongs to health: playing facilitates growth and therefore health; playing leads into group relationships; playing can be a form of communication in psychotherapy' (Winnicott 1971, p.41).

The group chose pages from sketchbooks to display in the glass cabinets. This became a personal reflective experience for each participant as they looked back on the life of the group via their own sketches and record of thoughts and ideas. One participant asked if he could display sculptures that he had created previously, before the *Creative Dialogues* project, as he was keen to share his artistic skills with the public again having not done so for several years due to substance misuse. The group agreed that this was a great idea once they had seen the work and heard the story behind its creation.

An invitation list was created and one of the students created a flyer which was emailed out and printed. The image on the flyer (Figure 6.3), a photograph from a charcoal workshop, was chosen from a selection by the group as it was an example of a whole-group element of the project and one of the most enjoyable art materials that the group worked with. It was felt that the charcoal workshop was an important bonding experience for the group. This was the messiest workshop, and the group cleared up together with enjoyment and laughter at the mess that they had created. The importance of this workshop was perhaps connected to this messy element, reflecting a shared experience of their inner worlds which might include emotional trauma from the past (O'Brien 2004).

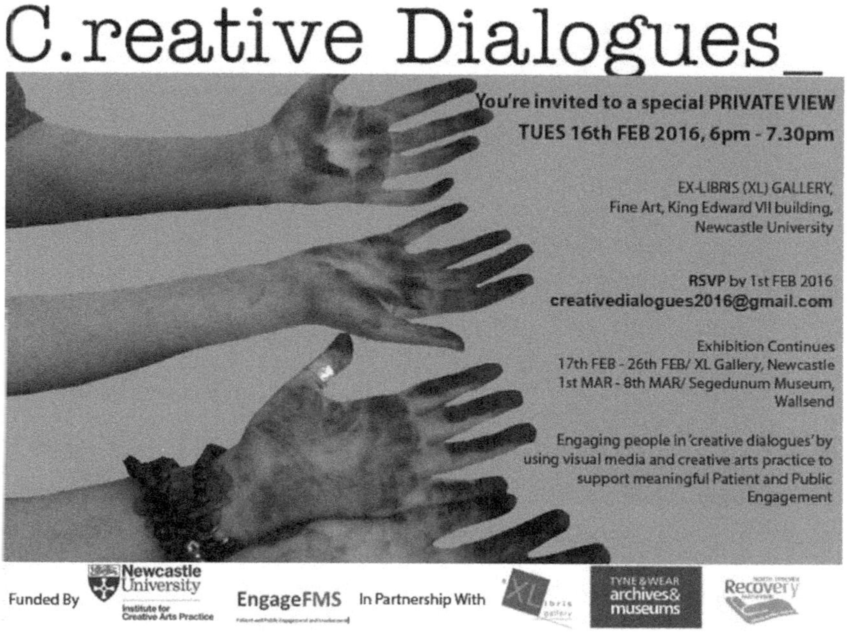

Figure 6.3 The flyer invitation

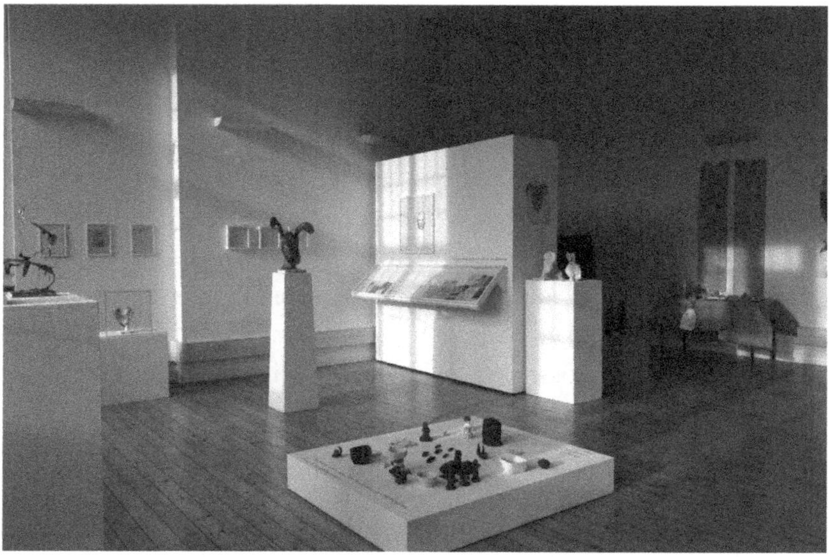

Figure 6.4 The exhibition

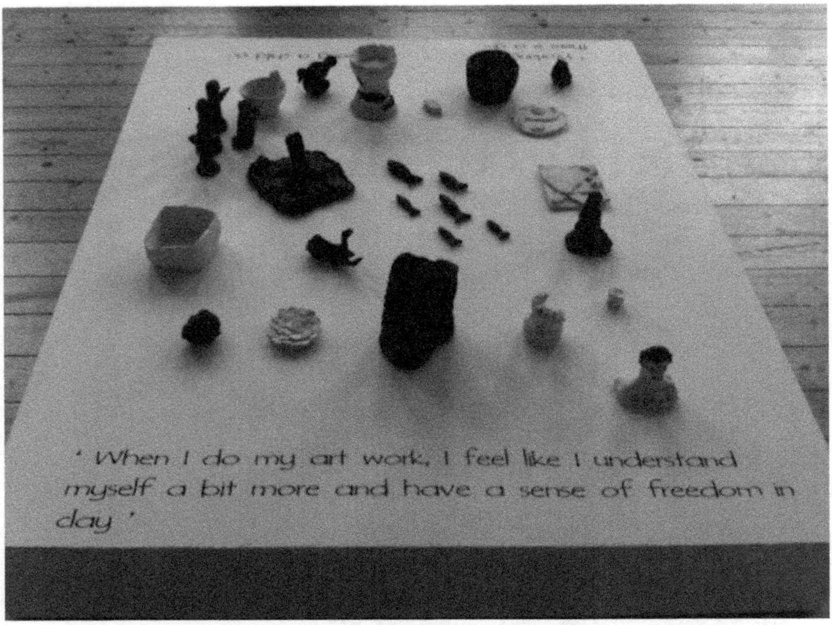

Figure 6.5 The exhibition: detail

The participants distributed the flyers to friends, family, local libraries and other recovery project participants. The group discussed the preview opening of the exhibition and decided on having a non-alcoholic drinks reception, a short welcome speech to describe the project and a performance by the charity Streetwise Opera (an award-winning national charity that uses music to help people who are, or have been, homeless to make positive changes in their lives).

Some of the opera performers knew some of the group, and they had performed in many museums and galleries throughout the UK so were in a good position to support the participants and help them to feel more at ease. It was hoped they would be an inspiration by showing how other vulnerable adults can enter the museum and gallery environment and overcome their fears.

Quotes from participants included (Creative Dialogues 2016):

> I am feeling grateful for the experience I have had and all the learnings I have taken from the *Creative Dialogues* art group.

> I can't believe how many people came to the exhibition opening and to see my work, I never thought that would happen.

> I have found my time at *Creative Dialogues* both challenging and engaging. It has pushed me creatively and personally. This has been more than I initially expected.
>
> I felt so proud to show my friends and family my artwork on the walls in the exhibition. Can't believe how professional it looked.
>
> Thank you so much for putting up the exhibition, it looked amazing, I was quite overwhelmed.
>
> I was so proud to see so much of my work on the walls and see how great all our work looked together. I loved our quotes stuck to the walls as well.
>
> It was lovely having Streetwise Opera there to sing, made it feel special and was great as I knew some of them too.

'It's not about recovery, it's about discovery'

Two female and one male participant attended the end-of-project focus group after the exhibition. The focus group was scheduled to happen the day after the exhibition so that they had an opportunity to join together at a time when they might have felt low because the project was coming to an end. The small number of attendees for this focus group did bring into question whether the ending felt too difficult for some participants. In hindsight, allowing more time between the end of the exhibition and a project reunion for the focus group might have produced a higher turnout. The aim of the focus group was to explore the impact of the project and to share our reflections with funders and partners of the project, Newcastle University and Tyne and Wear Archive Museums.

We were surprised to discover in our focus group that there was an absence of 'recovery talk' from group members and they did not discuss their substance use or attempts to change. Rather, members discussed their experience of art, both the doing and the viewing of it, talking about the impact of this on their values and perceptions and, importantly, what they learned about themselves along the way. One group member summed this up by saying, 'It's not about recovery, it's about discovery.' The people in the focus group told us that *Creative Dialogues* was welcoming and encouraging, a safe space for people with a shared experience of using drug and alcohol recovery services.

In the *Creative Dialogues* project blog, group members said that the project had also benefited their social relationships with others outside the group. People spoke about being able to 'disappear into their art', providing them with a welcome break from anxieties, concerns and cravings to use substances. This 'disappearing into their art' was an experience that happened within the museum and gallery spaces as they entered and became immersed in the objects and artwork on display and sat down to create art within these quiet spaces. People spoke about immense pride in themselves and each other during the exhibition. They appreciated the time and effort that others had committed to preparing the exhibition, including the professional presentation of their work in frames. The high-quality environment provided by the gallery as well as the attendance of Streetwise Opera on the opening night all contributed to a greater sense of self-worth. While visiting the gallery space during the site visit, one participant talked about her envy of students at Newcastle University Fine Art Department. At the *Creative Dialogues* exhibition opening night, she talked with pride at being able to show her own artwork within this same space. The group as a whole spoke of the positive impact on them of the exhibition being in such a 'prestigious building' within Newcastle upon Tyne.

Health and wellbeing are increasingly understood as tied up with, and not separate from, learning, creativity and connectedness, and thus are part of what museums have always offered to their communities, even if not articulated in these terms (Desmarais, Bedford and Chatterjee 2018). Lackoi *et al.* (2016) suggest that museums and heritage venues bring people together at the heart of their communities, which helps both their physical and mental health at every stage of life. One *Creative Dialogues* participant said:

> I've found my time at *Creative Dialogues* both challenging and engaging. It has pushed me creatively and personally. This has been more than I initially expected. Continuing this group will be a great journey. I feel I've grown... I'm looking forward to continuing this journey. (Creative Dialogues 2016)

This quote was a direct indication of the achievement of one of the goals of the project, which was to have a legacy of the art group continuing after the project. The outreach team at TWAM agreed to support the participants by facilitating the group to continue meeting on a weekly basis and providing museum staff and museum artists to support the art-making. This continued for several months after the project ended before the group progressed towards discovering further interests within their lives. Some members of the group started socialising outside the group and joined a debating group together. Other members set up a visit to BALTIC contemporary art gallery for their recovery group. As the project developed, some participants arranged meeting points to travel to visit museums and galleries together.

Discussion

We started with some questions:

- Does engaging in a 'creative dialogue' add something to people's recovery from drug and alcohol problems?
- How do we engage people meaningfully in arts and cultural practice when they are in recovery, through using museum and gallery spaces and artefacts?

Participants of *Creative Dialogues* reported that the workshops, museum and gallery visits, and exhibition did add something to their recovery – a sense of discovery and personal growth through valued, shared experiences. Participants demonstrated meaningful engagement in arts and cultural practice, gaining confidence in receiving from and contributing to cultural activity. They came to see themselves as people who could and should access museums and galleries and began to value their own creative expression.

Through linking people's experience to the *Creative Dialogues* themes informed by concepts of recovery capital (Cloud and Granfield 2008), we can see that the project seemed to enhance human, social and cultural capital. The group members' newly found knowledge of art had developed their human capital (Cloud and Granfield 2008), as was apparent in the focus group when members spoke articulately and in depth about their artwork and that of their peers in the group. Membership of the group generated reciprocal obligations and social capital 'stock' (Bourdieu and Wacquant 1992). These social bonds seemed to benefit individual group members (Laub and Sampson 2003) through forming relationships with others who were supportive of recovery (Longabaugh *et al.* 2010). In addition to the interpersonal relationships within the group, members developed art skills. In doing so, group members enhanced both their human and cultural capital (Granfield and Cloud 1999; Cloud and Granfield 2001).

Participation in and creative engagement with museums and galleries has great potential to support people who are in recovery from substance misuse. Art therapists can play a central role in providing a safe framework for the participants, and enable artists, museums staff and recovery staff to collectively support the social needs, mental and emotional wellbeing and personal growth of participants in projects of this kind.

Acknowledgements

Creative Dialogues was funded by Newcastle University's Faculty of Medical Sciences and the Newcastle Institute for Creative Arts Practice EngageFMS fund. Special thanks to Fine Art staff Tracy Tofield, Bridget Kennedy, David Butler and LifeWorkArt Fine Art students Charlotte Cook, Lydia London, Anna Skulczuk and Clare Townley from the School of Art and Culture, Suzanne Prak-Sandilands and Zoe Brown from Tyne and Wear Archives and Museums, Changing Lives staff at North Tyneside Recovery Partnership, and XL Gallery staff.

References

Aletraris, L., Paino, M., Edmond, M.B., Roman, P.M. and Bride, B.E. (2014) 'The use of art and music therapy in substance abuse treatment programs.' *Journal of Addictions Nursing 25,* 4, 190–196.

Bourdieu, P. and Wacquant, L. (1992) *An Invitation to Reflexive Sociology.* Chicago, IL: University of Chicago Press.

Brooker, J. (2010) 'Found objects in art therapy.' *International Journal of Art Therapy 15,* 1, 25–35.

Cloud, W. and Granfield, R. (2001) 'Natural recovery from substance dependency: Lessons for treatment providers.' *Journal of Social Work Practice in Addictions 1,* 1, 83–104.

Cloud, W. and Granfield, R. (2008) 'Conceptualizing recovery capital: Expansion of a theoretical construct.' *Substance Use and Misuse 43,* 12–13, 1971–1986.

Creative Dialogues (2016). *Project Blog.* Accessed at www.creativedialoguesproject.wordpress.com.

Desmarais, S., Bedford, L. and Chatterjee, H.J. (2018) *Museums as Spaces for Wellbeing: A Second Report from the National Alliance for Museums, Health and Wellbeing.* Accessed at www.museumsandwellbeingalliance.wordpress.com.

Edwards, D. (2004) *Art Therapy.* London: SAGE.

Granfield, R. and Cloud, W. (1999) *Coming Clean: Overcoming Addiction Without Treatment.* New York, NY: New York University Press.

Hackett, S., Ashby, L., Parker, K., Goody, S. and Power, N. (2017a) 'UK art therapy practice-based guidelines for children and adults with learning disabilities.' *International Journal of Art Therapy 22,* 2, 84–94.

Hackett, S., Taylor, J.L., Freeston, M., Jahoda, A. *et al.* (2017b) 'Interpersonal art psychotherapy for the treatment of aggression in people with learning disabilities in secure care: A protocol for a randomised controlled feasibility study.' *Pilot and Feasibility Studies 3,* 1, 42.

Hennessy, E.A. (2017) 'Recovery capital: A systematic review of the literature.' *Addiction Research and Theory 25, 5,* 349–360.

Kurimanzutto (2018) Accessed on 12/7/2018 at www.kurimanzutto.com/en/artists/gabriel-orozco.

Lackoi, K., Patsou, M. and Chatterjee, H.J. *et al.* (2016) *Museums for Health and Wellbeing. A Preliminary Report from the National Alliance for Museums, Health and Wellbeing.* Museums for Health and Wellbeing.

Laub, J.H. and Sampson, R.J. (2003). *Shared Beginning, Divergent Lives: Delinquent Boys to Age 70.* Cambridge, MA: Harvard University Press.

Lloyd, B. and Kalmanowitz, D. (2005) *The Drawing Shed.* Accessed on 24/7/18 at www.thedrawingshed.org/bobby-lloyd.

London, L. (2016) 'LifeWorkArt External Projects – Creative Dialogues.' (Unpublished master's dissertation). Newcastle University.

Longabaugh, R., Wirtz, P., Zywiak, W. and O'Malley, S. (2010) 'Network support as a prognostic indicator of drinking outcomes: The COMBINE study.' *Journal of Studies on Alcohol and Drugs 71,* 837–846.

McNiff, S. (1998) *Trust The Process, An Artist Guide to Letting Go.* Boston, MA: Shambhala.

O'Brien, F. (2004) 'The making of mess in art therapy: Attachment, trauma and the brain.' *Inscape 9,* 1, 2–13.

Putnam, R. (2000) *Bowling Alone: The Collapse and Revival of American Community.* New York, NY: Simon & Schuster.

Rothwell, K. and Hackett, S. (2018) 'Violent Acts and Creative Responses: Resilience Building Through Art Psychotherapy.' In J. Adlam, T. Kluttig and B.X. Lee (eds) *Violent States and Creative States: From the Global to the Individual. Volume II – Human Violence and Creative Humanity.* London and Philadelphia, PA: Jessica Kingsley Publishers.

Schaverien, J. (1999) *The Revealing Image: Analytical Art Psycotherapy in Theory and Practice* (second edition). London: Routledge.

White, W. and Cloud, W. (2008) 'Recovery capital: A primer for addictions professionals.' *Counselor 9*, 5, 22–27.

Winnicott, D.W. (1971) *Playing and Reality*. London and New York, NY: Routledge.

CHAPTER 7

The Caring Museum/ Le Musée qui soigne

Art Therapy at the Montreal Museum of Fine Arts

Stephen Legari, Marilyn Lajeunesse and Louise Giroux

Introduction

Entering the International Atelier for Education and Art Therapy Michel de la Chenelière at the Montreal Museum of Fine Arts (MMFA) you are greeted by a broad corridor with dark tiled floors and walls that climb to a vaulted glass ceiling more than 20 metres high. The effect is cathedral-like and inspires the gaze to wander up. There you will find Betty Goodwin's sculpture *Triptyche*, featuring a massive bronze ear and a bifurcated reflection that, along with its accompanying text, speaks of the perils of language. This is a space conceived for creative human activity.

With more than 3500 square metres dedicated to the activities of the Department for Education and Wellbeing (DEW), the Atelier is the largest of its kind in a museum setting in North America. There are 12 studios, two venues for exhibitions, a community open studio, a group dining area, and spaces to relax. This is also where the art therapy programme is housed. The programme includes various therapy groups, workshops, exhibitions, student placements, the

Art Hive, several research partnerships, and a full-time art therapist in residence. It is the culmination of nearly 20 years of engaged community practice and stands as a bold response to a society's needs that are only growing in number and complexity.

On a given week, the Atelier is abuzz with school groups, specialised visits for wellbeing, workshops, and museum art therapy. As it is one of Quebec's major cultural institutions, French is the common language of exchange, but the MMFA enjoys a multilingual energy reflecting Montreal's multicultural population and the one million plus annual visitors. It is an ever-evolving hub that draws the attention of educators, benefactors, researchers and those seeking to connect through art. This chapter will report on the theory, practice and evolution of art therapy at the MMFA. We will identify the confluence of professionals, partners and stakeholders who germinated a handful of pilot projects into a fully integrated and sustained museum-based art therapy practice. We hope to inspire both the international museum community and art therapists worldwide to expand and develop museum art therapy.

A humanist fine arts museum

In 2016, Nathalie Bondil, Director General and Chief Curator of the MMFA, published a Manifesto for a Humanist Fine Arts Museum. She wrote:

> Rethinking the nature of our public means, above all, to consider our visitors as living, experiential beings. The human need for 'beauty,' or at least for aesthetic sentiment, is physiological, not just philosophical or cultural... We now have to think about art as a force for social cohesion and individual wellbeing. (Bondil 2016, p.20)

Congruent with this manifesto, the orientation of the education and art therapy team is Rogerian. Present-focused, empathic, authentic, relationship oriented and unconditionally positive in regard are the humanistic principles which guide the practice of the museum's DEW. When the team encounters the public, whoever that may be, the regard is one of understanding, acceptance and welcome (Rogers 2003). This theoretical framework allows for cohesive intention across the disciplines of group art therapy, open studio, mediation, gallery visits and supervision.

The humanistic approach, however, is not practised to the exclusion of other orientations. The museum's full-time art therapist is systemically and psychodynamically trained and oriented. While the here and now informs the general practice of art therapy, exploration of early experience, attachment, family of origin and systemic stressors can be mobilised for the benefit of the participant, when appropriate. Additionally, the art therapy training programme at the MMFA accommodates the approaches of collaborating universities, whether psychodynamic/eclectic (Concordia University), or gestalt/existential/humanistic (Université du Québec en Abitibi-Témiscamingue/UQAT).

Museum art therapy

The international literature on art therapy in museums and galleries has been instrumental in illuminating the diversity of this specialised practice and has inspired the art therapy programme at the MMFA. While the exploration of the fine arts museum as a setting for art therapy began to emerge in earnest in the 1990s (Alter Muri 1996; Parashak 1997; Stiles and Mermer-Welly 1998), recent literature details the increasing range of therapy activities possible in a museum setting and the populations they can reach (Bennington *et al.* 2016; Jury, Landes and MagSIG 2015; Spraggins Rochford 2017).

Art therapists have developed the notion that museums can be therapeutic spaces (Coles and Harrison 2018; Hamil 2016; Ioannides 2016). The fine arts museum, historically a bastion of privilege, has become a venue offering wellness and respite to those marginalised by factors of race, gender, socioeconomics, intersectionality, sexuality, mental health and physical illness. Museum art therapy finds footing in this dynamic as a bridge to include marginalised communities in museum programming (Canas 2011; Thompson 2012), as therapeutic benefit for people living with long-term illness such as cancer (Deane, Carman and Fitch 2000) and for those living with psychosis and severe mental health difficulties (Colbert *et al.* 2013; Coles and Harrison 2018; Marin 2015; Thaler *et al.* 2017), as well as their caregivers (Shaer *et al.* 2008).

Research in the arts and health has proliferated in recent years (All-Party Parliamentary Group on Arts, Health and Wellbeing 2017; National Institute for Arts in Health 2017). Within this momentum, art therapy and wellbeing programming can be found sharing the same venue in a museum. This is true for the MMFA, the Memphis Brooks Museum of Art and the Indiana University Eskenazi Museum of Art (Keller n.d.; Memphis Brooks Museum of Art n.d.). This co-habitation of programming offers a collaborative resource and can at times contribute to confusion for both the public and staff alike. For instance, wellbeing as a concept is widely employed by the cultural sector but evades common definition (Thomson *et al.* 2012). Van Lith and Spooner (2018) report on important differences in practice and expertise to delineate art therapy from wellbeing activities. Their findings suggest that programmes share common ground in seeking to improve the lives of participants, with art-making as an essential ingredient, but differ in terms of objectives, facilitation and qualification. Wellbeing projects are often facilitated by educators or artists, and activities are associated with increased feelings of enjoyment and happiness. Art therapy projects focus on individual client objectives and treatment outcomes, and must include the presence of a qualified art therapist (Van Lith and Spooner 2018).

Art therapy at the MMFA

In 2017, the MMFA launched a fully integrated art therapy programme as a branch of the DEW. The department hired a full-time art therapist, Stephen Legari, as programme officer. Based on available research, this was the first time internationally that a museum had created a full-time position for an art therapist. This position has a mandate to develop programming, facilitate groups, collaborate on research, supervise students and manage the museum's Art Hive. While innovative in its scope and implementation, the programme benefits from nearly two decades of community outreach and programme development in the DEW.

When developing new art therapy projects, steps are taken to guarantee the ethical treatment of each participant, with emphasis placed on co-creation with partnering organisations. Each project is

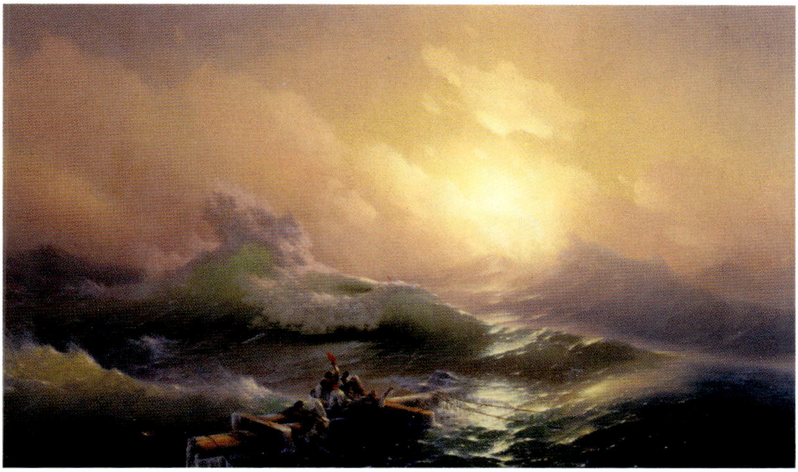

Figure 4.1 Ivan Aivazovsky, 'The Ninth Wave' (1850), oil on canvas, © State Russian Museum, St Petersburg

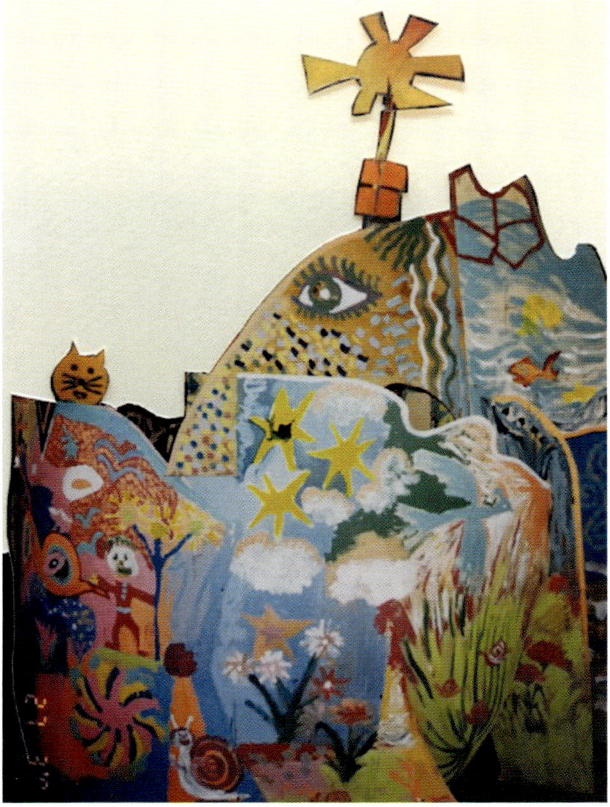

Figure 4.2 Painted sculptures. 'From monologue to dialogue' workshop (1997)

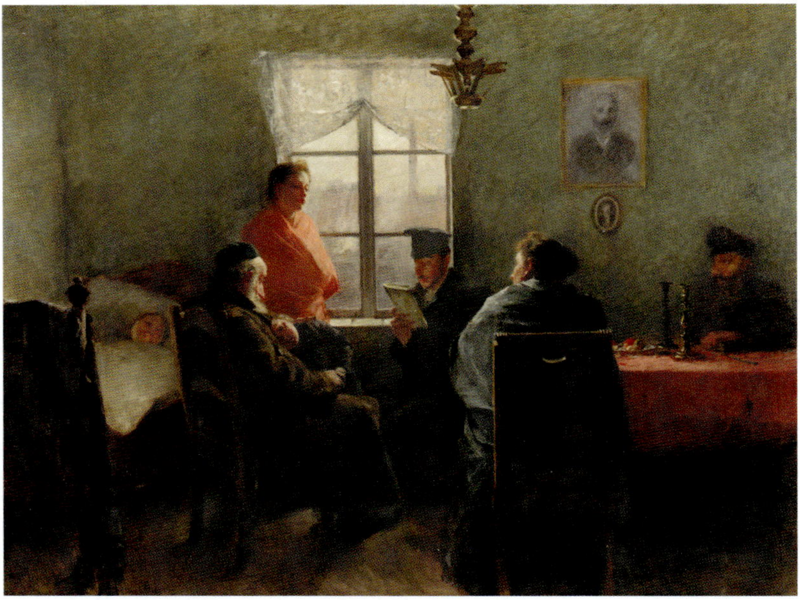

Figure 5.1 Samuel Hirszenberg, 'Sabbath Rest' (1894), oil on canvas. Ben Uri Collection

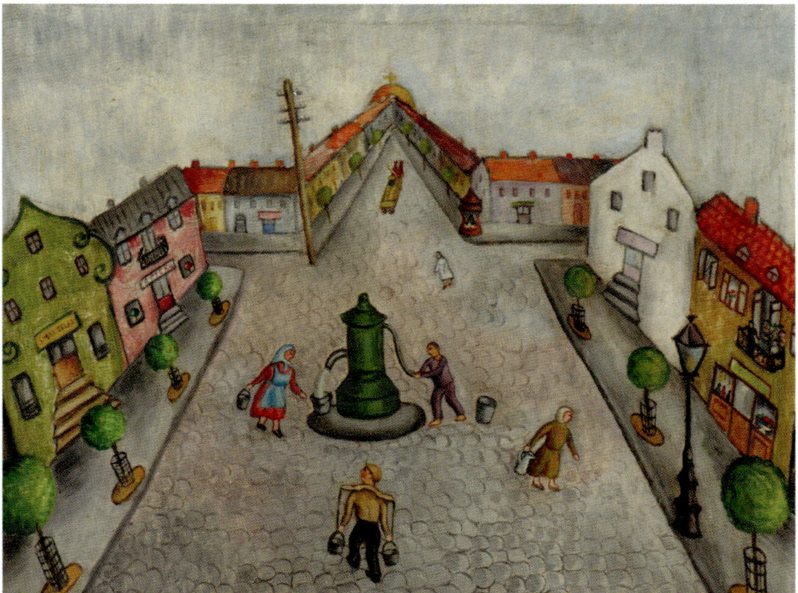

Figure 5.2 Chana Kowalska, 'Shtetl' (1934), oil on canvas. Ben Uri Collection

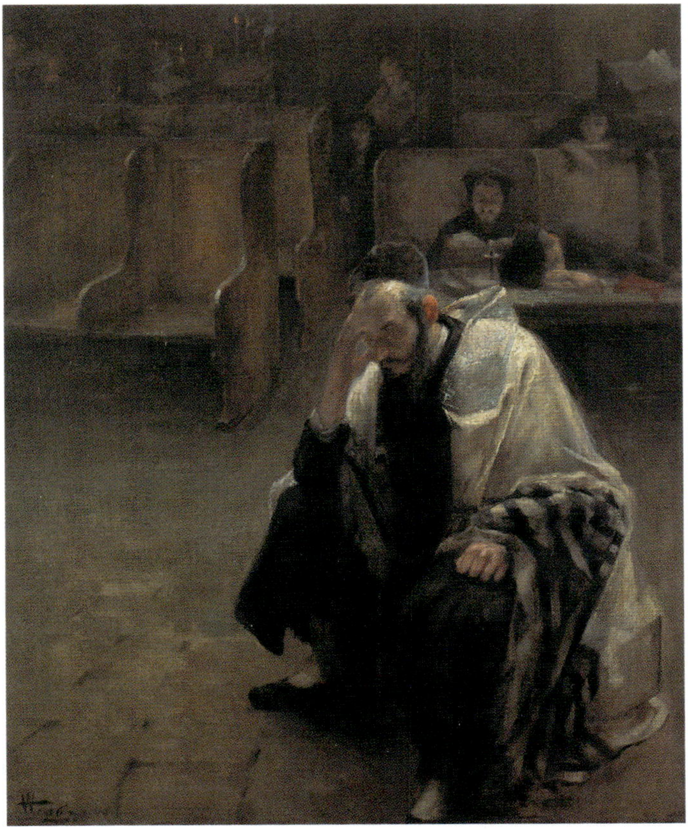

Figure 5.3 Alfred Wolmark, 'In the Synagogue' (1906), oil on canvas. Ben Uri Collection

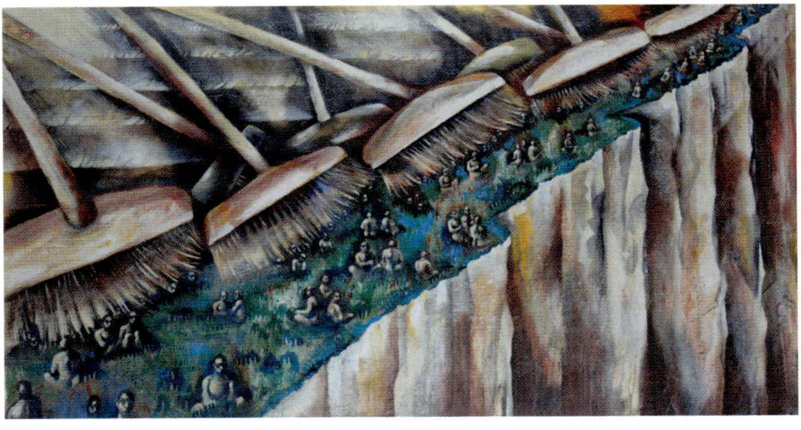

Figure 5.4 David Breuer-Weil, 'The Edge' (2007), oil on canvas. Ben Uri Collection

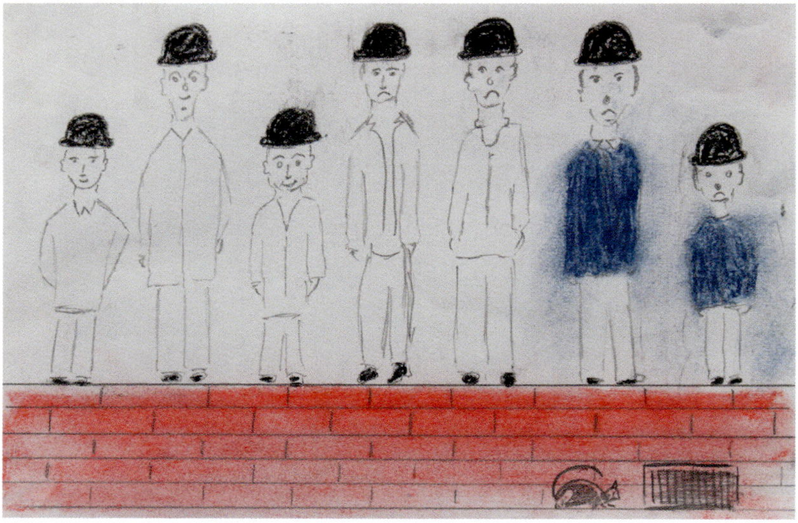

Figure 5.5 Albert, 'Waiting in Line', pencil and pastel drawing

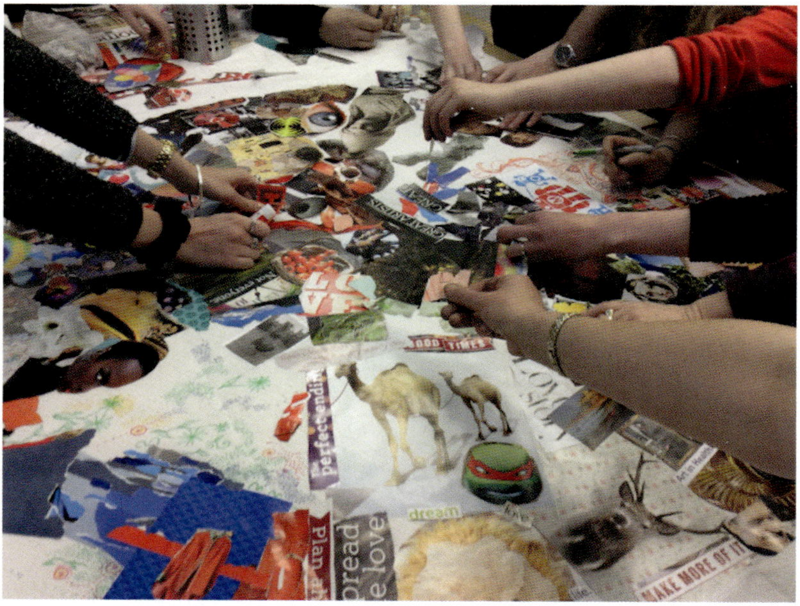

Figure 6.2 Collective collage workshop

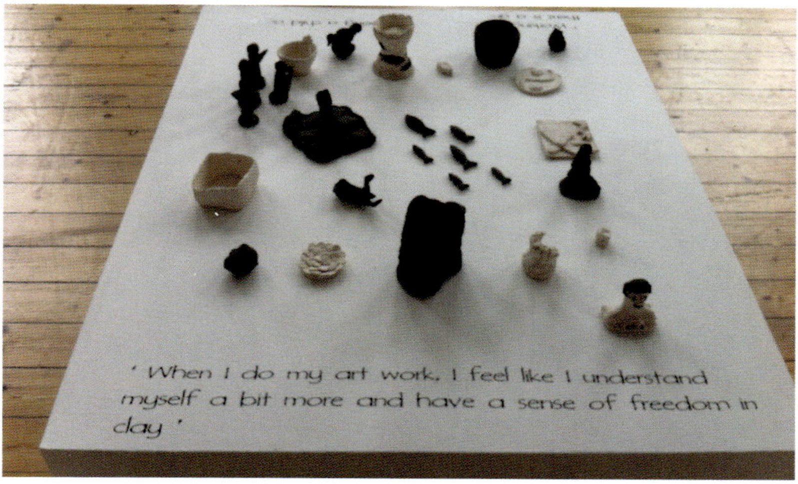

Figure 6.5 The exhibition: detail

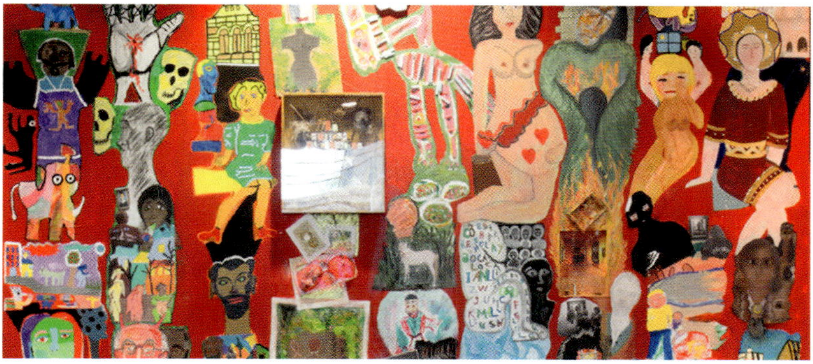

Figure 7.2 'Totem-Muses', collective artwork by participants from Le Cap

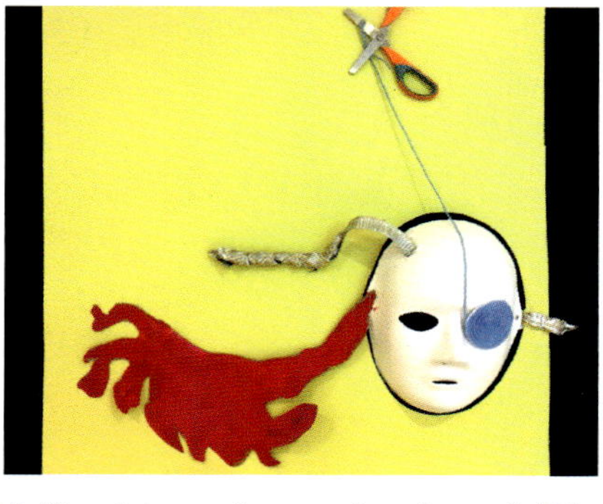

Figure 7.3 'Expérience de mort imminente' ('Near Death Experience'), part of the contrasts *project. Participant artwork portraying experience as a patient with traumatic brain injury*

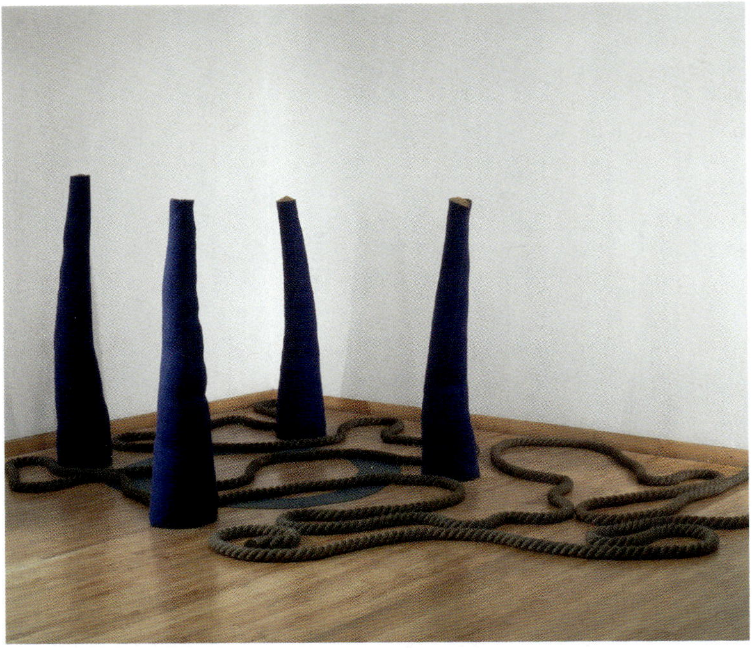

Figure 8.1 (detail) '4 casb 2 '67', 1967; Barry Flanagan (1941–2009). Purchased 1976; © The estate of Barry Flanagan/ Bridgeman Images; Photo © Tate, London 2019

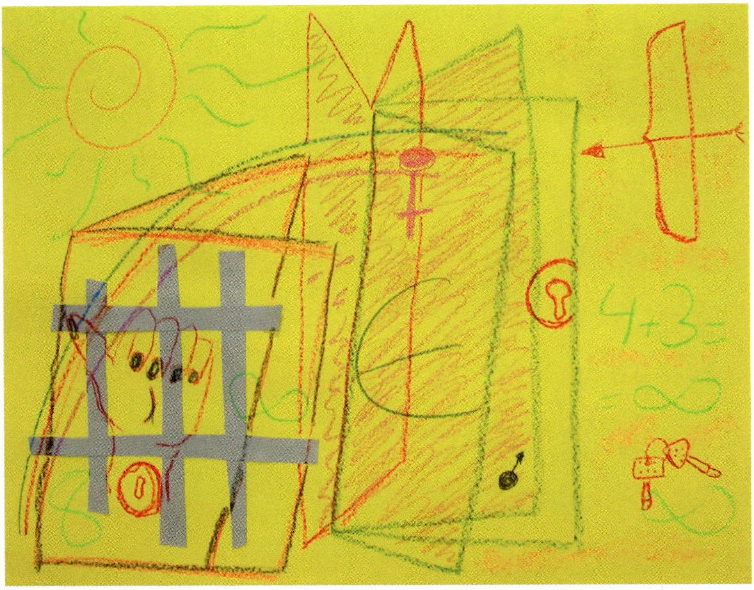

Figure 9.1 Participant artwork after viewing 'The Rape of Europa'

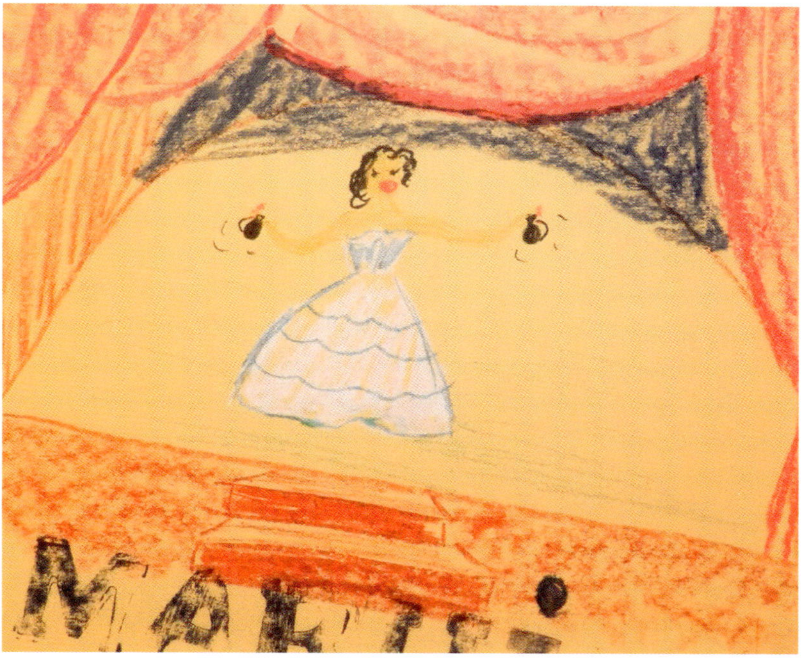

Figure 9.2 Participant artwork after visiting the 'Messages from the Wall' exhibition

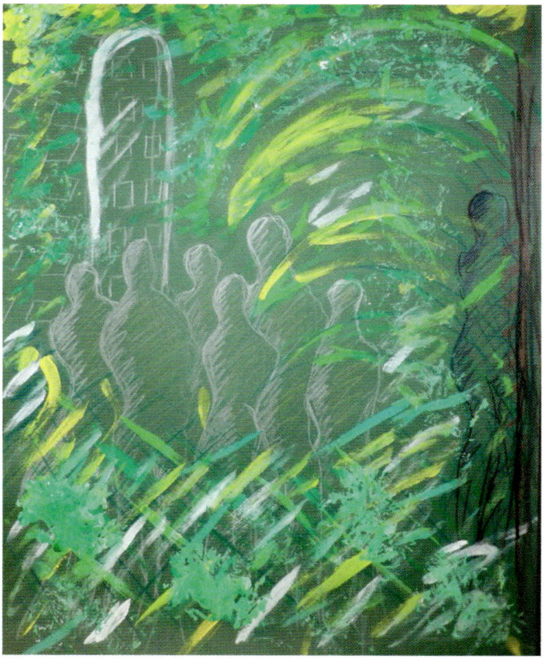

Figure 9.3 Participant artwork after viewing 'Albia'

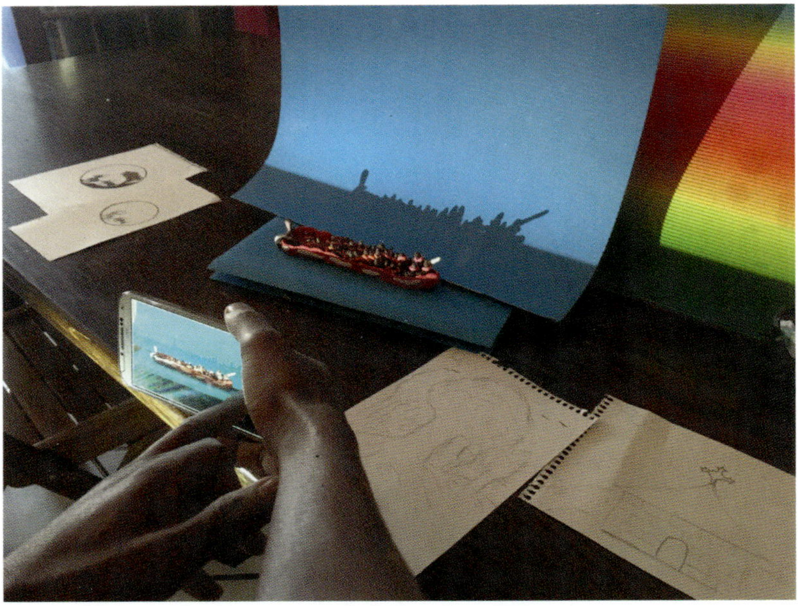

Figure 12.2 Stage-managing the boat

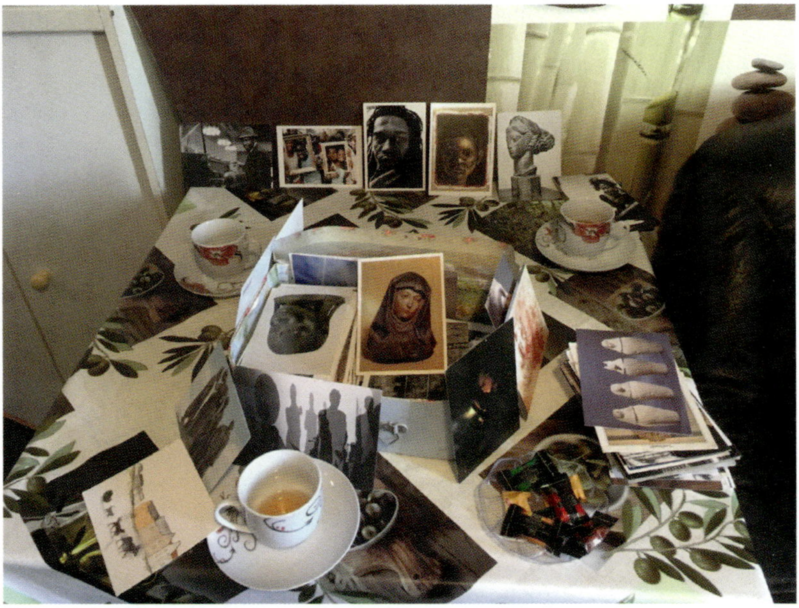

Figure 12.3 Postcard exhibition on the table

planned according to objectives, theme(s), frequency, materials and human resource. Projects might benefit from collaboration with other professionals including museum mediators and health or mental health care professionals. However, the art therapy component of each session is always facilitated by an art therapist and all projects are built on the foundation of art therapy practice. In the dynamic of this therapeutic relationship, the art-making and the encounters with works of art, a participant may experience an improvement in health alongside a recovery/discovery in their sense of self, and/or a respite from burdens of chronic illness. The following is an outline of the best practice tenets for art therapy projects at the MMFA, developed from programme evaluations in community partnerships, which are discussed later.

Co-creation

Each project is treated as a stand-alone collaboration requiring the expertise of the partnering organisation. Their knowledge and understanding of their membership help the museum team understand the motivations, needs and abilities of participants. The process begins with important questions for the partner that include previous experience with art therapy, previous experience with the MMFA, participant needs, frequency of sessions requested, and whether the museum setting has been fully considered. This is followed by a series of meetings at the museum and the partner's setting. As the partnership develops, the museum relies on the partner to recruit, typically, eight participants per therapy group. When a project is in pilot stage, it is clearly stated so that the participants know they are contributing to something new and can impact its development. Standard practices of informed consent are conducted when the group begins.

Roles

The roles, field of expertise and limitations of each stakeholder are made clear at the outset of the project. Responsibilities are defined both at a logistical level (e.g. transport for participants), and at a professional level (e.g. facilitation of group art therapy). Initial meetings help to establish these roles, serving to limit miscommunication between team members when the art therapy project is under way.

The museum collection

Projects are related to artworks in the MMFA's collection. Art therapy at the MMFA takes as its point of departure that interacting with works of art in the gallery adds a unique dimension to the art therapy process and is believed to enhance participant experience.

Evaluation and record keeping

Feedback, evaluation, and debriefing are essential tools for resolving problems and improving delivery of the programme. Team members must communicate about the project's progress throughout in order to serve the participants well. This includes celebrating successes and planning for subsequent sessions. Similarly, paying careful attention to participants' feedback is essential. Written reports are produced and maintained by the art therapist and programme officer. While reports on participants' therapeutic progress are not shared as they are confidential clinical material, reports on the project's progress are, thereby respecting the confidential boundaries of the project.

Exhibitions

Exhibition of participants' artwork must be preceded by fully informed consent by all participants at the outset of a project. This begins at the recruitment stage when partnering agencies communicate the motivation, potential benefits and risks involved in exhibiting work made in an art therapy context. Not every project will result in an exhibition, but the experience of exhibiting in the fine arts museum milieu can be validating for participants and educational for the public.

Early collaborations

In 2014, a regional community mental health centre (Le Centre d'Apprentissage Parallèle de Montréal[1]) that provides services to adults living with psychological or emotional difficulties proposed a collaboration with the MMFA. The centre emphasises artistic creation as a means of personal recovery and socio-professional reintegration, and includes art therapy with the pioneering Quebec art therapist, Yvon Lamy.

For this pilot project, ten participants made ten visits of two-and-a-half hours to the museum, including visits to galleries facilitated by a museum mediator and art therapy workshops facilitated by Lamy. Themes, which ran for two weeks each, were co-developed and included: the self-portrait, the artist and his/her environment, symbols and what they represent, and 'a work that fascinates me'. The project culminated in a 12′ x 7′ collective mural that was exhibited in the museum's education pavilion and a short video filmed at intervals, with the full consent and voluntary participation of the participants.

The objectives of the project were congruent with the centre's own strengths-focused approach. The centre's programme includes the regular exhibition of work in its gallery space that highlights the work of its members. The centre also makes regular use of video to educate the public, destigmatise mental health problems, and offer testimonial opportunities to its members. The video filmed at the MMFA was made available to the centre for its purposes.

While the gallery visits were theme-based, participants were encouraged to identify works that resonated with their personal experience. One participant identified with proto-surrealist Alberto Martini's 'Self-Portrait' (1929) (Figure 7.1). The participant likened the darkness and nude figures to her experience of incest. She later incorporated these themes into her own work, which showed stacked figures in a totemic style. She reported:

> It needs to be talked about because it happened to me…the way that I imagined my project was in stages. That's my life. The adult [figure], she suffered. Up higher we find the child. That's to show that there is more to come than what she survived. (MMFA 2014)

1 www.ateliersducap.org/en/who-are-we/mission

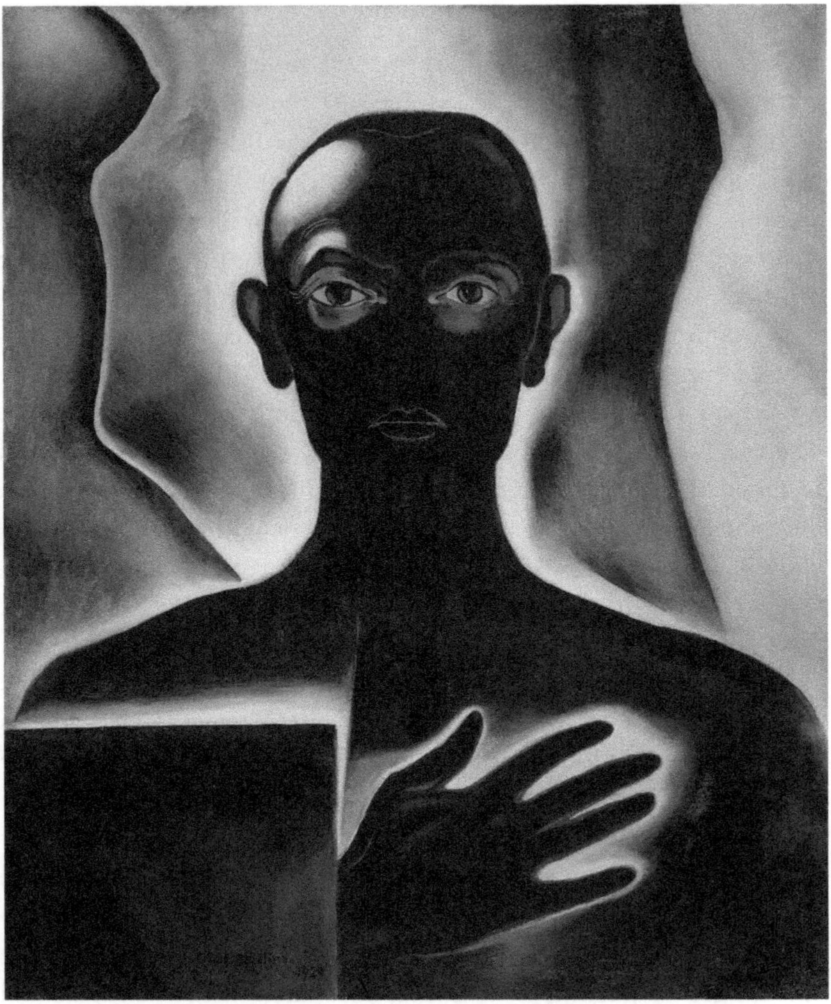

Figure 7.1 Alberto Martini, 'Self-Portrait' (1929), oil on canvas. The Montreal Museum of Fine Arts, purchase, Horsley and Annie Townsend Bequest. Photo MMFA, Brian Merrett

The exhibition of the collective mural would be the museum's first presentation of work done in an art therapy context. Work produced in art therapy can often be raw, unrefined, honest and devoid of the constraints of an academic approach. These qualities were a challenge to the previous administration of the education department, who were not accustomed to the process-orientated nature of art therapy art-making. This tension necessitated collaboration and education between partners. In the end, the work was prominently displayed in a public space joining the educational pavilion and the galleries. An art opening was held and the participants were invited to speak.

Attested by art therapist Yvon Lamy, for many participants the experience was transformative: 'There were people who were in crisis during the process, who continued the process despite everything... An experience like this is a support, a means of survival, in the midst of profound difficulty' (MMFA 2014). Thus, the opportunity to exhibit their work and speak publicly about their lived experience was an opportunity of validation for the participants (Figure 7.2).

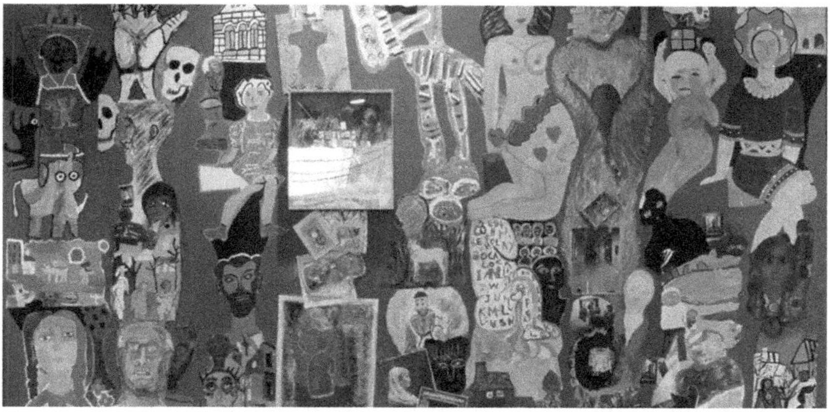

Figure 7.2 'Totem-Muses', collective artwork by participants from Le Cap

Another project which informed the development of the art therapy programme was a research collaboration between the MMFA, the Eating Disorders Program of the Douglas Mental Health University Institute, and the Art Therapy Graduate Program in the Department of Creative Arts Therapies at Concordia University (Baddeley *et al.* 2017; Thaler *et al.* 2017). The groups are closed, but to accommodate the structure of the clinical programme, returning participants join those coming to the museum for the first time. In addition to the art therapist and mediator, the group is accompanied by two psycho-educators who are responsible for the continuity of the behavioural clinical protocol, including the monitoring of breaks and calorie intake.

Each session begins with research questionnaires (Thaler *et al.* 2017) that include scales rating eating preoccupation and urges, body satisfaction changes and mood. Another scale for museum visit satisfaction is completed at the end of the day. Snacks and check-in follow the questionnaires before the mediator guides the group through the gallery, where she elicits the personal associations of the participants while providing historical and anecdotal information on the works of art. As with all art therapy groups at the MMFA, the visits take place during regular museum hours. Many agencies have a social integration objective for their populations which the visits can help to fulfil. Participants consent to visits ahead of time and all groups remain unidentified. Feedback on the visits is incorporated into future sessions.

Themes are chosen based on the evolving goals for the group, whether to encourage respite from preoccupying thoughts (e.g. *the imaginary*) or issues closer to the group's shared experience (e.g. *the female figure*). Themes are believed to help contain an experience that can otherwise be anxiety-provoking. Themes are also flexible enough to allow for a variety of associations. The clinical goal of normalising eating together in a public space means that following the visit, lunch is shared by both participants and staff.

After lunch, the art therapist reintroduces the theme by inviting links between the morning's visit and the choice of materials provided. If working with a theme such *as the container and the contained*, the art therapist might provide craft boxes and a variety of materials to explore the inner and outer world of the participants. On other occasions, non-directive, media-focused approaches are used, such as working with clay, natural materials and fluid media. It has been observed that semi-structured interventions provide a container that helps to minimise anxiety. Participants are always encouraged to explore the materials in any way they choose.

Shared reflection on personal process follows the art-making. Moments of ease can be hard won by these participants, who contend with the psychological impact of distorted self-image, anxiety, depression, fatigue and other symptoms. Qualitative data suggests there are discernible benefits to the museum art therapy programme.

As Thaler *et al.* (2017) report, 'patients often noted that visits helped distract them from troublesome thoughts and feelings. In addition, many patients noted enjoying the exposure to an alternative way of letting feelings out, or of being more present in the here and now' (p.5). Further findings are discussed later.

2017 to present

The art therapy programme has enjoyed a robust development, with opportunities to collaborate with community organisations, clinics, agencies and universities. The following is a sample of the projects realised since its full-time inception.

The programme ran a weekly two-month pilot project for women living with breast cancer. Following the group, voluntary feedback was sought from participants through an anonymised questionnaire. The results were predominantly positive, and the comments helped refine themes and length of components. One example of the feedback received was from 'Claire' (pseudonym):

> The project has helped me significantly with the ordeal of my breast cancer, and each week has allowed me to regain the serenity and acceptance of illness needed to get through these difficult times. In addition, sharing with women with similar experience was extremely important and provided me with significant moral support. The eight weeks passed too quickly and I would have needed more to continue to benefit from the therapy.

A collaboration with the Centre de Services de Justice Réparatrice (Centre for Services in Restorative Justice)[2] is structured as a monthly semi-closed group for adults whose lives are impacted by violent crime. A theme is chosen each month (e.g. *reconciliation, navigating the storm*) and one or more artworks from the collection are selected. Up to eight participants are recruited for the three-hour group, which includes check-in, reflection on the theme and artwork, art-making, and reflection on the process.

2 https://csjr.org/en

Another partnership, with Autisme Sans Limites,[3] an organisation supporting young adults with high-functioning autism, runs a weekly group focusing in equal parts on psycho-education and art therapy, with the time divided between the galleries and the studio. The 24-week programme emphasises the exploration, identification and experience of emotions and their nuances, and strives to help the participants reduce social barriers. This project is now in its second year.

The art therapy programme was invited by an association of Francophone doctors, Médecins Francophones du Canada (MFdC), to present an exhibition of client artwork at their annual conference. To respect client confidentiality, a project was conceived in collaboration with the Centre for Excellence in Patient Partnership with the Public,[4] with the express purpose of communicating patient experience through art to a community of physicians. The participants co-designed the project with the art therapist and included the theme of *contrasts* (life before and after diagnosis), and consented to an exhibition of artwork. Inspired by the benefits of museum-based social prescribing (Chatterjee and Camic 2015; Chatterjee *et al.* 2018), this project coincided with the development of a collaborative pilot project between the MFdC and the MMFA (MMFA-MFdC n.d.) (Figure 7.3).

The art therapy programme also collaborated with an agency providing end-of-life care and bereavement services (Welcome to NOVA Montreal[5]) to create a museum-based, eight-week, art therapy and bereavement support group pilot project. The group followed a certified bereavement protocol that included viewing artworks and tailored art therapy interventions. The group was co-facilitated by the MMFA's art therapist and an agency social worker and is scheduled for relaunch following a project evaluation.

3 www.autismesanslimites.org/en

4 www.ceppp.ca/en

5 www.novamontreal.com

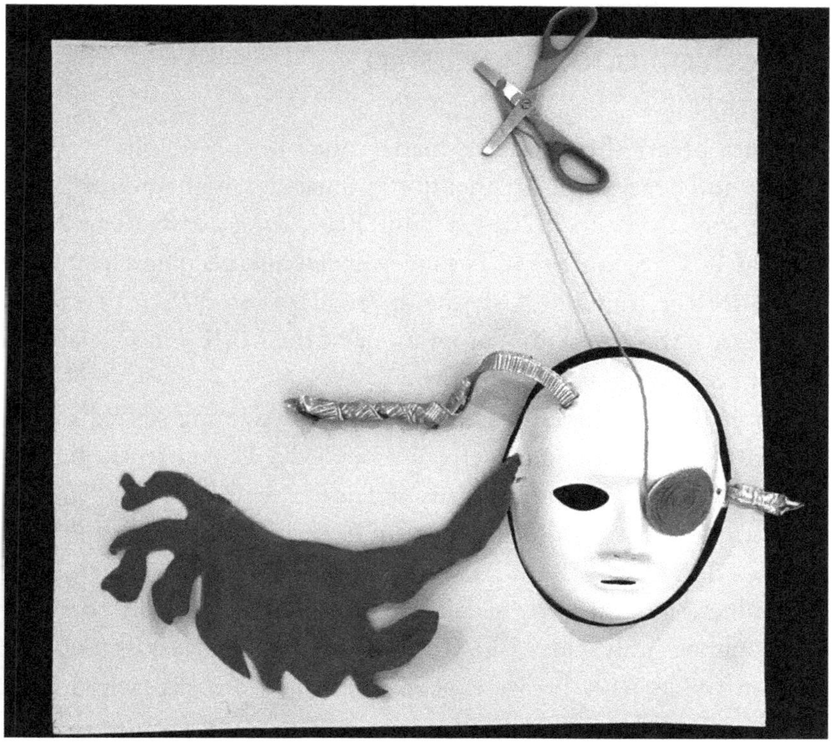

Figure 7.3 'Expérience de mort imminente' ('Near Death Experience'), part of the contrasts *project. Participant artwork portraying experience as a patient with traumatic brain injury*

Other ongoing projects include a monthly group for young adults living with language and communication difficulties (Installation Raymond-Dewar[6]), retreat workshops for healthcare providers, a dance movement therapy collaboration for people living with Parkinson's (Parkinson en mouvement[7]), and collaborating art therapists' facilitated groups for young adults living with cancer, and another for trans and non-binary youth.

6 www.fondationrea.ca/en/ird

7 www.parkinsonenmouvement.org

Museum art therapy: training, education and scholarship

Training

Students of art therapy have made valuable contributions to the theory and practice of art therapy in museums with several theses on the subject (Babock 2011; Hamil 2016; King 2018; Klein 2015; Moreau 2017; Sloan 2013). The museum has also become a legitimate milieu for the training of art therapists (Treadon 2015). In its full-time status, the art therapy programme of the MMFA has welcomed both student scholars and interns.

In 2017, the MMFA was recognised as a training setting for art therapy, with two students from Concordia University beginning an eight-month placement. This included facilitating two groups weekly, one with women living in transitional housing (Y des femmes de Montréal[8]) and a second with young adults living with high-functioning autism. In February of 2018, a student from the francophone university UQAT facilitated a ten-week group for women living with breast cancer. Students were supervised both on-site and at the university.

For training purposes, the students from Concordia University also follow one individual in art therapy during the school year, referred by a collaborating agency. Individual art therapy in a museum setting is both of interest and problematic. While those who participated may have benefited from a therapy they could not otherwise access, the resources to provide such a service to a larger public do not yet exist. For the time being, individual art therapy will remain within the practicum frame.

Art therapy courses at the museum

In 2017, the MMFA housed its first master's course in art therapy. Taught by Dr Janis Timm-Bottos, the course titled *Symbolic Imagery and Art Therapy* benefited from the museum setting to provide access to both the studios and collections, for experiential learning. In her syllabus, Timm-Bottos writes: 'through experiential art workshops

8 www.ydesfemmesmtl.org/en

and readings, symbols and the symbolic/metaphoric function are examined with reference to various psychological models, including Freudian psychoanalysis, Jungian analytical psychology and Hillman's archetypal/imaginal psychology' (Concordia University 2017). The course in symbolic imagery is a core course of the master's curriculum (Concordia University n.d.).

Art therapy research at the MMFA

The Art and Health Advisory Committee of the MMFA is helmed by Quebec's Chief Science Officer, Rémi Quirion, and comprises recognised researchers, philanthropists, museum and departmental directors, and art therapists. The role of the committee is to guide and advise research projects developed for the museum, which includes art therapy research. For each project, qualified researchers and art therapists are responsible for the holding of participant experience, therapy frame, data analysis and sharing of findings. Whether arts-based, qualitative or mixed-methods, the projects employ the same protocol of co-creation as other art therapy groups.

Concordia University Creative Arts Therapies Associate Professor Yehudit Silverman brought the challenging research project, *Seeds of Hope: An arts-based approach to raising awareness about suicide and fostering resiliency.* Silverman, who had previously produced both literature and a film on the subject of suicide (Silverman and Firm 2014; Silverman, Smith and Burns 2013), invited 20 adult participants, including those from the Inuit community, to explore the impact of suicide on their lives through guided museum visits and mask-making. The project culminated in a group exhibition.

Beginning in 2017, Vera Heller, Professor of Art Therapy at UQAT, employed the myth of the hero's journey as a foundation for her heuristic research project, Imagined Journeys. Working with a group of adult individuals who had migrated voluntarily from their home nation, the group explored the existential complexities of migration and hybrid identity. The group was led through various eras of the museum's collection to explore the personal, the symbolic and the metaphoric by museum mediator Sayeh Sarfaraz who drew upon her own lived experience of migration as well as her expertise as a contemporary artist. Over 20 sessions, Heller invited the group to enter the realm of the imaginary to bring transformation to their real-life journeys. A group exhibition at the museum completed the project.

In 2017, two articles were published on the project with the Douglas Mental Health Institute (Baddeley *et al.* 2017; Thaler *et al.* 2017) looking at the museum experience as an adjunct for people living with eating disorders. The first evaluated the potential for art therapy to produce short-term benefits in self-image and mood. Data was collected during each visit, with a total sample of 78 patients. Measurements included the Profile of Mood States (POMS-BI) (Lorr, McNair and Fisher 2010), eating disorder preoccupations and urges using a visual analogue scale, as well as body image concerns using the Body Satisfaction Scale (Slade *et al.* 1990). The participants also completed a questionnaire at the end of the day for thematic analysis. Questions included: 'How did you find your experience of being at the museum?', 'What could be improved?' and 'How was your experience during the art therapy workshop at the museum?' (Thaler *et al.* 2017).

The study found that art therapy was a suitable adjunct for adults with eating disorders with no significant short-term impact on eating preoccupations or body image, either positive or negative (Thaler *et al.* 2017). The qualitative data suggested nearly uniformly positive support for the museum protocol, with participants reporting increased calmness following the art therapy sessions. A sampling of participants' comments included, 'I love the opportunity to let out my emotions in another way than speech or writing' and 'I liked the therapy workshop as it helped me change my mind and be more present' (Thaler *et al.* 2017, p.3).

Complementary to this study, Professor Laura Evans from the University of North Texas reported on the project design from a museum education perspective (Baddeley *et al.* 2017), conducting interviews with the museum team, including the programme officer, mediator and art therapist. From the interviews, she identified salient thematic challenges for constructing such a project in a fine arts museum setting. These included the necessity of careful collaboration, developing strategies for responding to participants' experiences, appreciating the challenges of the population, and the intersection of museum education and art therapy (Baddeley *et al.* 2017).

Art therapy graduate student Ellen Smallwood developed a museum-based protocol for adolescents and young adults living with epilepsy, inspired by the approach of the art therapists of Studio E (Stafstrom, Havlena and Krezinski 2012). Smallwood's mixed-methods study followed a group over eight weeks at the MMFA. The protocol included four theme-based visits to galleries, art therapy, and before-and-after testing at the Sheldon Memory Lab of McGill University (Sheldon Memory Lab[9]). Smallwood's data for the attend group showed decreased scores of depression and stress and increased scores in quality of life compared to the no-attend group, with interviews revealing themes of social connection and the externalisation of the impact of epilepsy (Smallwood 2019).

In 2019, the art therapy programme conducted a research collaboration with UQAT art therapy Professor Jacinthe Lambert in collaboration with the Quebec Breast Cancer Foundation. Lambert, who is both an art therapist and psychologist with an expertise in positive psychology (Lambert and Ranger 2009), serves as lead researcher looking at the lived experience of women living with breast cancer. Existing literature supports the positive impact of art therapy for women with breast cancer (Collie Bottorff and Long 2006; Thyme *et al.* 2009). There is, however, little literature exploring a museum-based art therapy programme (Deane *et al.* 2000). The study followed two consecutive groups of eight women over ten weeks with sessions lasting three hours per week and gallery visits on every other week.

The Art Hive of the MMFA

Art therapists at the MMFA are also active in non-clinical work at the Art Hive. This community studio, the first of its kind in a museum setting in the world, is a partnership with Concordia University and builds on the applied research of Art Hive founder and art therapy professor Janis Timm-Bottos. With a mandate of arts-based social

---

9 www.sheldonmemorylabatmcgill.com

inclusion, the Art Hive opens its doors twice weekly to the general public and provides free access to materials, space, the support of an art therapist and a museum mediator, and the opportunity to freely explore art-making and social connection. At the time of writing, there were 135 art hives worldwide with more than 30 in Montreal alone.[10]

At first glance, the Art Hive appears to be the synthesis of both open studio and community practice (Deco 1998; Hosea 2006). Studio practice is sometimes conceived of as a polarity to clinical art therapy practice (Wadeson 2002) with its emphasis on the art-as-therapy process and its recognition of participants as artists rather than patients or clients (Allen 1995; Malchiodi 2007). In Timm-Bottos's vision, the Art Hive transcends its association with the psychiatric milieu to truly connect with its roots in community organising, and takes its place as a co-constructed, community-driven third space (Timm-Bottos 2006, 2016; Timm-Bottos and Reilly 2014). While the Art Hive is often facilitated by art therapists, Timm-Bottos calls for an egalitarian dynamic wherein the professional is as much a learner, art-maker and community member as those who make the hive their public *homespace*. The Art Hive of the MMFA occupies a unique space at the intersection of the museum, the community, education and art therapy. The number of visitors varies each time the Art Hive opens, with an average of 20 participants. In its first year, the Art Hive of the MMFA welcomed more than 3000 participants.

Programme origins: sharing the museum

Several art therapy projects have enjoyed development through their affiliation with museum educators (Deane *et al.* 2000; Parashak 1997; Rochford 2017; Treadon, Rosal and Thompson Wylder 2006). This is true of the art therapy programme at the MMFA. The following describes the expansion of the MMFA's educational activities between 1997 and 2017 and its impact on the education department's identity and public role. We hope that through this description, other museums and art therapists will find ingredients to realise their own ambitions in museum art therapy.

10 www.arthives.org

In 1997, the MMFA embarked on a humanist mandate to broaden its educational and cultural mediation reach to the widest possible audience. The foundation of this initiative, entitled *Sharing the Museum (Le Musée en partage)*, was built on the following tenets: to establish a programme of free, ongoing activities for the public that included access to both the museum's collections and creative activities; to develop and provide specially designed projects, both short and long term, to community groups; and to adopt a socially progressive approach based on openness, attentiveness and action. The programme became the foundation for the co-creation of community partnerships at the MMFA and is the template on which the art therapy programme was later built. Programme Officer Marilyn Lajeunesse has been *Sharing the Museum*'s steward since its inception and remains so today.

In its first five years, the programme mobilised the reach of the MMFA's collection and expanded the presence of community exhibitions through co-created partnerships. These diverse groups included children from disadvantaged neighbourhoods, young families on limited incomes, people with disabilities, at-risk youth, older adults, immigrants, literacy groups and various ethnic communities from across Montreal. The breadth of these projects demonstrated a move towards the inclusion of wellbeing objectives as opposed to strictly traditional educational ones.

In 2002, a major five-point evaluation of the programme was launched consisting of interviews with administrators, focus groups, a series of in-depth interviews with a sampling of participants, and the distribution of 1000 free tickets to a sampling of those who had participated in group activities in order to evaluate individual return visits. The entire education team was involved in this process. The results yielded invaluable feedback from partners and participants and produced salient themes that came to inform the future of all community collaborations. These included: the quality of welcome and the closing process of each group are important; the programme is congruent with other community work and complements the work in holistic health management/prevention; the arts are not a luxury – they are a means to feed spiritual and emotional health; exhibits offer other perspectives and important links to history.

By the end of 2004, an average of 38,154 individuals had participated in the programme. From 2004 onwards, the wellbeing dimension of the activities expanded as did the populations that were involved. These included children with terminal illness, various mental health associations, major hospitals, participants with autism spectrum disorder and others with pervasive developmental disorders, people impacted by homelessness, people with Alzheimer's, indigenous groups, and senior citizens groups which eventually took the form of weekly free activities for those 65 and over.

As the number of partnerships expanded, a new position was created in 2014 to coordinate them. Louise Giroux, now Programme Officer for Well-Being, is a former museum educator at the MMFA herself and develops and implements partnerships with several communities, hospitals and populations (Figure 7.4).

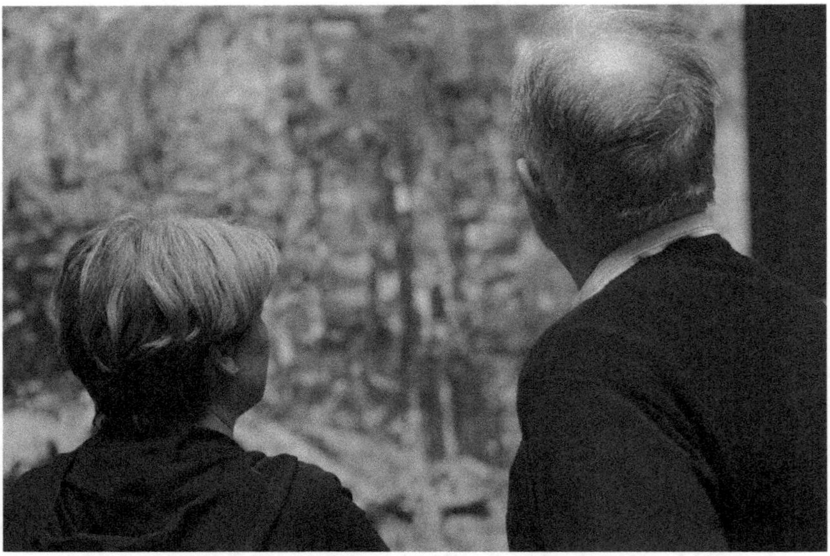

Figure 7.4 Sharing the Museum (Le Musée en partage) *(Photo: Pierre Arsenault)*

Philanthropy

Philanthropy has been the lifeblood for the development and expansion of the MMFA's education, wellbeing and art therapy initiatives. Increasingly, family foundations, corporations and individuals have sought to direct their funding towards programmes that are impact oriented and socially conscious. The art therapy programme owes its sustainability to the relationship between donors and the museum's foundation, which are charged with communicating the programme's activities and ambitions.

Conclusion

As a unique model of fully integrated art therapy in a fine arts museum, the MMFA's programme continues to innovate and expand its activities in therapy groups, research, training and new partnerships. New students arrive every autumn to begin their placements, research projects help to expand both our appreciation and understanding of the art museum as a legitimate milieu for art therapy, and the expanding presence of collaborating creative arts therapists contributes invaluable expertise to the programme's development. The programme has gained attention in the press both locally and internationally, and the future of art therapy at the Montreal Museum of Fine Arts looks flourishing.

References

Allen, P.B. (1995) 'Coyote comes in from the cold: The evolution of the open studio concept.' *Art Therapy 12,* 3, 161–166.

Alter Muri, S. (1996) 'Dali to Beuys: Incorporating art history in art therapy treatment plans.' *Art Therapy 13,* 2, 102–107.

All-Party Parliamentary Group on Arts, Health and Wellbeing (2017) *Creative Health: The Arts for Health and Wellbeing* (second edition). Accessed on 15/7/19 at https://www.culturehealthandwellbeing.org.uk/appg-inquiry/.

Babock, J.L. (2011) 'Art Therapy in a Museum Setting: The Emotional Expression of Seven to Ten Year Old Girls in Response to Established Work.' Hofstra University.

Baddeley, G., Evans, L., Lajeunesse, M. and Legari, S. (2017) 'Body talk: Examining a collaborative multiple-visit program for visitors with eating disorders.' *Journal of Museum Education 42,* 4, 345–353.

Bennington, R., Backos, A., Harrison, J., Reader, A.E. and Carolan, R. (2016) 'Art therapy in art museums: Promoting social connectedness and psychological well-being of older adults.' *The Arts in Psychotherapy 49,* 34–43.

Bondil, N. (2016) 'Manifesto for a Humanist.' In N. Bondil (ed.) *Michal and Renata Hornstein: Pavilion for Peace.* Montreal: Montreal Museum of Fine Arts.

Canas, E. (2011) 'Cultural institutions and community outreach: What can art therapy do?' *Canadian Art Therapy Association Journal 24,* 2, 30–33.

Chatterjee, H.J. and Camic, P.M. (2015) 'The health and well-being potential of museums and art galleries.' *Arts and Health 7,* 3, 183–186.

Chatterjee, H.J., Camic, P.M., Lockyer, B. and Thomson, L.J.M. (2018) 'Non-clinical community interventions: A systematised review of social prescribing schemes.' *Arts and Health 10,* 2, 97–123.

Colbert, S., Cooke, A., Camic, P.M. and Springham, N. (2013) 'The art-gallery as a resource for recovery for people who have experienced psychosis.' *Arts in Psychotherapy 40,* 2, 250–256.

Coles, A. and Harrison, F. (2018) 'Tapping into museums for psychotherapy: An evaluation of a pilot group for young adults.' *International Journal of Art Therapy 23,* 3, 115–124.

Collie, K., Bottorff, J.L. and Long, B.C. (2006) 'A narrative view of art therapy and art making by women with breast cancer.' *Journal of Health Psychology 11, 5,* 761–775.

Concordia University (n.d.) *Art Therapy Sample Course Sequence.* Accessed on 29/11/18 at www.concordia.ca/finearts/creative-arts-therapies/programs/art-therapy-ma/sequence.html.

Concordia University (2017) *ATRP 603 Symbolic Imagery & Art Therapy Workshop/Studio.* Montreal: Janis Timm-Bottos.

Deane, K., Carman, M. and Fitch, M. (2000) 'Le rapprochement entre l'art-thérapie et l'éducation muséale dans le contexte du vécu.' *Canadian Oncology Nursing Journal 10,* 4, 143–146.

Deco, S. (1998) 'Return to the Open Studio Group: Art Therapy Groups in Acute Psychiatry.' In S. Skaife and V. Huet (eds) *Art Psychotherapy Groups: Between Pictures and Words.* London: Routledge.

Hamil, S. (2016) *The Art Museum as a Therapeutic Space.* (PhD thesis). Expressive Therapies Dissertations, Lesley University. Accessed on 30/5/17 at https://digitalcommons.lesley.edu/expressive_dissertations/31.

Hosea, H. (2006) '"The brush's footmarks": Parents and infants paint together in a small community art therapy group.' *International Journal of Art Therapy 11,* 2, 69–78.

Ioannides, E. (2016) 'Museums as therapeutic environments and the contribution of art therapy.' *Museum International 68,* 3–4, 98–109.

Jury, H., Landes, J. and MagSIG (2015) 'Re-viewing museums: Innovative art therapy practice in museums and art galleries.' *British Association of Art Therapy Newsbriefing December 2015*, 26–28.

Keller, M. (n.d.) *IU Eskenazi Museum of Art.* Accessed on 30/11/18 at www.news.iu.edu/stories/2018/11/iub/02-eskenazi-art-museum-hires-new-art-therapist.html.

King, L. (2018) *Art Therapy and Art Museums: Recommendations for Collaboration.* Indiana University. Master of Arts in Art Therapy, Herron School of Art and Design, Indiana University. Accessed on 30/11/18 at http://hdl.handle.net/1805/16338.

Klein, D. L. (2015) The Art of War: Examining Museums' Art Therapy Programs for Military Veterans. Master of Arts in Museology, University of Washington. Accessed on 15/9/17 at http://hdl.handle.net/1773/33420.

Lambert, J. and Ranger, D. (2009) 'L'art-thérapie et la psychologie positive: Ensemble pour favoriser le déploiement des forces de vie' ['Art therapy and positive psychology: Working together to allow life forces to flourish']. *Revue Québécoise de Psychologie 30*, 3, 57–70.

Lorr, M., McNair, D.M. and Fisher, S. (2010) 'Evidence for bipolar mood states.' *Journal of Personality Assessment 46,* 4, 432–436.

Malchiodi, C. (2007) *Art Therapy Sourcebook*. New York, NY: McGraw Hill.

Marin, A. (2015) *Quand le musée soigne. La Lettre de l'OCIM*. Accessed on 15/6/17 at https://journals.openedition.org/ocim/1471?lang=fr.

Memphis Brooks Museum of Art (n.d.) *Art Therapy Access Program*. Accessed on 20/12/2018 at www.brooksmuseum.org/art-therapy-access-program.

MMFA (2014) *Totem-Muses: Un atelier en art-thérapie*. Accessed on 15/8/2017 at www.facebook.com/306619919368966/videos/796740687023551.

MMFA-MFdC (n.d.) *Museum Prescriptions: Museum Visits Prescribed by Doctors*. Accessed on 29/11/18 at www.mbam.qc.ca/en/news/museum-prescriptions.

Moreau, A. (2017) 'Art-thérapie et musées: Rencontres et relations entre espace muséal et processus de soin.' Diplôme Universitaire de l'université Paris Descartes, spécialisation en Art-thérapie.

National Institute for Arts in Health (2017) *Arts, Health and Well-being in America*. Accessed on 28/12/18 at https://thenoah.net/wp-content/uploads/2019/01/NOAH-2017-White-Paper-Online-Edition.pdf.

Parashak, S.T. (1997) 'The richness that surrounds us: Collaboration of classroom and community for art therapy and art education.' *Art Therapy 14,* 4, 241–245.

Rochford, J.S. (2017) 'Art therapy and art museum education: A visitor-focused collaboration.' *Art Therapy 34,* 4, 209–214.

Rogers, C. (2003) *A Way of Being*. New York, NY: Houghton Mifflin Harcourt.

Shaer, D., Beaven, K., Springham, N., Pillinger, S. *et al.* (2008) 'The role of art therapy in a pilot for art-based information prescriptions at Tate Britain.' *International Journal of Art Therapy 13,* 1, 25–33.

Silverman, Y. and Firm, K. (2014) *The Hidden Face of Suicide*. Accessed on 30/6/17 at www.dev.kanopystreaming.com/node/115094.

Silverman, Y., Smith, F. and Burns, M. (2013) 'Coming together in pain and joy: A multicultural and arts-based suicide awareness project.' *The Arts in Psychotherapy 40,* 2, 216–223.

Slade, P.D., Dewey, M.E., Newton, T., Brodie, D. and Kiemle, G. (1990) 'Development and preliminary validation of the body satisfaction scale (BSS).' *Psychology and Health 4,* 3, 213–220.

Sloan, L. (2013) 'Your Brain on Art: Art Therapy in a Museum Setting and its Potential at the Rubin Museum of Art.' Master of Art, City College of New York. Accessed on 26/10/17 at https://academicworks.cuny.edu/cc_etds_theses/398.

Smallwood, E. (2019) 'Group Art Therapy for Young-Mid Adults with Epilepsy: A Psychosocial Inquest into Multiple Ways of Knowing.' Concordia University. Accessed on 21/5/19 at www.spectrum.library.concordia.ca/985282.

Spraggins Rochford, J. (2017) 'Art therapy at the John and Mable Ringling Museum of Art.' *The Journal of Art for Life 9,* 2, 1–17. Accessed on 3/1/2018 at http://journals.fcla.edu/jafl/article/view/90781/100997.

Stafstrom, C.E., Havlena, J. and Krezinski, A.J. (2012) 'Art therapy focus groups for children and adolescents with epilepsy.' *Epilepsy & Behavior 24,* 2, 227–233.

Stiles, G.J. and Mermer-Welly, M.J. (1998) 'Children having children: Art therapy in a community-based early adolescent pregnancy program.' *Art Therapy 15,* 3, 165–176.

Thaler, L., Drapeau, C.-E., Leclerc, J., Lajeunesse, M. *et al.* (2017) 'An adjunctive, museum-based art therapy experience in the treatment of women with severe eating disorders.' *The Arts in Psychotherapy 56,* 1–6.

Thompson, G. (2012) 'The social work of museums.' *Art Therapy 29,* 1, 46–47.

Thomson, L.J.M., Ander, E.E., Menon, U., Lanceley, A. and Chatterjee, H.J. (2012) 'Quantitative evidence for wellbeing benefits from a heritage-in-health intervention with hospital patients.' *International Journal of Art Therapy 17,* 2, 63–79.

Thyme, K.E., Sundin, E.C., Wiberg, B., Öster, I., Åström, S. and Lindh, J. (2009) 'Individual brief art therapy can be helpful for women with breast cancer: A randomized controlled clinical study.' *Palliative and Supportive Care 7,* 1, 87–95.

Timm-Bottos, J. (2006) 'Constructing creative community.' *Canadian Art Therapy Association Journal 19,* 2, 12–26.

Timm-Bottos, J. (2016) 'Beyond counseling and psychotherapy, there is a field. I'll meet you there.' *Art Therapy 33,* 3, 160–162.

Timm-Bottos, J. and Reilly, R.C. (2014) 'Learning in third spaces: Community art studio as storefront university classroom.' *American Journal of Community Psychology 55,* 1–2, 102–114.

Treadon, C.B. (2015) 'Bringing Art Therapy into Museums.' In D.E. Gussack and M.L. Rosal (eds) *The Wiley Handbook of Art Therapy.* Accessed on 12/5/2018 at www.doi.org/10.1002/9781118306543.ch47.

Treadon, C.B., Rosal, M. and Thompson Wylder, V.D.T. (2006) 'Opening the doors of art museums for therapeutic processes.' *The Arts in Psychotherapy 33,* 4, 288–301.

Van Lith, T. and Spooner, H. (2018) 'Art therapy and arts in health: Identifying shared values but different goals using a framework analysis.' *Art Therapy 35,* 2, 88–93.

Wadeson, H. (2002) 'Confronting polarization in art therapy.' *Art Therapy 19,* 2, 77–84.

CHAPTER 8

Expanding the Frame

Developing and Sustaining a Long-Term NHS Art Museum Partnership Within a Workforce Development Strategy for Enhanced Quality of Care

Sheila Grandison

Introduction

The right to take part in cultural life is explicitly stated in Article 27 of the *Universal Declaration of Human Rights* (United Nations 1948): 'Everyone has the right freely to participate in the cultural life of the community, to enjoy the arts and to share in scientific advancement and its benefits.' It is perhaps surprising then that some 70 years later widening access to cultural institutions and diversification is seen to be in need of urgent attention at a policy level. The report *Equality, Diversity and the Creative Case* (Arts Council England 2018, p.40) asserts:

> In our strategy we acknowledge that there are significant differences in how much people engage with arts and culture – and the opportunities they have to do this. Those most actively involved tend to be from the most privileged groups; engagement is heavily influenced by levels of education, socio-economic background and where people live.

This chapter discusses a long-term NHS art museum partnership that appears to contradict these assertions. It considers the development of the opportunity for an underprivileged and vulnerable group of people to access modern and contemporary art in an art gallery setting, in a way that diversified visitor demographics to an iconic London gallery. It also advanced an NHS workforce directive for delivering compassionate care, and expanded the contextual frame of art therapy. Art therapy and museum education are both rooted in practices promoting dialogue when looking at art objects and artefacts. These two specialised fields have come together in this innovative partnership to bridge the different environments of hospital ward and art gallery in a way that has benefited NHS patients and staff of both institutions alike.

The partnership between the East London NHS Foundation Trust and Tate Modern (the ELFT/Tate partnership) enables access to a major London public art gallery for adult mental health service users resident in three areas of east London that fall within the five per cent of most deprived areas of England, namely Newham, Hackney and Tower Hamlets (Greater London Authority n.d., p.515). Many of the service users are first-time visitors to an art gallery and the partnership enables them to engage directly with the collection displays in one of the largest galleries of modern and contemporary art in the world. The ELFT/Tate partnership is ongoing, but the time-frame considered here is 2007–2017. During this period, significant policies from the health and culture sectors helped shape the partnership's flexible working model for delivering gallery-based groups with service users in line with recovery-focused practice, alongside training workshops for nursing staff, arts therapists, specialist psychiatric registrars and consultant psychiatrists.

Reclaiming the rights of people with mental health problems drives recovery-focused practice in its shift away from recovery in the narrow sense of receiving treatment for symptoms, to the recovery of values defined by individuals themselves. When drawn from a common sense of humanity, these values include expressing the right to culture. Cultural rights are embedded in human rights and what it is to be human. Supporting access to art and culture, Michael Rosen, the children's author, states (Arts Council England 2013, p.11):

> The arts are a means by which we can investigate and understand the past and the present, our world and our feelings. We can do this by 'doing' it or by 'spectating' it or both... This is one of the ways in which we can discover the history and shape of humanity and where or how we fit into it.

Additionally, through its capacity to create connections between individuals and groups, the museum director Diane Lees (Arts Council England 2013, p.37) refers to art and culture as providing 'the context for the richest of social interactions'. These reported effects concerning 'how we fit into', within a context of social interactions, chime with the desired psychotherapeutic goals of group art therapy when reflecting on cultural difference, expressions of social identity and power relations in group process.

The art therapy context

In 2007, before the Olympics came to east London in 2012, and as an art therapist working in acute clinical settings at the Newham Centre for Mental Health, I found that reflecting on clinical practice in this specific geographic location raised a particular issue: how to connect service users to the collections of an art gallery or museum, given neither a gallery nor a museum existed in the borough at that time.

Newham, a deprived outer London borough in east London, is an area characterised by immigration, which is mirrored in the local population of mental health service users. For inpatients, the group art therapy table could function as a symbolic hospitable space, around which people were enabled to express themselves through sensory engagement with art materials to start a process of defining their worlds. Through making, using and learning from the artworks made, new forms of seeing and understanding were made possible. Being with, and being curious about, cultural diversity was a live dynamic in the group matrix. Openness and tolerance may not have matched the lived experience of group members from incoming communities, so looking first to the immediate environment of the ward community, and how to engage service users more fully in their social relations with ward-based staff (also a culturally diverse group), was an important first step for building the ELFT/Tate partnership.

The 2011 Census showed Newham to have the most diverse population in the UK, with higher rates of patients recorded with diagnoses of schizophrenia, bipolar affective disorder and other psychoses (Aston-Mansfield 2017). Hand-in-hand with ethnic diversity is a high turnover of the local population, mirrored in a rapid changeover of service users in the throughput of admissions and discharges to and from the inpatient wards. While English continues to be the main language spoken, many in Newham report they cannot speak English well, or at all. With 103 different languages identified, Bengali, Urdu, Gujarati, Lithuanian, Tamil, Polish, Punjabi, Romanian, and more, can all be heard on the streets, in the shops and in the local mental health centre.

Despite no local art gallery to draw on in Newham, it was the steadfast belief in the capacity of art to connect, contain difference and promote cultural understanding that guided the strategic development of the ELFT/Tate health and culture partnership, with diversity at its core. How might engagement with the community resource of Tate Modern, an art gallery some eight miles away, assist in vitalising socialisation between service users and staff working alongside them in the East London NHS Foundation Trust? What bridges, symbolic and concrete, would need to be crossed?

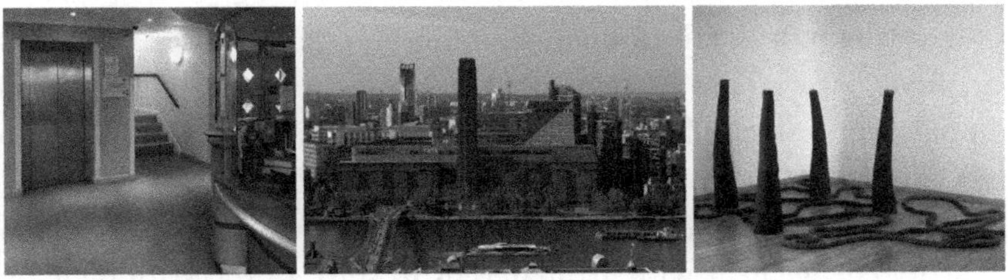

Figure 8.1 Connecting: Art as a bridge across site and context
Left: Entrance to the Newham Centre for Mental Health. Supplied courtesy of East London NHS Foundation Trust. Photo credit: © Sheila Grandison, 2012
Centre: Tate Modern from St Paul's, 2016, Tate Photography. © Tate, London 2019
Right: '4 casb 2 '67', 1967; Barry Flanagan (1941–2009). Purchased 1976; © The estate of Barry Flanagan/Bridgeman Images; Photo © Tate, London 2019

The three photographs in Figure 8.1 show the ELFT/Tate partnership in compressed visual form. On the left is the reception area of the

Newham Centre for Mental Health, the middle image is a view of Tate Modern from St Paul's looking across the River Thames with the Millennium Bridge in the foreground, and the image on the right shows a gallery installation at Tate Modern, with the floor sculpture '4 casb 2 '67', 1967, by the Welsh sculptor Barry Flanagan (1941–2009). If the four, over life-size, conical shapes of Flanagan's artwork were transposed from gallery space to the entrance space of the mental health centre, their identity would no doubt shift from artwork to objects of risk. A further, imaginative shift is also possible – from risk to curiosity – about these unexpected and unusual objects formed of blue canvas sacks filled with sand. The affect of interest comes into play, transcending the confines of site and context. How are the disparate materials of canvas and sand related? Helen Delaney (2002) refers to their mutual support 'by which the sand holds up the canvas, while the canvas contains the sand'. For the viewer, this intriguing interchange arouses curiosity and inquisitive interest. Choosing to look at contemporary artworks, not so much for determining their place and value within the cultural establishment, but for their provocative open-endedness for stimulating engagement, enquiry and reflection and the exchange of ideas, was central to the ELFT/Tate partnership.

In the early stages of developing the partnership, 2007–2009, the role of the arts therapies in inpatient care was coming to the fore at ELFT, with art therapy and music therapy recognised as contributing to high-quality care and good practice on the wards in a rigorous programme of standards known as AIMS (Accreditation for Inpatient Mental Health Services), regulated by the Royal College of Psychiatrists (2017). Also, the National Institute for Health and Care Excellence (NICE) included, first in 2009 and again in 2014, the recommendation: 'Consider offering arts therapies to assist in promoting recovery, particularly in people with negative symptoms' (NCCMH 2014, 9.3.8.4, p.221) in clinical guidelines for psychosis and schizophrenia in adults.

Group art therapy was being practised at the time in the inpatient clinical settings, offering a regular safe space for service users for whom the capacity to be with others, their families and communities, had broken down. Therapeutic focus was on restoring interpersonal relating, informed by the group analytic objective to achieve a healthier integration of individuals in a network of relationships. The ELFT/Tate partnership provided an opportunity to expand the network beyond the boundaries of inpatient group art therapy, to the larger group of staff and service users in the immediate ward community and beyond – to social groups with members of the public at Tate Modern.

In group art therapy on the wards, the group size was small (six to eight service users), allowing people to express themselves and promote individuation. While on the ward, the daily lives of service users and staff are inextricably linked. It was envisaged that to increase the size from a small group in a clinical ward setting to a median group in a public gallery space (with a membership of at least 13, composed of service users and ward-based staff), would be a means to promote an atmosphere of social interaction and participation, involvement and sharing. Pisani (2009, p.287) describes the median group's objective as: 'not so much to socialize the human individual as *to humanize the socio-cultural context*' (my italics), and cites the essence of the median group in this endeavour to be 'free floating dialogue'.

Through the visual and verbal dynamics of inpatient group art therapy, issues of loss through the trauma of social upheaval, instability of identity formation, and the abjectness of social isolation were being explored. People from different parts of the world were making connections to the personal lived experiences of others, with the felt loss collectively shared. International, contemporary visual art is often produced in contexts of conflict and trauma, with the art used to offer reflections and bring people together. By maintaining the relationship between the individual and the group, and the essentially social nature of human experience, the question was how a partnership with Tate Modern might contribute to understanding trauma empathically. Also, by expanding the therapeutic frame to include the social space of a public art gallery, whether it was possible to look at the quality of relationships with others in relation to the reported benefits of 'improved social functioning and improved mental health' (Crawford and Patterson 2007, p.70) evidenced in group art therapy for people diagnosed with schizophrenia. The combined membership of service users and staff in an off-ward group would reflect the wider norms of society, not only the conventions of role while on the ward.

The selection of artworks from Tate Modern's collection was key to reflecting on these questions in the ELFT/Tate groups. In their pre-group preparation and dynamic administration, curator and art therapist, as co-facilitators of the groups, identified artworks specifically for their potential to enhance the engagement process for first-time viewers, and to resonate with contemporary social concerns. One such work was 'No Woman, No Cry', 1998, by Chris Ofili (born 1968), the British Turner Prize-winning artist. The title is taken from the song by Bob Marley, the Jamaican reggae musician, where the persuasive, repetitive chant of the lyrics urges an unseen female listener not to be sad. In Ofili's painting, the female made visibly manifest is the mother of Stephen Lawrence, the black teenage boy murdered in an unprovoked racist attack in London in 1993. At the centre of the tears falling from her eyes, Ofili has collaged a small photograph of her son's face and written the words 'RIP Stephen Lawrence 1974–1993' across the canvas.

Access to cultural rights and the right to freedom of expression underpins Tate's commitment to achieving equality and diversity. Viewing Ofili's painting prompts awareness of the findings of the judicial inquiry into the teenager's tragic death that exposed professional incompetence in police conduct and institutional racism (Macpherson of Cluny 1999). An overhaul of Britain's race relations followed the inquiry's recommendations. The viewer engages in the gravity of the social content through the range of unexpected mixed media used. Resting on two large lumps of elephant dung placed on the floor, the painting leans against the gallery wall, inviting the viewer to look ever more closely at the detail and into the pale blue tears, which is what the groups did. The group dialogue that developed around viewing contemporary artworks was as much about the curiosity of seeing work that stretched personally held definitions and stereotypes of what art might look like, to the enjoyment of finding intriguing visual details, to exploring cultural resonances pertinent to both personal lived experiences and wider social issues evoked in the narrative of artworks such as 'No Woman, No Cry'.

The opportunity to experience the alternation of spatial, psychological and cultural displacement and transformation in a gallery setting, as a viewer was made possible by looking at large-scale sculptural environments in particular. Personal memories of the South Korean artist, Do Ho Suh (born 1962), are conveyed through his artworks based on the architectural spaces he has occupied at different times. In 'Staircase-III' (2010), the memory of the space of his parents' traditional Korean house in Seoul is fused with his Western-style living as an adult. Using diaphanous red material, a replica of the staircase in his New York apartment is suspended from the ceiling but does not reach the floor – it is dreamlike. Suspended, too, is the theme of migration and cultural displacement specific to the artist, and the feeling of estrangement he associates with a divided cultural background. As an installation that occupies an entire room at Tate Modern, the staircase floats in gallery space. In psychological, in-between space, the viewer is invited to connect with the staircase as an object of transition, captivated by the multitude of associations it conjures up.

The policy context

Significantly, the ELFT/Tate partnership is focused on acute adult mental health, involving service users and staff from inpatient wards, rather than community outpatient services. This deliberate choice was to address the state of acute mental health care in the mid-2000s and to work innovatively with a representative cross-section of the multicultural local population and the multiple psychosocial dimensions associated with it. Policy reviews from this period, for example from the Sainsbury Centre for Mental Health (1998, 2005), had highlighted widespread difficulties in acute inpatient mental health care, neglected as a consequence of prioritising community services. Service users were reported as describing a lack of regular and meaningful engagement with ward-based staff and feelings of not being treated with due respect, dignity and understanding during acute admissions. A strategic swing to address concerns regarding standards of care in inpatient mental health settings was shown to be pressing.

During the same period, the culture sector was looking to engage a broader audience in recognising that national cultural institutions belong to everyone. In *Culture on Demand*, the Department of Culture, Media and Sport (2007) had confirmed the challenge to cultural engagement in three identified priority groups: disabled people (covering both physical and mental disability, or infirmity), black and minority ethnic people and people from lower socio-economic backgrounds (Department of Culture, Media and Sport 2007, p.6). From the outset, the ELFT/Tate partnership was clear that its work together would not consist of 'tick-the-box', one-off days out for service users to an art gallery which, although they might well be enjoyed, could perhaps be forgotten and therefore were of no real consequence. Furthermore, we wanted ward-based staff to be integral to the partnership's work.

What started in 2007 as a local initiative within the context of group art therapy practice at the Newham Centre for Mental Health, has over ten years become integrated into a Trust-wide workforce development strategy intent on delivering creative approaches for compassionate care by all, and for all. Art therapy remains central to the ELFT/Tate partnership and as the initiating art therapist, I remain actively involved in my role as Trust-wide Training & Development Lead for Arts Therapies. Facilitation of the ELFT/Tate partnership groups is held jointly by me and the Curator of Public Programmes at Tate Modern, currently Michèle Fuirer, and formerly Liz Ellis (then Curator, Community Programme, Tate Learning), with invaluable support from Assistant Curator, Emily Stone.

Another key colleague in the partnership was Barbara Rice, a former Borough Lead Nurse for Newham. She first endorsed the partnership's visual arts programme as continuing professional development for ward-based nursing staff to enhance reflective thinking and promote new ways of relating to service users. Through her innovative recruitment programme in Newham, 2007–2010, the promotion of creative approaches to mental health treatment and recovery became integrated into the job plans of nursing support staff. These new staff members worked alongside nurses and arts therapists at the Newham Centre for Mental Health in supporting creativity-based solutions for service user engagement in daily one-to-one contact.

Pioneers from the first recruitment cohorts, and in particular, Rose Hall, Stephanie Hands, Aimee Neale, Claire Vestergaard and Jamie Williams, were colleagues actively involved in the ELFT/Tate partnership groups who contributed to promoting the partnership with staff and service users on their respective wards. Support for the working model of the ELFT/Tate partnership to develop creative initiatives in staff development programmes continues at a strategic level with the Lead for Nurse Development Programmes (Rebecca Lingard), the Professional Lead for Allied Health Professions (Stephen Sandford) and colleagues in the People & Culture directorate.

The ELFT/Tate partnership has three phases. *Thinking about Looking*, 2007–2014, was funded through the East London NHS Foundation Trust, with Tate Modern Public Programmes providing curatorial staff expertise and material resources for use in the workshops. Groups were limited during this first phase to nursing support staff and adult service users from the Newham Centre for Mental Health. The second phase, *Creative Approaches to Compassionate Care*, 2014–2017, was scaled up as a training model for nursing support staff across the Trust, with external funding received through Health Education England. The current phase continues enquiry into how creativity fits with compassionate care, with the McPin Foundation, a specialist mental health research charity, undertaking an external evaluation of the ELFT/Tate groups with nursing and medical staff in the period 2015–2019.

Following the public inquiry into the scandal and failings of care at the Mid Staffordshire NHS Foundation Trust (Francis 2013), the Cavendish Review (Cavendish 2013) flagged attention to training, finding that training and development of healthcare assistants and support staff was often not consistent or good enough. It was similarly noted (Health Education England 2015, p.39) that in providing approximately 60 per cent of hands-on care, healthcare assistants 'must be a significant focus for investment because they are so important to patient safety and wellbeing', noting 'yet often have little access to training or personal development'.

ELFT/Tate Creative Approaches to Compassionate Care training workshops for developing observation and empathy skills are now included in ELFT's Care Certificate for nursing support staff, life skills recovery workers and social therapists working across the Trust in adult, MHCOP (mental health care of older people), CAMHS (child and adolescent mental health services), forensics, and other specialist services. What started as a localised art therapy initiative has developed into a Trust-wide training initiative, at the centre of which is looking together at artworks in a gallery. The use of art materials in response to what has been seen, and in relation to the process of spectator participation – of noticing, recognising, connecting, taking-in and reflecting – remains paramount throughout the programme. The partnership holds central the potential for art to make a difference to the individual and the collective through an intensive and subtle process of making meaning from art. Enhanced observation and listening ability and the exchange and exploration of ideas in group dialogue are transferable skills to take back to the workplace.

Improving the experience of inpatient care is a key target for all. For service users in acute states of mind, communication can often be through challenging behaviours, including verbal abuse, withdrawal and apathy, unpredictability of mood, and self-neglect. Staff can feel devalued and helpless, finding it difficult to think and reflect in the face of resistance and the cross-fire of projections. Nevertheless, delivering compassionate care is paramount. With a view to supporting staff to maintain the capacity to be resourceful and reflective with service users, the partnership aims to encourage creative approaches and new ways of relating. The East London NHS Foundation Trust is committed to testing out innovative training opportunities and considering creative ways to expand and support the existing workforce through the fusion of arts and health skills.

One question for ELFT is how being together with service users in a group in the gallery might help with risk management and working with resistant behaviours on the ward. Overall, we found that the experience of speaking more freely in groups at Tate promoted better communication back on the ward – for all involved.

Clinical vignettes written by nursing support staff include both pre- and post-group information. They include the anxiety of multi-disciplinary team colleagues regarding the suitability of service users to attend the ELFT/Tate groups, as well as the positive feedback from the staff and service users after attending. Vivid accounts of how service users stayed focused, contributed to group dialogue, shared their own artwork and made personal links with the artworks seen in the gallery are reported. Important too, are the reports of increased cooperation in the care planning process back on the ward. For example, a service user struggling with personal hygiene may be more receptive to assistance from nursing staff, in contrast to being previously aggressive or resistant to support.

As the partnership looks ahead to the next five years, its focus will be on the area of staff retention, as much as on direct service user benefit. Patient care and workforce development go hand-in-hand. In her response to the recent report, *Leading Change, Adding Value: A Framework for Nursing, Midwifery and Care Staff* (NHS England 2016), Karen Deeny from the NHS England Patient Experience Team pertinently asked in her blog (Deeny 2017):

> When we talk about staff and about patients, should we think of them as separate groups of people delivering care and groups of people receiving care? Do we need to make better connections between the two sides of the coin, the two sets of experiences, in order to make better sense of how they relate and what this means for our work together to improve them?

Deeny's (2017) question envisages patient experience and staff experience as a co-creation. For improvement of each to be possible she advocates looking purposely at 'the two sides of the coin together'; holding the two-way tension, rather than considering each side separately. For the ELFT/Tate partnership, conceptualising enhanced quality of care *as a relationship*, seeing two different sets of experiences and holding in balance their meaningful relatedness, has always been central to the partnership's development.

Providing opportunities for mental health service users and health staff to be together in a public art space was the keystone for bridging two very different environments of psychiatric ward and art gallery.

Exploring what it means to embed patient groups in the delivery of staff training programmes was made possible by this bridge. The patient voice is integrated through service users reporting on the positive impact of the public gallery space, with its rich sensory stimulation of the artworks, in contrast to the starker environment of wards. Reports from service users feeling respected when viewing art with ELFT and Tate staff corroborated this, as did their feelings of being nourished, symbolically through group dialogue and the transformative power of art, as well as through good food at Tate.

Collaboration between experts of experience and experts by training – co-production – is a means for transforming mental health care and the direction towards which the ELFT/Tate partnership is moving. In supporting new collaborative relationships between frontline professionals and service users, the ELFT/Tate partnership actively contributes to this significant attitudinal shift by innovatively engaging the resources of both groups in an off-ward environment.

The ELFT/Tate working model

The ELFT/Tate partnership looks to bridge the worlds of two very different public service institutions, to connect and break down barriers to contribute to the better understanding and functioning of each. From a health perspective, the ELFT/Tate working model addresses the needs of service users and staff from inpatient mental health settings. For service users, the need for more direct time with staff had been flagged, and for ward-based staff, innovative staff development training programmes were required to meet national standards for compassionate care. From a cultural perspective, there was the opportunity to develop links with the healthcare sector and consider an audience-engagement initiative for diversity and inclusion in relation to current issues and practice in the field of mental health. Both the East London NHS Foundation Trust and Tate Modern could consider the impact of cultural access and patient care from the partnership's working model.

Tate Modern had been running the workshop programme *Art into Life* since the gallery opened in 2000, offering free gallery introductions that attracted a wide range of adult groups from social and health settings. The aim of the ELFT/Tate partnership was to develop a bespoke programme that fostered a two-way bridge between psychiatric ward and art gallery. An inquiry into diversity policy and practices in the cultural sector was undertaken between 2007 and 2009 by Dewdney and colleagues in the extensive research project *Tate Encounters: Britishness and Visual Culture* (Dewdney, Dibosa and Walsh 2013). The recommended direction for cultural policy regarding diversity was to move closer to a model of relational reflexivity, rather than educational pedagogy. The combined thinking of gallery educator and art therapist could move creatively between these two conceptual frames of reflexivity and pedagogy.

From a psychotherapeutic stance, Burnham (2005, p.4) describes relational reflexivity as how therapists and clients 'explicitly engage one another in coordinating their resources so as to create relationships with therapeutic potential'. Reflecting further, he states: 'it takes hard work as well as imagination to coordinate the resources of client and therapist to create and maintain a relationship that is experienced as therapeutic for the client'. Exploring ways of relating to service users that could be '*experienced as therapeutic*' (my italics), and as co-created with ward-based staff, has defined the ELFT/Tate working model.

Tate, with its expertise in museum and gallery education, and informal learning programmes for including multiple voice perspectives, and ELFT's expertise in understanding the remit of inpatient care and group dynamics, came together to dissolve rather than reinforce boundaries associated with imbalances of power between service users and ward-based staff. The groups did not aim to work with service users as practised in small group art therapy in a clinical setting. The objective was to enhance curiosity, thinking and dialogue through engaging with contemporary artworks in a gallery setting, for a richer understanding of sense of self and others, by experiencing how anxieties and social issues may be revealed and aesthetically reconciled in contemporary artworks.

Group dialogue

The ELFT/Tate partnership looks to the everyday to understand better how to balance the opposites of site and context. The performance artist Naomi Kashiwagi asserts (Arts Council England 2013, p.57):

'The arts have the potential to show that the everyday can be reinvented and that the ordinary is usually extraordinary and that the extraordinary can become part of or intervene and wonderfully interrupt everyday life.'

To conceptualise and bridge art gallery and mental health settings, the link to the everyday is pivotal. Referring to visitor participation in museums, the American Museum director Nina Simon urges us to 'Imagine looking at an object not for its artistic or historical significance but for its ability to spark conversation.' (Simon 2010, p.127). Such an ethos chimes with the aims and objectives of the ELFT/Tate partnership. The gallery displays, the public spaces and the collection at Tate offer a unique social space for participatory learning. Opportunities are made for group members to reflect together in the shared public space, building connections together through imaginative thinking and high-quality art-making activities.

The transformation of everyday, commonplace materials taken from natural and industrial worlds made for new connections between art and life. In response to 'Tree of 12 Metres', 1980–82, by Giuseppe Penone (born 1947), an Italian artist of the Arte Povera group, group dialogue ranged between curiosity about the enormous scale of the sculpture, the dwarfing of their human scale next to it and how that felt, to thinking about wood as a material in everyday objects around them – the doors they walked through, the tables they sat at, the paper drawn on, and books read. Through making connections with different materials and moving between general and personal associations, group dialogue held new and embodied narratives. Participants travelled imaginatively through associations, memory, hopes and dreams.

Central to the ELFT/Tate groups were visual art dialogues and creative interactions facilitated in the gallery with the nursing staff and service users, for building forms of shared meaning. These dialogues were developed through looking at and making artworks together, then exported to the wards for further one-to-one development in the context of the care planning process and so work which began at Tate Modern continued back on the wards in a cooperative and collaborative way. For the service user participants, the Tate groups were destigmatising, providing the opportunity to be in a public space as equal members of the public. For the nursing support staff, the groups challenged preconceived ideas about contemporary art and questions concerning what, if anything, partnership with an art gallery could achieve. By interacting with service users away from the risk-averse environments of the ward, nursing staff came to experience the ELFT/Tate groups as an example of positive risk management in providing an opportunity to be with, experience and understand service users anew. For both service users and nursing staff, talking freely and discussing artworks together was experienced as optimistic and constructive.

In the first phase of the ELFT/Tate partnership, *Thinking about Looking*, four group days were facilitated annually at Tate Modern. In-between, nursing support staff received group supervision from an art therapist in relation to their work with service users on the wards, and follow-up sessions at the Newham Centre for Mental Health were arranged with the Tate curator. Service users who had participated in the ELFT/Tate groups helped facilitate an inpatient group for service users who had been unable to make the journey to Tate Modern. By projecting large-scale slides of artworks during the cross-ward *Living Gallery Group*, service users were able to share their experiences and continue discussion of artworks they had seen at Tate Modern with others who had not been there on the day.

The role of the facilitators in the ELFT/Tate groups was to work with the many projective threads and resonances in the group, to facilitate group cohesion and the development of group narrative. The fluidity of the free association conversations, and interest taken in the personal and subjective responses of all, enabled marked changes in levels of engagement, concentration and articulation. In enabling connections to be made, the co-facilitation of museum educator and art therapist provided a sense of security for participants to develop dialogue. Positive experiences relating to being in a group featured prominently in the thematic analysis of post-group feedback forms. When working with people with histories of psychosis it was found that the simplicity of a statement such as, 'I was part of a group', speaks loudly of achievement in awareness of self and orientation to others. Feedback also referred to the joy of being in a group and recognising that coming to an art gallery on one's own would not be the same. Being in a group with different people raised awareness, cooperation and patience. Seeing more through looking and talking about art together in a group increased confidence and self-esteem.

Some ELFT/Tate groups in the second phase of the partnership, *Creative Approaches to Compassionate Care*, were designed specifically as training workshops for staff. Keeping the emphasis on creative responses to the everyday, nursing and medical staff were asked to make use of a range of throwaway, abject – or found – objects picked up from everyday clinical environments. Examples included tops of biros, perforated tear strips from salary slips, paperclips, coffee cartons, empty food containers, elastic bands, straws, dried up whiteboard pens; an eclectic variety of objects not regarded as having creative potential. The staff group's task was to transform abjectness through creative responses. While working concretely with the found objects and playing with them creatively, language used in response to these objects could be worked with metaphorically. A vocabulary describing the discarded, abandoned, broken, overlooked and forgotten objects could then be linked to what it is to work with powerful projections of worthlessness and rejection, unconsciously communicated by service users and experienced negatively by staff in their daily lives in clinical environments. Seeing and discovering how artworks displayed at Tate Modern could be as much about small-scale gesture as about large-scale physical presence was significant for building the confidence of nursing and medical staff to make use of everyday and commonplace things in their conversations and interactions with service users back on the wards.

Metaphorical resonances to mental health care informed the selection of artworks for use in the staff training workshops. 'Babel', 2001, by the Brazilian artist Cildo Meireles (born 1948) (Figure 8.2) speaks of interference, conflict and the inability to hear, listen and communicate with one another. Constructed of radios, lighting and sound, it is playful, yet disturbing in its cacophony. Hundreds of radios are stacked together in layers, each radio tuned to a different wavelength frequency and volume. The mix of voices and music emits a confusion of sound information as they compete with each other to be listened to. Links were made in the group dialogue to what it is like to work on often chaotic psychiatric admission wards, and the phenomenon of hearing voices in psychosis. With its immersive multimedia of sight and sound, this installation repels communication, yet simultaneously invites touch and participation to tune in.

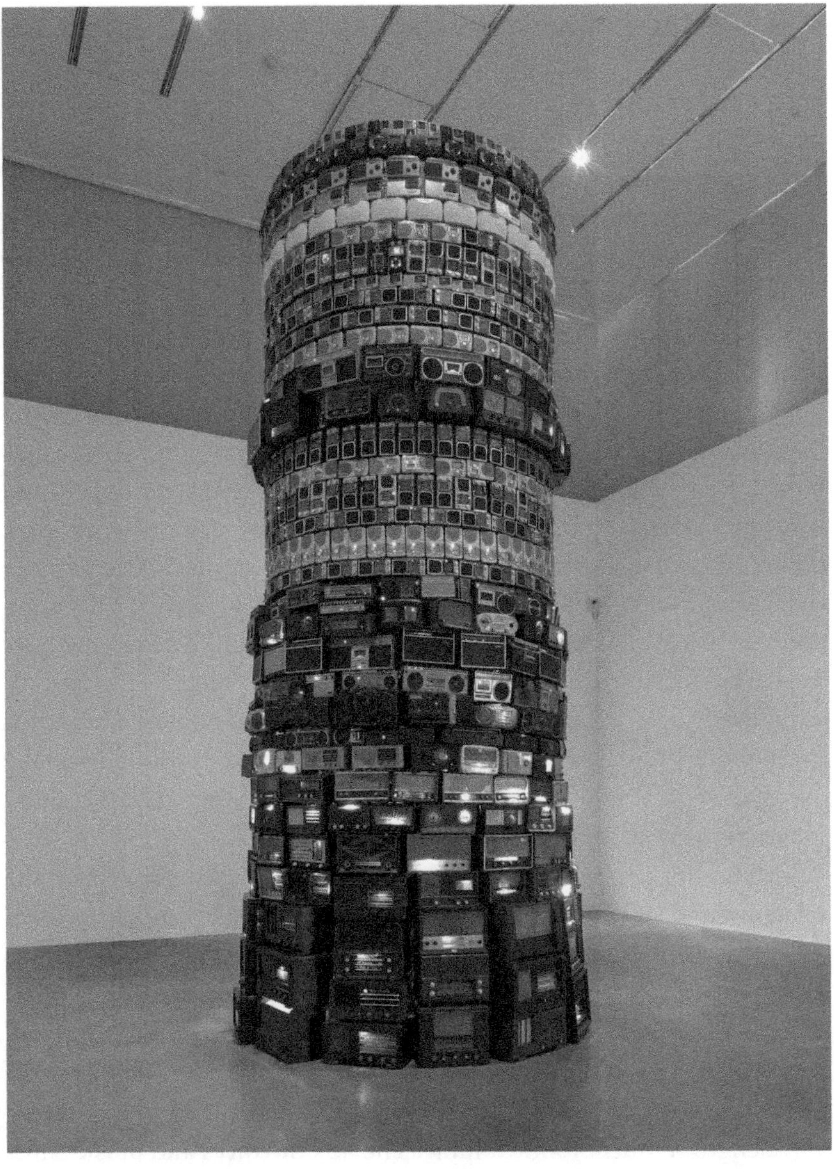

Figure 8.2 'Babel' 2001; Cildo Meireles (born 1948). Purchased jointly by Tate, London (with the assistance of the Latin American Acquisitions Committee) and the D. Daskalopoulos Collection, 2013, as a promised gift to Tate; © Cildo Meireles; Photo © Tate, London 2019

In contrast to thwarted attempts at attunement set up in 'Babel', the 2015 Hyundai Commission for Tate Modern's Turbine Hall, entitled 'Empty Lot', by the Mexican artist Abraham Cruzvillegas (born 1968), was more hopeful. Describing his artwork in terms of hope, Cruzvillegas explained: 'everything is usable, nothing is dead – everything is alive' (Cruzvillegas in Tate 2015). Included in this installation is soil collected by the artist from different parks across London and discarded materials from building sites. Cruzvillegas refers to the possibility that something might grow as well as not grow in the plots of soil, affording opportunity for hope. An artist's capacity for patience in tolerating both possibilities, of new growth or not, resonates metaphorically with what it is to be with people in disturbed states of mind, and to be in relation with them hopefully, respectfully, and creatively.

Conclusion

The challenge of supporting adults experiencing complex presentations of mental ill-health in ways which recognise the individuality and cultural context of each person at a time of shrinking budgets, raises significant issues. The policy briefing *The Role of Arts and Cultural Organisations in Health and Wellbeing* (All-Party Parliamentary Group on Arts, Health and Wellbeing 2017) confirms:

> Museums and galleries offer a non-clinical, non-stigmatising environment in which to undertake journeys of self-exploration… and the case is being advanced for them to be considered part of the public health landscape. Cultural institutions could do much more to address health and wellbeing.

Galleries and museums are spaces in which subjective experiences of diversity are made manifest, held in the artworks by a diverse range of international artists as well as in the diversity of the audience viewing them. Delivering small group art therapy for service users at Tate Modern was not a part of the ELFT/Tate partnership, but facilitating median groups, with a combined membership of service users and ward-based staff, and Tate gallery staff, was central to it. Trust, confidence, knowledge and relationships have been built with gallery staff, health staff and service users over the long duration of the partnership. The opportunity developed for Tate to more fully belong to the neighbourhood of London, and be part of the lives of adults in east London who would not previously have been aware of the gallery.

The ELFT/Tate partnership looked to emphasise the potential for social engagement through conversational enquiry in front of artworks, with a view to enabling humanising experiences and dialogue to find their way back into the working life of busy inpatient wards of acute mental health units. Understanding playful, interactive and improvisational ways of establishing hopeful and compassionate emotional contact with service users, how to be with them and how to be in relation with them creatively, was the work we did together.

References

All-Party Parliamentary Group on Arts, Health and Wellbeing (2017) *Creative Health: The Arts for Health and Wellbeing* (second edition). Accessed on 15/7/19 at https://www.culturehealthandwellbeing.org.uk/appg-inquiry/.

Arts Council England (2013) *Great Art and Culture for Everyone: 10-Year Strategic Framework 2010 – 2020* (second revised edition). Accessed on 11/8/19 at https://www.artscouncil.org.uk/sites/default/files/download-file/Great_art_and_culture_for_everyone.pdf.

Arts Council England (2018) *Equality, Diversity and the Creative Case: A Data Report, 2016–2017*. Accessed on 16/12/18 at www.artscouncil.org.uk.

Aston-Mansfield (2017) *Newham: Key Statistics 2017*. Accessed on 16/12/18 at www.aston-mansfield.org.uk/wp-content/themes/aston_mansfield/uploads/Newham_Statistics_2017.pdf.

Burnham, J. (2005) 'Relational Reflexivity: A Tool for Socially Constructing Therapeutic Relationships.' In C. Flaskas, B. Mason and A. Perlesz (eds) *The Space Between: Experience, Context, and Process in the Therapeutic Relationship*. London: Karnac.

Cavendish, C. (2013) *The Cavendish Review: An Independent Enquiry into Healthcare Assistants and Support Workers in the NHS and Social Care Settings*. Accessed on 11/8/19 at https://assets.publishing.service.gov.uk/government/uploads/system/uploads/attachment_data/file/236212/Cavendish_Review.pdf.

Crawford, M.J. and Patterson, S. (2007) 'Arts therapies for people with schizophrenia: An emerging evidence base.' *Evidence Based Mental Health 10*, 69–70.

Deeny, K. (2017) Blog 13 March 2017. Accessed on 16/12/18 at www.england.nhs.uk/blog/karen-deeny.

Delaney, H. (2002) Tate catalogue entry for B. Flanagan '4 casb 2 '67'. Accessed on 20/12/18 at www.tate.org.uk/art/artworks/flanagan-4-casb-2-67-t02061.

Department of Culture, Media and Sport (2007) *Culture on Demand: Ways to Engage a Broader Audience*. Accessed on 20/12/18 at www.culturehive.co.uk/wp-content/uploads/2013/04/Culture-On-Demand-full-report1.pdf.

Dewdney, A., Dibosa, D. and Walsh, V. (2013) *Cultural Inequality, Multicultural Nationalism and Global Diversity: Tate Encounters: Britishness and Visual Culture*. Third Text Project. Accessed on 16/12/18 at www.thirdtext.org/cultural-inequality.

Francis, R. (2013) *Report of the Mid Staffordshire NHS Foundation Trust Public Inquiry*. London: The Stationery Office. Accessed on 11/8/19 at https://webarchive.nationalarchives.gov.uk/20150407084231/http://www.midstaffspublicinquiry.com/report.

Greater London Authority (n.d.) 'Economic Evidence Base for London 2016', GLA Economics, p.515. Accessed on 11/8/19 at https://www.london.gov.uk/sites/default/files/economic_evidence_base_2016.compressed.pdf.

Health Education England (2015) *Raising the Bar: Shape of Caring: A Review of the Future Education and Training of Registered Nurses and Care Assistants*. Accessed on 20/12/18 at www.hee.nhs.uk/our-work/shape-caring-review.

Macpherson of Cluny, W. (1999) *Report of the Stephen Lawrence Inquiry*. Accessed on 20/12/18 at www.gov.uk/government/publications/the-stephen-lawrence-inquiry.

National Collaborating Centre for Mental Health (2014) *Psychosis and Schizophrenia in Adults: The NICE Guideline on Treatment and Management*. National Clinical Guideline Number 178. Accessed 11/8/19 at www.nice.org.uk/guidance/cg178/evidence/full-guideline-pdf-490503565.

NHS England (2016) *Leading Change, Adding Value: A Framework for Nursing, Midwifery and Care Staff*. NHS England Publications Accessed on 11/8/19 at https://www.england.nhs.uk/publication/leading-change-adding-value-a-framework-for-nursing-midwifery-and-care-staff.

Pisani, R. (2009) 'The Median Group.' *Group Analysis 42*, 3, 286–289.

Royal College of Psychiatrists (2017) *Standards for Acute Inpatient Services – Working-Age Adults (AIMS W-A)* (sixth edition, first edition 2006). Accessed on 20/12/18 at www.rcpsych.ac.uk/improving-care/ccqi/quality-networks-accreditation/assessment-and-triage-wards-aims.

Sainsbury Centre for Mental Health. (1998) *Acute Problems: A Survey of the Quality of Care in Acute Psychiatric Wards*. London: SCMH Publications.

Sainsbury Centre for Mental Health (2005) *Acute Care 2004: A National Survey of Acute Psychiatric Wards in England*. London: SCMH Publications.

Simon, N. (2010) *The Participatory Museum*. Santa Cruz, CA: Museum 2.0.

Tate (2015, August 12) *Abraham Cruzvillegas – Empty Lot | TateShots* [video file]. Accessed on 30/8/19 at www.youtube.com/watch?v=BtIZxSwjW1w.

United Nations (1948) *Universal Declaration of Human Rights*, 10 December 1948. Accessed on 31/7/18 at www.un.org/Overview/rights.html#a27.

CHAPTER 9

Art Therapy at the Bilbao Fine Arts Museum

A Gaze Through Emotions, Culture and Social Integration

Karen Lund

Background and basic principles

The intention of this chapter is to show the interrelation between art therapy and social projects in a museum context through the design, setting up and execution of the programme *Let's Include the Museum*, carried out by the Bilbao Fine Arts Museum (BFAM), which has shown a continued interest in creating a participatory meeting space for people at risk of social exclusion. The programme began with a three-month pilot project in January 2011 and has continued ever since.

Art therapy in a museum context offers a therapeutic approach to help enhance the individual and social integrity of socially excluded groups in relation to their community (and in this case, to the BFAM as an institution at the service of society). By mediating through artistic appreciation and process in the presence of an art therapist and providing a secure 'holding' setting, it facilitates and contains the expression of emotions. Without the support of a therapist to contain these emotions there is a potential risk that the activity would be experienced as destabilising or disturbing, as argued by Shaer *et al.* (2008). The presence of an art therapist helps to establish a confidential setting of trust, an important ethical consideration when working with these groups. Additionally, throughout the programme, particular attention has been paid to understanding and adapting to the clients' emotional needs, for example by choosing paintings in the gallery that will most interest them and will help to foster their personal, emotional and social responses so that they might have the opportunity to be transformed by the experience. The importance of the role of a professional art therapist in creating an appropriate setting and carrying out suitable interventions with these specific groups cannot be understated and is explored further later.

In 2010, meetings were held between me, as an independent art therapist with prior experience of working with diverse groups, and the BFAM to explain exactly how art therapy works (something the institution was unfamiliar with), with a view to creating a programme proposal based on the considerations already mentioned above. The mutual interests of both parties led to a working agreement whereby the museum took me on as a member of their staff to develop the project and carry out the future programme.

The programme, *Let's Include the Museum*, was structured around two fundamental aspects agreed between the Department of Education and Cultural Action (DECA) of the BFAM and the art therapist. First was the museum's desire to be seen as a public space for the benefit of the whole community and its interest in creating a collaborative resource that encourages centres working with groups at risk of exclusion to make use of art as a means of personal growth and integration. This was achieved through programmes such as *Let's Include the Museum* that prioritise the active participation of socially less considered groups and help to fulfil the museum's commitment to combatting stereotypes and social isolation. Second was the importance of the incorporation of an art therapist to design and co-ordinate interventions based on an understanding of the emotional and interrelational needs of the group, as well as knowledge about art and its creative processes. By focusing on non-verbal and mainly visual language and communication, art therapy offers a valuable alternative to the written and spoken word, as argued by Dalley (1987). The dialogue that is established through symbolic, metaphorical and creative processes facilitates understanding because it allows the artistically expressed contents of the artwork to sometimes become accessible to both the participant and the group long before they are consciously recognised. This process, mediated through the art object, facilitates contact and the expression of feelings or thoughts, at times difficult to verbalise (Dalley 1987). The art therapist plays an important part in helping to open up an individual's creative process, accompanying them in the process and accepting the outcome in a non-judgemental way, so that both the creative process and its product occur without outside influence, opinion or preconception. This neutrality helps encourage spontaneous creative expression and offers a secure environment for exploration of both the process and the finished artwork.

Objectives of the programme

Considering the fundamental aspects mentioned, the main objectives of the ongoing programme can be summarised as follows:

- To bring these groups to the museum to enable them to discover its artistic heritage, and to allow them to respond to the artworks themselves through the group's own artistic expressions.
- To empower these groups by welcoming their personal contributions through contemplation and dialogue concerning the artwork displayed.
- To provide opportunities for people to give their own voice to their feelings and opinions through the creative expression in the workshop.
- To aid personal growth.
- To promote the integration of these groups in public life, counteracting a tendency towards isolation, and emphasising the relationship between the individual and their environment to promote a path towards healthy emotional development.

Once the basic principles and objectives of the programme were established, between me, as the art therapist in charge of the project, along with the Director of the DECA who acted as a co-facilitator in its setting up, we agreed to start the programme with a pilot project for a period of three months focusing on individuals with mental health difficulties.

First, we held meetings with: Osakidetza, the mental health network of the Basque Public Health System; Lantegi Batuak, the organisation that generates job opportunities for people with cognitive and physical disabilities and those with poor mental health; and Avifes, an association of people with mental health problems and their families. We explained the idea of the programme and the institutions contributed with their opinions and experience. Our proposal was novel because their existing extra-clinical activities focused on occupational workshops, leisure workshops or recreational outings, and did not in most cases involve any psychological therapy outside the institution. They were particularly interested in the idea of both opening up the museum to their users and providing them with the opportunity to actively participate through their own artistic creation. In their own words, the programme was seen as 'innovative, interesting and necessary'.

Implementation of the programme

The pilot project, as a first step in the overall programme, started in January 2011. The BFAM allocated funds from its budget, and for the first time incorporated into its team, formed of historians, educators and artists, an art therapist as a professional in charge of planning the practical details of the programme in cooperation with the DECA.

It was agreed that the activities of the programme, starting with the pilot group, would be carried out every fortnight for a minimum of three months, unlike the one-day activities usually offered by the museum. This frequency was established in order to obtain better results in terms of encouraging deeper engagement in the activity by the groups and to promote interrelation within the individual groups. As Case and Dalley (2006) argue, group therapy enables members to improve their interpersonal skills; participants can try out new roles and through mutual support discover new aspects of themselves, especially in terms of taking their own initiative and discovering a new sense of independence. At the same time, the feeling of being accompanied by the art therapist and the whole group helps to encourage members to see change as a real possibility. In short, the interactive group experience can help members to internalise positive group experience.

It was agreed that each session would be two hours in length and the number of participants would be no more than ten. Case and Dalley (2006) argue that the size of group is important so that everyone can maintain visual and verbal contact with each other. In addition, a small group provides an opportunity for each person to have an adequate share of time in discussion, reflection and exploration. At the same time, the DECA prepared an organisational chart regarding schedules, availability of halls and workshop rooms, and any necessary artistic materials. The participating institutions committed themselves to collaborating by taking into consideration the characteristics of the programme and informing their users clearly about the creative and therapeutic nature of the project. They also explained that participation was voluntary.

Since all of the participants were referred to the programme by the participating organisations, it was impossible for me, as the art therapist, to organise prior assessments, request consent forms or consider the make-up of the groups prior to their formation, as might have been customary in a clinical setting. Consequently, before the commencement of the project I did not know the participants personally, and so meetings were held between me and one professional from each institution (psychologist or social worker) to better understand the profiles of future participants, to understand and consider their emotional presentation and diagnosis, their capacity to tolerate and carry out work in a group and their level of compatibility, motivation and commitment. This information was necessary before we decided the final configuration of each group, to ensure maximum group cohesion. In this way, we achieved agreements that respected the criteria and the professional objectives of both parties, which during the course of the programme has turned out to be particularly enriching through the interchange of professional knowledge and shared views.

The details of the programme were then explained again by me and the Director of the DECA in the first meeting with the groups to highlight the voluntary, therapeutic and cultural nature of the programme, the importance of confidentiality and the timing of the programme, and to offer an opportunity for individuals to ask questions. The participants gave their verbal consent to take part in both the project and the evaluation at the end. As we did not have written consent from the participants before the start of the programme pilot, appropriate consents were requested before the end to conform with data protection. It was made clear to all individuals that their comments would be recorded and might be used, for example, in internal reports and academic articles or publications, their confidentiality and anonymity being maintained at all times.

In addition, as requested by the centres, it was agreed that there would be one accompanying professional from each institution (psychologists, social workers) for each group of a maximum of ten people. This was part of the institution's policy to monitor the participation of their users in activities outside the centre to ensure their safety. The importance of establishing the role of the person accompanying the group as a non-participating observer was emphasised. Since from my personal experience I knew that their presence would influence the activity, as argued by Kislev (2015), it was essential to try to minimise the possible effect of their role on the participants' responses to the group, and on development of creative processes in the workshop. For me, as the art therapist, this aspect was fundamental to create a sense of trust and a strong bond with the group in order to facilitate their emotional expression. In this respect, the way the art therapist facilitates the group plays a key role in the nature of the group, as argued by Waller (1996). Lack of clarity in the role of the observer, resulting in observers making interventions contrary to the art therapist, can result in ambiguity and confusion. In particular, comments about the art-making process, or passing aesthetic judgement on the artworks, can feel intrusive and inhibit group members from voicing their feelings and opinions through their creative process. 'If the interventions of the facilitator help the group to achieve their tasks, we could say that the group is going in the right direction' (Ramos i Portas 2003, p.4).

It was also agreed that the professional accompanying the group would submit a written report after the workshops, providing additional information for the art therapist by observing what went on before and after the workshops. For example, the professional might note any changes in the emotional state of the participants, observations or knowledge about the participants that could affect the group work, or anything they noticed during the activity which they considered to be important, bearing in mind their understanding of the participants.

Structure of the activity

Each meeting of two hours was divided into three phases:

1. Visiting the gallery: contemplation of a previously selected artwork within a thematic selection chosen by myself and bearing in mind the characteristics of the group.
2. Creative-experiential workshop: non-directive workshop where the group could freely explore their own interests and resources, inspired by their visit to the gallery.
3. Sharing session within the group: time for group reflection, always voluntary, on their artwork and the feelings evoked.

The activity, both in the pilot and in the subsequent programme, began by going to the museum gallery to contemplate a single artwork. The purpose of viewing a single artwork was to create a space for focused visual attention in order to facilitate free associations, especially for groups not used to visiting museums. Bearing this in mind, I considered it important to adjust the museum visit to the participants' needs. Many people feel excluded from museums, thinking that they are only for people who know about art, to the extent that a museum visit may be intimidating. In order to minimise these effects, the experience of viewing art needs to be as accessible and comfortable as possible to motivate the group participants to view the work with confidence, to feel relaxed about their reaction and comments, and to feel that these are as relevant as any theoretical understanding of the artwork. For this reason, our approach has been to not influence the group with prepared comments about the artwork so that the engagement with it can be as free and spontaneous as possible. Seated in silence, observation was invited with questions such as: 'What do we perceive in it? What emotions are awakened? What impression does it make on you?' This first contact with an artwork, as Gilroy (2007) argues, is an aesthetic moment where there is a non-verbal state, a fusion between subject and object. Works of art are dynamic entities that allow the viewer to project their feelings and thoughts while exploring the meanings and narratives to explain private and social experiences.

In the observation and dialogue, various processes occur, as mentioned by Maclagan (2005). First is the description that allows us an initial contact to discover and get to know the object of our attention. Then there is the elaborative process when we begin to relate to and expand on what we see, when the observed image invites us to form different associations and create new narratives. This is followed by interpretation, when we make connections between the artwork and individual or collective symbolism. These processes tend to be mingled so that 'what might appear as merely suggestive or indecisive can have the advantage of keeping things open and preventing meaning from being foreclosed' (Maclagan 2005, p.27).

The viewing process in the activity relates to heuristic theory by proposing practical or informal strategies that guide the act of discovery. As Mahony (2001) says, 'the direct experience of the process being investigated strengthens the validity of the findings' (p.52). In this case, and in order to clarify this idea, the investigation or discovery is understood in terms of the personal appreciation of the artwork by the members of the group, based on their own discoveries which then validate the artistic process later. In the viewing process, the observer projects their experiences and perceptions onto the artwork and finds meaning in what is being observed. Starting from their own emotions, the viewer resonates with what they feel they see in the artwork. The viewer involves the whole self in the process, identifying personally with the artwork and at times seeing aspects of the self, or personal experiences, reflected in the artwork. When this process is shared in a group, not only is the perception of the work enriched, but also the viewer's self-perception. In this sense, understanding the artwork represents an encounter with the self. This process of personal and group connection also occurs with artworks created in the past. These artworks can become relevant to a contemporary understanding, opening up to new interpretations as the observers confront themselves and their reality in a new context. Despite the historical time lapse, the observer appropriates the artwork and brings it closer to their own life.

After visiting the gallery, we moved to a museum workshop to carry out our creative activities. The well-illuminated space was equipped with tables and chairs, a great diversity of artistic material, access to water, and nearby bathrooms, and cupboards to keep the participants' artwork safe as these were not works for visual exploration by others, but were treated as clinical work. This space had no external interruptions, allowing the art therapist to foster an environment of trust and security so that the participants could express personal feelings and thoughts. This process was framed by confidentiality, understood as the ethical commitment to protect the privacy of the individual/group. As the accompanying worker was present here too, it was important that they remain outside the group process, purely as an observer and respectful of the confidentiality of the setting so that they did not compromise the free expression of the participants. Despite my initial reservations as the art therapist, I was able to ensure that the presence of outside observers did not impede the free creative expression nor the verbal interventions of the participants.

The artistic creation in the workshop was one of free expression. The purpose was for the group to explore what interested them, to express their own personal concerns, which may or may not have been connected to the experience lived in the gallery. It represented a space for the participants where their images could 'create clarity of expression, especially with regards to certain difficult things to say' and at the same time, could 'make such feelings become less threatening' (Dalley 1987, p.16). On occasions, repressed memories, painful emotions, or past traumas may appear in the artworks. In art therapy, 'the ensuing art object may act as a container for powerful emotions that cannot be easily expressed' (Waller 1996, p.3) and, unlike verbal descriptions which can be too direct, artistic language permits a more indirect communication where 'the most important thing is for the creator to find his or her own meanings' (Liebmann 2000, p.14). The art therapist provides containment based on her capacity to tolerate and hold with empathy any overwhelming feelings expressed by patients. Casement (2013) argues that when the patient is met by the response of the therapist, their initial painful emotions become more manageable because the therapist witnesses them and contains them. For this reason, the art therapist needs to be authentically in touch with what the other person is feeling and with what is being expressed, but at the same time maintain neutrality towards preconceived ideas to ensure they do not influence the process.

Workshops also provide a time for reflection on the artwork produced, where the participants can enter into a dialogue both with their artworks and with the group. The resulting images act as intermediaries, favouring communication between the unconscious and the conscious mind; between the participant, the art therapist and the group. It is a moment to distance oneself and view the artwork objectively, letting it speak for itself and allowing a time of internal dialogue. It also provides a time to use words, to express oneself verbally, and through which the participant and the group as a whole can continue associating with dimensions of new senses of self.

Evaluation

At the end of the pilot project, anonymous surveys were conducted with the participants to compare their opinions with the assessment of the experience by the institutions (explored later), providing the museum as well as me with an internal qualitative evaluation.

The evaluation centred on two main aspects to assess the participants' level of satisfaction with the project. The first aspect centred on assessing the participants' perception of the museum in terms of accessibility and approachability. The second centred on analysing their appreciation and their experience of the visit to the galleries and the workshop.

On the first point, 90 per cent of the participants felt well received, and viewed the museum as being approachable. On the second point, the percentages were the same, with 90 per cent showing a favourable response. The viewing in the gallery was valued as being very interesting and participative; for example, participants commented that they enjoyed 'learning to look at a painting and interpret it from our own observations', that there was 'relaxed, good communication' and that 'I felt I understood and shared things, I didn't expect looking at art to be so interesting'. With reference to the creative workshops, which included both art-making and verbal exploration, they valued both the creative liberty and the subsequent personal and group reflection as being motivating, enriching and respectful: 'I really enjoyed it, it has helped me overcome a little my fear of drawing and painting'; 'I didn't expect that we would open up so much and talk about such personal things, I would definitely do it again'; 'Very positive, artistically and psychologically'.

As the art therapist, I prepared a report on the results at the end of the pilot project, which was evaluated with the museum. The conclusion was that the level of satisfaction was very positive in general, and that in particular the incorporation of the role of an art therapist had been very beneficial.

Formation of the ongoing group

In March 2011, we finished the three-month pilot project, during which we worked with three different groups from each of the three institutions already mentioned earlier in the chapter. The most relevant aspects of the assessments presented by the centres at the end of the experience were as follows. They highlighted the dialogue in the gallery that allowed 'deepening and expanding bonds among the group and with the artwork displayed'. Regarding the artwork, they valued with astonishment 'the emotional force and the personal meaning of the images produced and their reflection'. They also appreciated the great potential of the artistic production as a 'communicative means, demonstrating its value in the face of feelings of loneliness and isolation'. They assessed very positively 'the relationship they established with the art therapist and the atmosphere of trust and participation generated'. Above all, they appreciated 'the group work accomplished and the decrease of the anxieties in the groups when they were in a different space from their centres, which generated an increase of personal confidence and in the environment'.

Some of the participants who took part in the pilot project showed great interest in continuing, and due to the positive outcomes, the museum, the art therapist and the centres decided to create a group. For the structure of the new group workshops, I as art therapist outlined two changes: first, to do without the presence of personnel from the centres to enhance the personal autonomy of the group; second, to increase the number of biweekly sessions to a period of one year. These changes were based on the desire to deepen the cultural and therapeutic benefits by making the programme longer, and to assure the establishment of a safe and secure environment to promote a sense of trust, without the presence of an outside observer.

So that group members should benefit from the experience it was agreed that all participants must understand their condition and be in a position to manage their symptoms in order to be better able to cope with any stressful situations. For this reason, they needed to be in a period of relative stability to be able to take part in the museum activity. The group started in October 2011 and, with withdrawals and new members, it continues to this day (2019). It was formed of nine participants: men and women aged 30–55 years, most of them with paranoid schizophrenia, and some with social phobia and depression. They lived in family environments and all of them had jobs, as they worked in Lantegi Batuak, one of the participant institutions that offers job opportunities in their workshops for people with intellectual and physical disabilities, and those with mental health difficulties.

From contemplation to the creative response

The museum, with its artistic heritage, offers an unparalleled setting to introduce work of this type. Its atmosphere of tranquillity invites groups to move at a calm pace that predisposes a contemplative attitude and a direct and personal encounter with the artwork. This experience allows the participants to access a rich resonance between their own experiences and those communicated by, and contained within, the displayed artworks. As Gilroy (2007) describes, this process occurs when we face and contemplate an artwork, when we focus in on particular areas or aspects of the work, making conscious and unconscious choices about our interests. This depends on what we are looking for in our effort to find meaning. In addition, by being a large sensory space, the location also becomes an important alternative for enjoyment and exploration.

This programme within the museum setting is based on the post-modern vision of art, where 'the boundaries between product and process, individual and group creation and artist and viewer dissolve' (Alter-Muri and Klein 2007, p.82). In this sense, the viewers who contemplate the artwork are also creators of it and the creation of shared meanings is what confers the communicative value of art.

The idea of the programme is that the active engagement of the participant not only changes their perception of the museum space but also challenges the overall perception of the museum as an exclusive and elitist space. As López Martínez (2011) argues, the formal sense of curating the art of the institution, accessible mainly to specialists and researchers, has now developed further without losing the principles of conservation and research, to offer a much wider service to the general public and to open up access and social participation. Through a new approach, we can make these environments more accessible, helping to change the perception and the role of museums and art itself so that these groups, who may feel out of place and overwhelmed, lose their inhibitions and find a space with relevance to their own lives.

Experience with the group

The following vignettes of workshops illustrate the relation between the participants' personal associations and the meanings raised through viewing the artworks in the gallery and their discussion, with the thoughts and emotions evoked and expressed by the participants in the art-making in the workshops.

In this instance, two artworks were chosen from the museum's permanent collection and the third was a visit to a temporary exhibition. The first one, 'The Rape of Europa' (c. 1590) by Marten de Vos (BFAM n.d. a), is a painting from the High Renaissance, while the second one, 'Albia' (2002) by Mari Puri Herrero (BFAM n.d. b), is a contemporary figurative work. The third example is 'Messages off the Wall' (BFAM n.d. c), an exhibition about posters from 1886–1975, belonging to the BFAM collection.

'The Rape of Europa' represents the theme narrated by Ovid in his 'Metamorphoses', in which the god Zeus, in love with Europa, daughter of the King of Phoenicia, transforms himself into a bull in order to kidnap her and take her to Crete, while Hermes, surrounded by angels, watches from the sky.

The group perceived the distance between them and this centuries-old image that invited them to discover more about the image and the narrative it depicted. The participants explored the symbolic contents of the story and, from a contemporary perspective, opinions emerged about rape as an aggressive act; seduction and deceit; the feminine and masculine conditions in history; and the present struggle for equal rights. Although these themes could have been potentially distressing for the group, as an art therapist I was able contain any such unsettling emotions by keeping the focus on the symbolic and representative nature of both the artwork and the feelings that it evoked. In this way, the experience helped to foster the participants' own capacity to symbolise and to tolerate difficult emotions, a process argued by Shaer *et al.* (2008).

In the second part of the activity, we moved to the workshop. As the participants already knew the space, materials and its layout, they entered confidently. In the workshop, I as the art therapist aimed to encourage the participants' creative process, helping them to find their own unique expression and their experience with their own internal resources, so that the group grew to trust in its own artistic communication skills. I provided non-judgemental support to each participant's artistic process, giving equal value to everything that emerged.

When creative time finished, one participant shared her work with the group (Figure 9.1). She commented that the experience in the gallery had connected her with feelings of people's general lack of sensitivity and understanding which humanity continued to suffer from. She described that she had drawn doors that open and close representing the difficulties of the current working world and in the middle, the Euro, symbolizing the European economic crisis.

She continued explaining that the feminine and masculine symbols, as well as the bow and arrow of Cupid, represented conflicting relationships that begin and end. She wanted to express the impotence and the pain of these experiences through her drawing of the three crosses on Mount Calvary of the crucifixion of Jesus.

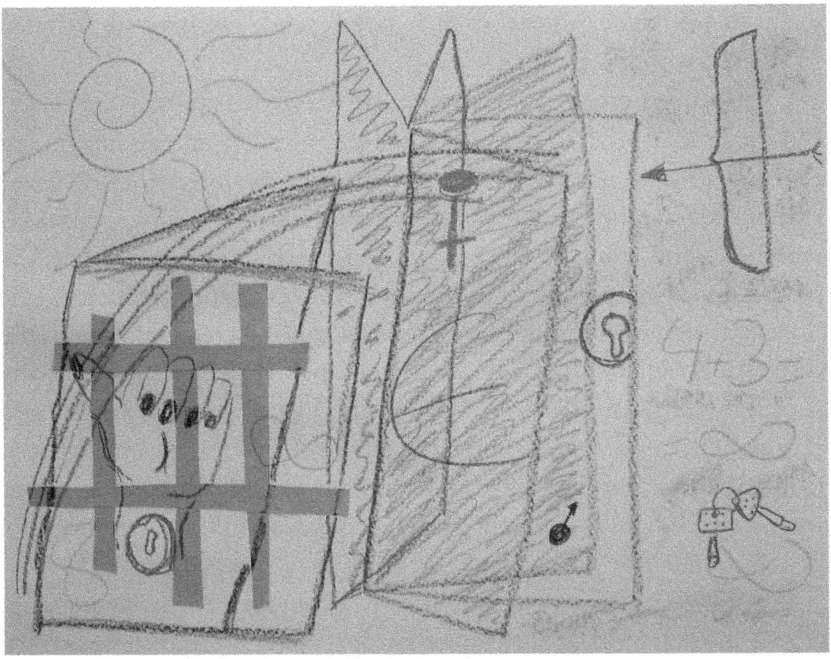

Figure 9.1 Participant artwork after viewing 'The Rape of Europa'

The group mentioned that 'the proximity between the crosses suggests bars, and the hand drawn on top of them looks like the gesture of someone hitchhiking'. After a moment of anguished silence, she said that she had not been aware of it while drawing but, when observing it, she suddenly connected with the accident and death of a student classmate that she had witnessed while hitchhiking. She told us emotionally that at that moment she had been in a crisis due to her illness and this event had shocked her a lot. In previous workshops, she had told the group that her illness appeared with intensity at 21 years of age, while studying at university.

At the end of her moving explanation, the group responded by helping her to contain her emotion, telling her that they understood her experience, and they recounted similar experiences that they had had themselves. For example, one member related how she had suffered cancer at a young age and had an operation which had led to a crisis. By being able to speak out and share such challenging topics, they were able to help each other manage difficult feelings. Both in the creative work and in the process of talking about it, the participants gained the ability to understand more deeply what was being expressed, and the feedback from the group could then be integrated by the creator of the image.

The following two examples demonstrate how the group explored viewing in the gallery in relation to their own life experiences. In the visit to the temporary exhibition on old posters 'Messages from the Wall' (1886–1975), one participant produced a creative work based on the aesthetics of the poster in tribute to her recently deceased mother. She commented that viewing the posters had aroused memories of her mother, with mixed feeling of both sadness and admiration. In her image, she painted her mother acting in a theatre (Figure 9.2). She told us that her mother had been a singer of some fame when she settled in Madrid at a young age. She stated proudly that, despite having the same mental condition as herself, her mother had achieved her goals. She demonstrated how important it was to share this with the group, since her family always avoided the issue in front of her for fear of a relapse in her illness and she felt that the members of the group would understand this. Revisiting these memories relieved her of her overwhelming feeling of emptiness.

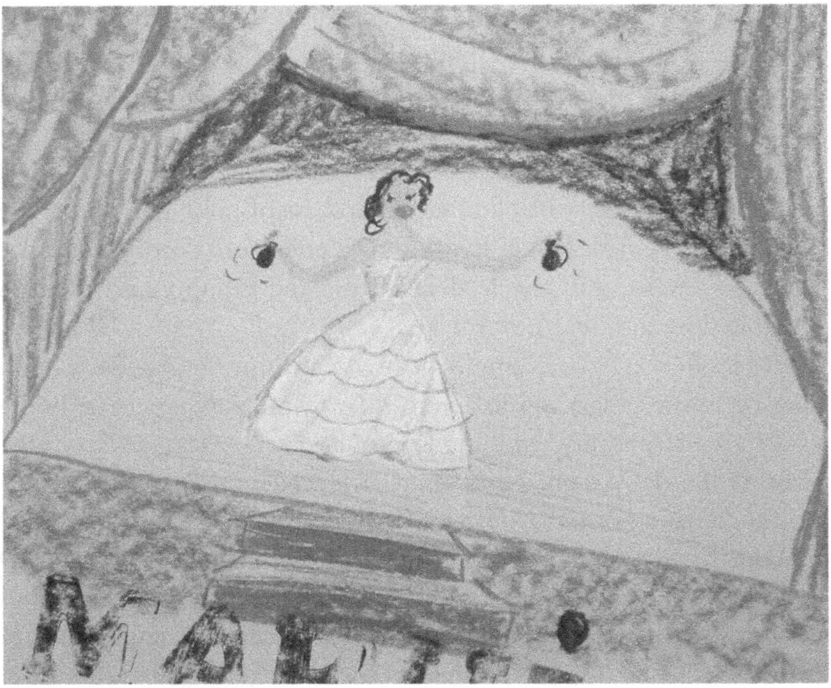

Figure 9.2 Participant artwork after visiting the 'Messages from the Wall' exhibition

On the occasion of the workshop about 'Albia', we looked at the painting in which groups of people walk through the trees in the gardens of a square in Bilbao. This figurative painting has a dream-like and symbolic quality associated with magical realism. One participant commented that observing the work of art in the gallery she felt at ease, and that the painting aroused pleasurable feelings. In her own creative work, the group participants are represented, and leafy, luxuriant vegetation seems to wrap the figures with care and protection (Figure 9.3). The art therapist appears in another colour on the right, accompanying the group. Reflecting on the connections that emerged in her creative work, she expressed how she had felt very welcomed by the group: 'This group has helped me to trust, I draw without thinking about the result, it is a liberating feeling.' Her creative work represented in some way the many achievements in the development and cohesion of the group.

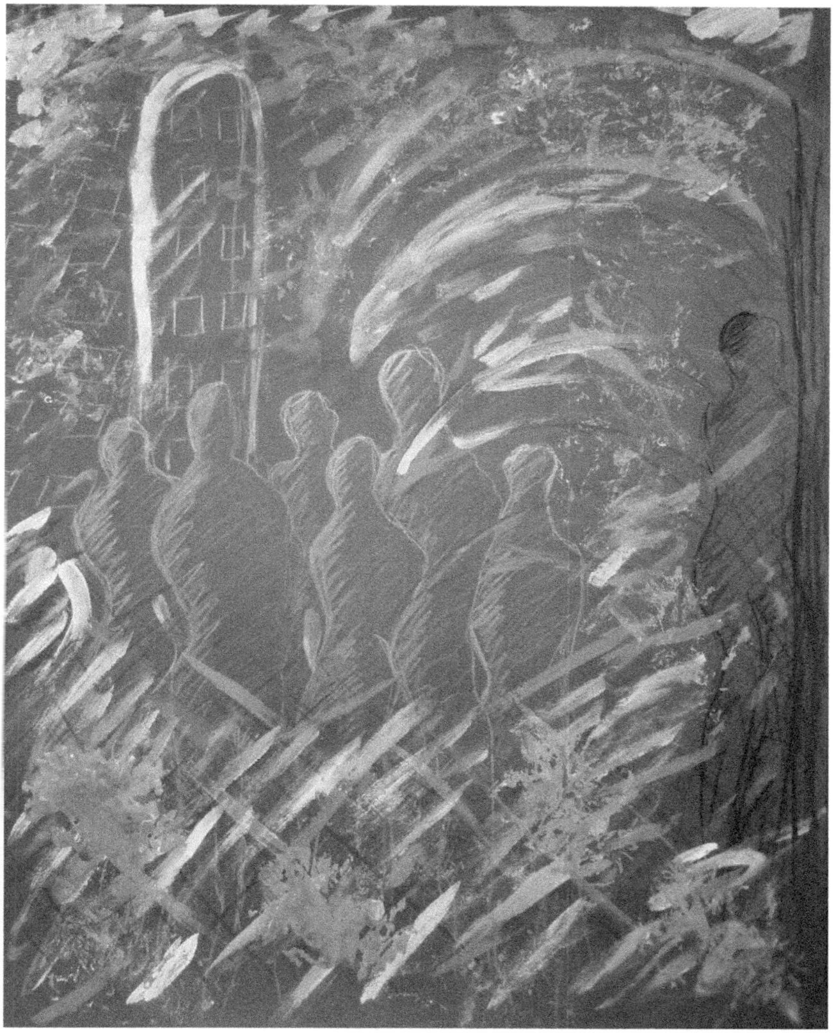

Figure 9.3 Participant artwork after viewing 'Albia'

From these examples, we can see how the experience, from the gallery to the workshop, helped to draw out feelings associated with relationships, mental illness or life experiences which were shared by the group. These images, linked to the contemplative experience in the gallery, led the way for a process of introspection and reflection. As in the potential space described by Winnicott (1971), the experience of the inner world is created through the internalisation of external experience; here, the artwork of the artist, the group, and the art therapist all encouraged insight and self-awareness and processes of transformation and constructive integration.

For the group members, going to the museum has become an important part of their lives. It is a place where they can share life experiences and escape from isolation. In their own words, as they gave feedback on the activities, 'We talk about our concerns and problems, about life, we get to know each other through the reflections about the creative works of the group'; 'They make us see things that we do not normally see'; 'Help to relieve the mind and to reflect on the moments you live'; 'I feel that this helps me to make personal changes'. In addition, the experience has activated their cultural interests and has improved their social lives.

Conclusions

The incorporation of art therapy in the design and development of the described programme has resulted in greater knowledge of the profession in the museum field. This has been established not only through the experience itself, but also through the continuous evaluations carried out with the groups and the participating institutions, as well as with the DECA and the art therapist. All of the institutions involved have assessed positively the results of this programme that happen outside the usual psychiatric and rehabilitation fields. They highlighted that the programme adds therapeutic benefits to the work carried out by these centres.

The following quotations are some of the positive feedback from staff at the centres involved in the project: 'It's an opportunity to observe and to get to know our users better from a different and deeper perspective: their emotions, their life histories and their childhood'; 'The participants are able to express and channel emotions in a way that wouldn't have been possible in their daily lives'; 'The project totally fulfils the objective of making the museum more inclusive; they are not seen as people with a mental illness but as a group of people interested in art.' The organisations involved also value the fact that the members of the groups have acquired expressive and communication skills from their experiences with the non-verbal artistic process. They recognise the determining role of the museum and of the art therapist in their integrative and supportive work, so that the members of these groups feel themselves to be an active part of the world to which they belong. Despite the length of time the programme has been running, it continues to surprise the staff at the DECA, as well as those involved from the participating centres, due to the power and intensity of engagement in the viewing process and in the creative art generated afterwards.

As a result of the positive assessment obtained for the pilot project, the programme has continued to thrive, resulting in its expansion to other groups. We now work with: offenders who are on probation; young people with learning difficulties or personal and family conflicts; unprotected minors who live in foster homes; people involved in conflictive adoptions; women who have suffered abuse; people with intellectual disabilities; and children and adolescents with special educational needs associated with mental health. The participating institutions are state organisations, such as the Youth and Family section of Social Services; the special needs section of the Department for Education; women's and family refuge centres and penal institutions, as well as diverse organisations and associations who work with socially excluded collectives.

Following the original three-month pilot project, the programme has been running for nine years. Throughout this period, the commitment of many professionals has been required, such as the team at BFAM, the art therapist, directors and support staff of the centres, psychologists, family therapists, social workers, educational therapists, special needs teachers and carers, as well as a multidisciplinary network made up of staff from the BFAM and the participating centres. All have worked together to collaborate and develop this resource for the benefit and the inclusion of the above groups.

To generate opportunities to enable groups of people to share their realities and their emotions, to hear themselves and be listened to by others, to value themselves and to be valued by others, means helping them to feel part of the society in which they live. The construction of this experience, based on feelings of trust and belonging, is our work as art therapists. By involving ourselves with museums and creating programmes such as *Let's Include the Museum*, we help to extend the use of art with therapeutic purposes and also help to provide broader perspectives of personal growth, while at the same time providing a cultural experience and an opportunity for social inclusion.

References

Alter-Muri, S. and Klein, L. (2007) 'Dissolving the boundaries: Postmodern art and art therapy.' *Art Therapy: Journal of the American Art Therapy Association 24,* 2, 82–86.

BFAM (n.d. a) 'The Rape of Europa.' Accessed on 16/2/19 at www.museobilbao.com/obras-maestras/martin-de-vos.

BFAM (n.d. b) 'Messages off the Wall.' Accessed on 16/2/19 at www.museobilbao.com/exposiciones/mensajes-desde-la-pared-238.

BFAM (n.d. c) 'Albia.' Accessed on 16/2/19 at www.museobilbao.com/catalogo-online/albia-02158.

Case, C. and Dalley, T. (2006) *The Handbook of Art Therapy*. London and New York, NY: Routledge. (Original work published 1992).

Casement, P. (2013) *On Learning from the Patient*. London and New York, NY: Routledge. (Original work published 1985).

Dalley, T. (1987) *El arte como terapia*. Barcelona: Editorial Herder S.A. (Original work: *Art as Therapy*, 1984, London and New York, NY: Tavistock Publications).

Gilroy, A. (2007) 'Taking a long look at art: Reflections on the context of production and consumption of art in art therapy.' *ATOL: Art Therapy Online 5,* 2, 1–36. Accessed on 20/10/15 at http://eprints.gold.ac.uk/113.

Kislev, E. (2015) 'The use of participant-observers in group therapy: A critical exploration in light of Foucauldian Theory.' *Group 39,* 1 (Spring 2015), 9–24.

Liebmann, M. (2000) *Art Therapy in Practice*. London and Philadelphia, PA: Jessica Kingsley Publishers. (Original work published 1990).

López Martínez, M.D. (2011) 'Arteterapia y Museos. Puntos de encuentro.' *Arte y políticas de identidad 4* (June), 127–136. Accessed on 19/4/12 at http://revistas.um.es/api:1989-8452.

Maclagan, D. (2005) 'Re-imagining art therapy.' *International Journal of Art Therapy 10,* 1, 23–30.

Mahony, J. (2001) 'Three commentaries: Looking experiences at three exhibitions.' *International Journal of Art Therapy 6,* 2, 51–62.

Ramos i Portas, C. (2003) 'The experiential art therapy group in the training of art therapists.' Paper presented at 1st Art Therapy World Congress, 30 March–2 April 2003, Budapest Convention Centre, Budapest.

Shaer, D., Beaven, K., Springham, N., Pillinger, S. *et al.* (2008) 'The role of art therapy in a pilot for art-based information prescriptions at Tate Britain.' *International Journal of Art Therapy 13,* 1, 25–33.

Waller, D. (1996) *Group Interactive Art Therapy: Its Use in Training and Treatment*. London, USA, Canada: Tavistock/Routledge Publications. (Original work published 1993).

Winnicott, D.W. (1971) *Playing and Reality*. London: Tavistock Publications.

CHAPTER 10

BALTIC Art Therapy Project

A Collaboration Between NHS Art Therapists and BALTIC Centre for Contemporary Art Gateshead

Michael Fischer and Whittaker Scott

Introduction

This chapter describes an eight-week pilot project developed by the art therapists in Northumberland, Tyne and Wear NHS Foundation Trust (NTW) Children and Young People's Service (CYPS) in conjunction with the BALTIC Centre for Contemporary Art and a practising artist. Northumberland, Tyne and Wear Children and Young People's Service is part of the National Health Service (NHS) in England and offers a mental health service for children and young people up to the age of 18 years old.

In this project, service users aged between 13 and 18 took part in a short-term art therapy group at the BALTIC Centre for Contemporary Art in Gateshead, which culminated in a public exhibition.

In the conception, planning and running of this project, a key question for us was: *What is it about the art gallery experience which can add to an art therapy group?*

Our chapter focuses on some of the practicalities of setting up and running this project that we hope will be useful to others planning, or engaged in, this type of venture.

We begin by outlining the background to the project, looking at relevant literature and describing the steps taken in setting the project up, from approaching the gallery to recruiting for the group. We then explore different aspects of the planning and delivery of the project, such as the experience of the art therapists working with an independent artist, some of the differences when providing an art therapy group in this setting, the group's experience of the gallery and public exhibition, and the opportunity for young people to exhibit their artwork in an internationally renowned venue.

Finally, we look at what we have learned from the project and at planning for future collaborations with BALTIC.

Background

The motivation for this project came about due to having a sub-optimal art therapy space in the Northumberland, Tyne and Wear CYPS provision, premises available that were not purpose specific, and on one site there being no creative therapy room at all. It also came from a conviction held by the art therapists that contemporary art galleries had something to offer the therapeutic process. This belief came from our own experience as artists and our involvement in community arts projects and exhibitions prior to becoming art therapists. We felt that the gallery environment and access to contemporary art that embraces different forms of expression could be inspiring for young people.

BALTIC is a major international centre for contemporary art in Gateshead, England. With no permanent collection, BALTIC has gained an international reputation for its distinctive and ambitious programme of exhibitions and events.

BALTIC's Learning and Civic Engagement Team works with a variety of different audiences throughout the region and nationally, and is committed to providing inclusive opportunities that enable individuals and communities to explore and exchange different perspectives and new ideas (BALTIC Centre for Contemporary Art 2018).

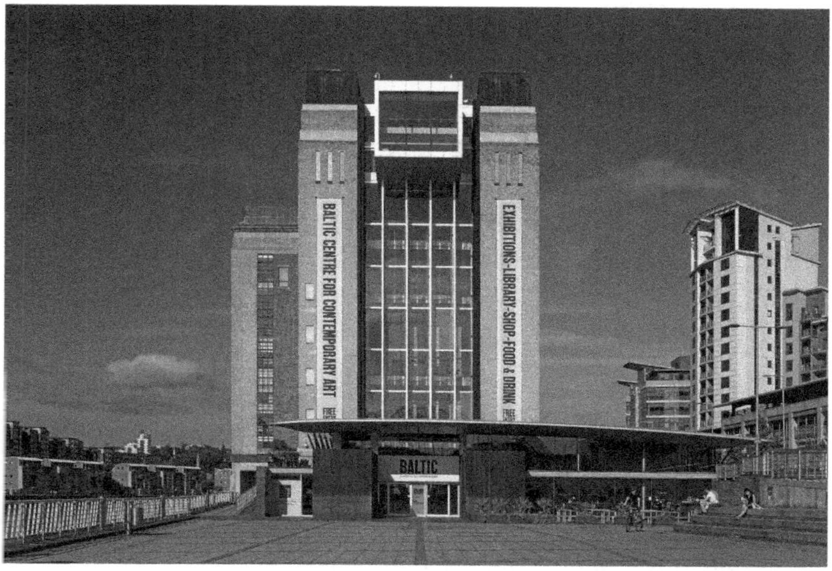

Figure 10.1 BALTIC

Our initial ideas were that the experience of group art therapy in a gallery could help to engage hard-to-reach adolescents who might find NHS premises stigmatising. We also thought that it could help participants who might have difficulties with confidence, low self-esteem and developing relationships, as it could provide an opportunity to work with others in an exciting gallery environment with access to various art media and potential to be involved in an exhibition at the end of the project. We felt that through exhibiting their own artwork, the project could give young people a voice and promote positive mental health awareness in the community.

The participants were not necessarily familiar with the centre of the city, as the catchment area for those taking part in the group included a large outlying suburban area, smaller towns, and rural areas. We were conscious that both the city environment and travel might be off-putting for some participants.

Literature

Group art therapy with young people

Offering group art therapy to adolescents experiencing mental health difficulties can be a helpful approach as it involves both self-expression and interpersonal learning through sharing, modelling and peer interaction (Linesch 1988; Waller 1993).

Adolescence is a time of rapid physical and psychological change. Young people are searching for new and meaningful relationships with their peers and other significant figures and there can be a tension between dependence on and avoidance towards adults (Anderson and Darlington 1998). The group setting can be a particularly relevant one but can also make running this type of group more challenging, where young people can test boundaries and there is the potential for the group to become counter-therapeutic. Linesch (1988) describes how careful planning and selection for adolescent group work is essential and how art can play an important part. 'Harnessing the adolescent's creativity and expressive potential, as is done in the art therapy modality, can direct and sustain group interaction' (Linesch 1988, p.134). In her work with adolescent male youths who have had backgrounds of adversity and trauma, Slayton (2012) discusses how making art and witnessing what is made in art therapy group work can help to engage young people, helping them to have meaningful and positive social experiences. Cole *et al.* (2018) describe how group art approaches involving self-expression and making connections with others can help to engage young adults in mental health services, and Riley (1999) describes how art therapy groups can seem less threatening than verbal group work, as young people can feel some control over what they choose to share in their artwork with their contemporaries. There are examples of group art therapy helping young people with difficulties – including eating disorders and mental health issues relating to epilepsy – to use art to express difficult-to-verbalise feelings to communicate with others (Pepper Goldsmith and Ben-Simon 2012; Congreave *et al.* 2017).

The visual nature of art can be useful in developing self-image, which can then be explored with others. Higenbottam (2004) describes how art therapy groups help female adolescents use art to express and develop a more positive body image and to improve self-esteem. Miller (2012) recommends offering a diverse range of art media and creative tasks that are sensitive to the needs and interests of the young people involved, to facilitate engagement. The art medium is also highlighted in outcomes in a group art therapy study with young people from low economic backgrounds in South Korea, where Jang and Choi (2012) suggest that the qualities of clay-making, through to the experience of seeing their artworks fired and completed, had a positive impact on young people's ego-resilience.

A recent review indicates that young people with mental health difficulties also show cognitive difficulties, especially those who have been homeless or in care, with some suggestion that these young people may be particularly open to interventions involving creativity (Fry, Langley and Shelton 2017).

Art therapy in museums and galleries with young people

There are examples of art therapy and art-based programmes with young people predominantly taking place in galleries and museums that support insight and awareness, improved self-esteem and social interaction. Silverman (1989) writes about structural family, art and play therapies for young people in the museum and how the setting can add to the therapy experience: 'Skilled in art history and techniques, art museum educators and curators can enhance an art therapy activity. Artwork in the collections can be used to stimulate discussion and creation' (Silverman 1989, p.141).

With reference to an art therapy project with middle school teenagers at the Museum of Tolerance in Los Angeles, Linesch (2004) describes how art therapy activities can also enrich the connection young people make with the collection and their understanding of the exhibits, and Kaufman *et al.* (2014) report a significant impact on self-concept in their research study of 176 children in an educational/youth development art programme at the Dali Museum in St Petersburg, Florida.

Treadon, Rosal and Thompson Wylder (2006) describe an art therapy pilot project with young people experiencing mental health and behavioural difficulties, involving seven 12–14-year-olds from an educational setting who visited a large state university art museum in the USA as part of a seven-week intervention. The focus was for young people to explore their feelings and relationships with family, and participants explored links between art exhibits, their own artworks and their personal lives. It was suggested that the experience had a positive impact on participants' engagement with their own artwork and with staff at school following the project. Schleien, Mustonen and Rynders (1995) describe structured group art activities with children both with and without autism at a children's museum, where results showed that social interaction of children without autism towards children with autism was boosted significantly during the intervention. Stiles and Mermer-Welly (1998) worked with young people from an early teen pregnancy programme where 13–15-year-olds were offered family therapy, individual and group therapy and museum visits. They found that through looking at museum artworks, the young people were able to reflect on themselves and feel more connected with the community, and that the experience had a positive impact on young people's self-esteem and other difficulties they were experiencing.

Malone (2017) reported empathic responses from visitors to a gallery exhibition co-created with young survivors of child sex exploitation in Dorset, England. This showed how personally sensitive material in the art is not necessarily a barrier to involving young people in a public exhibition. The young people selected had achieved some stability in terms of their difficulties and were seen in a small supportive group. Interestingly, Salom (2015) describes how a group of 15 internally displaced indigenous women aged between 12 and 40 took part in an art therapy programme at the Museo del Oro in Bogotá, Colombia, where a theme emerged of the museum acting as a safe and supportive environment and where personal and cultural experiences could be explored. Coles and Harrison (2018) describe evaluating a museum-based group with young adults aged 18–25 with severe mental health difficulties using mixed qualitative and quantitative methods; they report that participants found that the museum environment and objects were a helpful focus for ideas and social interaction.

The group

Initial networking

The initial idea for the project was conceived in 2012. The first contact was made by Whittaker Scott, Head of Art Therapies (CYPS North of Tyne Community) with a staff member at BALTIC's Learning and Civic Engagement Team. With a commitment to extend and deepen the engagement with contemporary art by diverse audiences and a track record in successful projects specifically for young people, this practice fitted with BALTIC's strategic objectives (BALTIC Centre for Contemporary Art 2018). Having worked with potentially vulnerable groups was particularly helpful and the gallery had an understanding of consent and confidentiality in this context. BALTIC suggested working with a member of its Freelance Artist Team and at these meetings the issue of financial cost was raised, for example for room use and participation of the BALTIC artist. This was significant as it meant funding from NHS CYPS and was one reason the project took time to come to fruition.

We thought the project might have a potential research aspect and contacted the NHS Trust Research and Development Department which oversees research projects and has experience and expertise significantly greater than ours was. In these discussions, proposing the project as research was mooted, and that the project fell between formal research and innovative practice evaluation. It was agreed to apply through the Integrated Research Application System (IRAS) process to obtain ethics approval to conduct the project as research. The committee considered the project's application, deciding it might not constitute research. Nevertheless, it was a useful learning experience for us and the project proceeded as a piece of innovative practice evaluation. BALTIC was also positioning the project as innovative practice, which was more in line with its strategic aims, as outlined above.

Discussions with NHS management and colleagues

Our NHS manager was aware of the BALTIC project through informal discussions and a case for it was presented to the management group; although the response was favourable, there were no funds at that time and the project was shelved. In 2015, funding was obtained and we were able to proceed, the manager visiting the exhibition before the group started, to review the content and check it was appropriate from a managerial viewpoint. This was important, because both the art therapists running the group and the BALTIC artist were trained artists familiar with contemporary art. Not everybody shares this position and set of assumptions – what might be seen as legitimately challenging in the art world might be seen as inappropriate for young people by those with a different perspective. Thankfully, she deemed it reasonable.

Through discussion with a consultant clinical psychologist it was suggested that a higher assistant psychologist from the NHS CYPS team would help facilitate the project. It was felt that the support this would bring (especially an understanding of theory and outcome measures) would be helpful. James Blacklock took on this role. Part of this was to offer support at the gallery in meeting and greeting participants and by being available in a nearby room for participants who might feel they needed to leave the group during a session – he could offer support and, if necessary, liaise with other CYPS team members. He also had the role of administering the outcome measures (see section below on 'Outcomes')

We liaised with various colleagues within our Trust to produce the information and consent forms for the participants and their parents/carers, giving consideration to our Trust's values and legal frameworks. Confidential storage of artwork made in the group was arranged at the NHS site in a locked cupboard.

Recruitment

Planning an art therapy group outside the NHS setting was a new experience with some challenges. Recruitment for the group took place over a few months as, when NHS funding became available, we needed to use it within a certain time frame while ensuring the group coincided with a suitable exhibition.

We identified potential candidates and they and their parents/carers were seen for initial individual assessment appointments on NHS Trust premises. Because the group would be taking place in a gallery, we needed to discuss with the service users and their parents/carers what risks might exist getting to and from the venue and being in a public gallery at this assessment stage, in order to manage and minimise these.

We recruited two male and six female participants. Presenting difficulties for the young people included disrupted childhood experiences, anger problems, low mood and anxiety.

Attendance

Attendance varied from one to all eight participants attending, with a 'core group' of three young people attending regularly. Sessions were one-and-a-half hours in length from 15:30–17:00 for eight weeks. The group was facilitated by art therapists Whittaker Scott and Michael Fischer and BALTIC artist Lesley-Anne Rose, with additional support from higher assistant psychologist James Blacklock.

Involving parents and carers

As with all CYPS interventions and supports, we aim to involve parents/carers where appropriate. A pre-group meeting was offered at BALTIC to meet the parents/carers of service users together with the art therapists and artist in attendance. The meeting aimed to build an alliance with parents/carers to support attendance at the group, and to consider parents'/carers' views of the suitability of exhibits and facilities their children would be seeing (e.g. they may have viewed some exhibits as potentially disturbing to their child). It offered the opportunity to involve them in refinement of risk assessments, our understanding of particular needs their children had, and any unforeseen transport issues.

An art therapy group with an artist

In the planning stages, Whittaker Scott met with the BALTIC artist Lesley-Anne Rose. Lesley-Anne had past experience of art projects with young people who had mental health issues. The principles of psychodynamic work, working with transference, counter-transference and relationships with therapists within the group were discussed. This raised the issue of how much, alongside a more directive approach, to address possible group processes such as awkwardness, silence and uncertainty. The artist saw these things as potential barriers to be overcome in order to proceed with a productive group, whereas the art therapist perspective saw difficult experience as part of a therapeutic process that can be worked with to help participants gain insights into themselves and relationships with others, benefiting the person in other situations in life. There is a history in some art therapy traditions of favouring spontaneous, non-directive art-making (McNeilly 1983), which can access unconscious material in a way directive work might not.

We settled on a combination of educational/directive and psychodynamic/reflective aspects. The artist would introduce techniques, and limited optional themes would be suggested, and there would also be room for difficult emotions and group processes to be acknowledged in the second part of the group sessions. Greenwood and Layton (1987) provide an example of combining theme-based and psychodynamic approaches in group art therapy with adult outpatients who have a history of psychosis.

Themes and directive activities were chosen by the artist and discussed with the art therapists. After setting some ground rules relating to mutual respect for group members, we reminded participants of the group structure: introductions/brief discussion at the start; looking at the exhibition/being introduced to materials; time for making artwork; a break; looking at artwork, and discussion. In initial sessions, optional themes and technical demonstrations from the artist appeared to reduce the young people's anxiety, providing structure and a starting point for ideas and discussion. These activities were followed by a shorter time towards the end of the sessions for looking at artwork and for discussion facilitated by the art therapists. We were keen to develop this space for reflection and to find a better balance between educational and reflective approaches. This was helped by regular post-group reflections with the artist, further planning, and supervision. In subsequent sessions, while maintaining the basic group structure of both making artwork and having time for showing and discussing it, we developed more flexibility, with some discussion and reflections during the art-making part of the group, extending the art-making time to enable participants to develop and complete work, alongside having some time to look at the exhibition together.

At times, the artist and art therapists also made artwork and we viewed this as therapists modelling the act of trying out materials and ideas to help the group's confidence. There is precedence for art therapists making art during sessions in the literature, specifically Havsteen-Franklin (2014) and Marshall-Tierney (2014). It was important to find and maintain a good functional relationship between the therapists and artist who have different roles and approaches, so that the group would work optimally. This was to give group members an experience of adult figures with different approaches and working together, like a functioning family.

The environment and facilities

While we thought BALTIC would be attractive to young people – a renowned gallery with a wide range of facilities – with the additional option of being part of an exhibition, we were aware that the experience might also be intimidating. Some young people could feel alienated by a gallery/museum environment due to personal, social and cultural attitudes based on each individual's experiences, views and attitudes of their family and social groups, and also the scale of this type of building. However, some participants were familiar with the gallery space either through family or from school visits in the past.

On arrival at BALTIC, the young people were asked to gather on the ground floor. The art therapists and the higher assistant psychologist were waiting to greet them. In retrospect, this situation may have increased self-conscious and anxious feelings, as it was a large space, with members of the public entering and leaving the building. Those attending appeared to get used to this, or chose to come straight up to the studio space. We later wondered whether this meeting arrangement might have been a factor for those who stopped attending, and that suggesting they went straight to the studio space might have been be a better idea.

The studio space was a relatively large space not open to the general public, containing two large tables, cupboards, sinks and equipment and a large wall area opposite to make larger work. Level 2 was accessed by glass-fronted elevators from the main hall below, and toilets were nearby. We were curious about what a wider range of art facilities and materials at BALTIC would bring to the art therapy group's experience. Alongside the more traditional art media associated with NHS site-based art therapy groups, such as pencils, pens, paints, collage and modelling material, the artist Lesley-Anne Rose introduced media such as print-making and animation. There was wariness about trying materials and equipment such as the camera to take part in an animation demonstration but by the end, when group participants had gained confidence, the access to technical materials and the space provided enabled different types of art production – for example, large-scale screen printing – which would have been difficult in art therapy in NHS-based therapy or clinical rooms.

The exhibition and its possible effects on the group

This project linked to 'DEPOT', a major new commission by Dutch artist and filmmaker Fiona Tan. 'DEPOT' made reference to the North East's whaling history, and Tan created an immersive installation especially for the gallery. Drawing on Newcastle's forgotten history as a principal whaling port in England from 1752–1849, 'DEPOT' re-imagined a fairground attraction, 'Jonah, the Giant Whale', a 76-foot long blue whale caught off the coast of Trondheim, Norway. Preserved in formaldehyde, the whale toured Europe from the 1950s to the mid-1970s, exhibited inside the 'longest lorry in the world', before being abandoned in Belgium. Tan rebuilt the vehicle, which spanned almost the entire width of the gallery, and which visitors could climb aboard. Instead of whale remains, the interior contained a cabinet of curiosities, including illustrations, archival photographs, a narwhal tusk and glass models of sea anemones by German glassmakers Leopold and Rudolf Blaschka (BALTIC Centre for Contemporary Art 2015).

Viewing this exhibition allowed the group to go physically out of the group room, the place for making and talking, into larger spaces for looking, which was a different experience to more typical art therapy groups where people remain in the therapy room during the session. We spent some time walking around the exhibition in the first two sessions. We noticed that participants at first seemed shy and withdrawn when back in the studio space, but that the experience of touring this exhibition appeared to help them to grow in confidence – perhaps because the focus was on looking at and talking about the artwork and less on each other. Isserow (2008), Scaife and Brunner (1975) and Huet (2011) describe how the joint attention of a therapist and client on an artwork echoes pre-verbal developmental steps of shared attention, recognition that the other's attention can be directed to something, and the ability to see the other's point of view. Looking at the exhibition together simultaneously reduced the direct focus on each other and created awareness of different knowledge, ideas and perspectives of the other, particularly at the beginning of the group's development.

In a pilot project of art therapy-based organisational consultancy within public healthcare, Huet describes how joint attention allows imaginative space to develop where participants explore possible meanings and stories relating to the artwork they are looking at (Huet 2011). We wondered if walking out of the art room into large spaces to look at unusual artworks would be intimidating or stressful for participants. How would group experience be affected by moving between public space and the more private art room? A possible disadvantage was disruption to group process. However, viewing the art in the gallery context was a key part of what might inspire the young people and it appeared to create no observable problems for group members: participants spoke to the therapists in the exhibition space and in the private studio space. The more emotionally challenging discussion topics happened in the studio space, facilitated by interventions from the therapists, with the participants able to judge for themselves (to some extent at least) what was appropriate to communicate, and in which context.

BALTIC positions gallery assistants, or Crew, in its exhibition spaces, who act as the frontline learning team, greeting and welcoming visitors, offering information about exhibitions, the building and local history, leading public tours and keeping both the artwork and members of the public safe (BALTIC Centre for Contemporary Art 2018). Crew were in a position to add to the group participants' experiences by answering questions about the featured artist and artwork, which group members took advantage of. Crew were not present in the studio space.

An NHS-based art therapy group would involve participants making artwork based on ideas and feelings from their imagination, rather than what they are looking at. In this project, features and themes from the exhibition appeared to develop in group artwork which were then explored in relation to group experience; for example, the BALTIC artist introduced the theme of whale and fish eyes, based on the exhibition, through photocopy and collage imagery as one optional directive in the first session. The artwork made in response built on this initial theme, using this material to express what we felt were strong feelings of people watching and being watched. This might be something expected in a group for young people where feelings of self-consciousness can be heightened, especially at the start of a group, but perhaps the feeling of watching and being watched was intensified by the public gallery experience where art is on display and where the group might also feel scrutinised. The eye motif taken from 'DEPOT' facilitated this expression in the group. The sea themes in 'DEPOT' also appeared influential in group artwork and whale, fish and sea-related imagery became a platform in the young people's artwork to communicate possibly frightening, frightened or painful feelings. The therapists commented on this in relation to how people might be feeling in the group.

Another idea that the art therapists noted from 'DEPOT' by Fiona Tan was the contrast in scale – there were some very large and some very small/delicate exhibits. We felt this may have been reflected in some of the participants' art, which ranged in scale from small, delicate sculptures to large-scale drawings and screen prints.

Outcomes

A combination of qualitative and quantitative measures was used. These were administered by the higher assistant psychologist. The quantitative measures proved problematic, largely due to poor return rates. Outcome measures included Young Person's CORE (Twigg *et al.* 2009) and Beck Youth Inventories (second edition) (Beck *et al.* 2001). The higher assistant psychologist contacted some participants after the group by letter and had conversations with some group members and their parents/carers to gather more qualitative information by phone to help us understand more of the participants' experience by offering the opportunity to speak with someone not directly involved in delivering the group.

Analysis was informal and looked for themes in the artwork, notes and processes. Of those who engaged with the telephone interview, the overall response was that the group was a positive opportunity, the feedback including positive comments about the location, and that it was interesting and enjoyable. Comments were made about feeling encouraged to try something different, art helping with self-expression, and having the opportunity to work with others. Some participants said they would consider returning to exhibitions at BALTIC at a later date, perhaps due to having positive associations as a result of their participation in the group there. A regular theme was the difficulty many had with the timing of sessions, with suggestions of how this could be changed – not having to travel through the city at a busy time, and not during work and school hours. Practicalities of getting to the city centre site were raised as problematic for some. Some participants also described feeling uncomfortable to begin with, but that this lessened as people got to know each other.

We thought about the possibility of having some more structured, guided art activities to facilitate initial engagement of participants. We also wondered about reviewing the timing of the project to a less busy time and increasing the session length from one-and-a-half to two hours. It was worth reviewing which outcome measures were best for this type of project: the Revised Children's Anxiety and Depression Scale (Chorpita *et al.* 2000) addressing low mood and anxiety, or the Rosenberg Self-Esteem Inventory (Rosenberg 1965) measuring self-esteem may be easier to administer than the Beck Youth Inventories, focusing on areas where the group proves helpful. It might be useful to consider if time at the start of the group could be used to complete these.

The group exhibition

The idea of the group having an exhibition was explained during the assessment before the group began, and also included in the consent form. It was explained that the exhibition would not contain names or identifying information.

The BALTIC Art Therapy Project Exhibition opening event took place six weeks after the last group session. The exhibition ran for two months and consisted of a film of still and moving images of artworks that were made in the group, and produced by the artist Lesley-Anne Rose. This was displayed on a wall-mounted TV monitor at BALTIC, with text describing the project. The opening event was attended by two participants and their parents, BALTIC staff, a member of CYPS management, the group artist Lesley-Anne Rose, and art therapists Whittaker Scott and Michael Fischer. Whittaker introduced the film on behalf of the group, putting it into context, and various agencies were thanked for their support. Group participants were asked if they wanted to be part of the speech and introductions, or to remain anonymous. The two young people who attended were happy to be identified as participants of the group but chose not to be part of the speech. They appeared pleased with the show. Their parents praised them and seemed impressed with the exhibit. It is possible that other group members visited the exhibition at other times, but we do not have specific information on this.

A note on artwork made in the group

Discussion with our NTW Trust Information Governance Department and the publishers led us to decide that the consent we had obtained to reproduce participants' artwork was not robust enough for us to use in this publication and it was not appropriate to seek further updated consent.

Conclusions

It is important to note that this pilot project and our ideas and conclusions drawn from it relate specifically to this group of young people, what they made and said, and the feedback obtained from them. The project was limited by a lack of data from outcome measures, but has represented a first step in our understanding of providing art therapy alongside an artist in a gallery setting, and has suggested what we could do differently next time.

The wider range of facilities available and large space to work in at BALTIC compared with NHS site-based art therapy created opportunity for different types of art production, such as large-scale screen printing. However, the wide choice of technical options such as animation and screen printing seemed to make participants wary to begin with. Screen printing was taken up later in the group. The presence of the artist in the art therapy group provided an educational component where the exhibition was described and facilities and materials were demonstrated, and this appeared to help engage young people in what was a relatively short-term project – only eight weeks. There was a learning curve for the facilitators, both art therapists and artist, in developing a flexible balance between educational and reflective aspects in this project.

From the experience of the initial sessions and feedback from participants, more structure, demonstrations of materials and equipment, and directive tasks at the start would be helpful. The exhibition and themes chosen by the artist based on the exhibition might have influenced the artwork made, and some themes in the exhibition, such as sea creatures and an eye motif, appeared to develop in group artwork. These were then explored in relation to the young people's experience in the group. Looking at the exhibition appeared to reduce group anxiety, and helped with a sense of being involved in something together, as well as fostering awareness of different ideas and views that developed in the group sessions. The experience of moving between the art room and the exhibition did not appear to intimidate participants, who largely appeared able to judge what to say where (i.e. not discussing more personal difficulties in the public space). Our view, along with positive feedback from some of the participants, was that the experience of being part of the exhibition at the end of the group project gave a boost to self-esteem and confidence. Young people's ideas and artistic self-expression were viewed by a large number of gallery visitors, which was an exciting prospect for the participants who attended the exhibition, the end result helping to promote mental health awareness to the wider public.

Areas to consider for future projects include how to reduce the drop-out rate. Attendance might have been helped by further liaison with parents/carers and schools in supporting and encouraging attendance. Some families lived outside the city, and so the distance and traffic congestion towards the end of the working day impacted on attendance, with feedback suggesting the location was difficult to get to. Options such as changing the day and time were looked at, as attendance can be affected by school exams and holidays. Arranging transport could also be considered in future. There were different views about the length of the group sessions: for some the one-and-a-half-hour sessions were too long at the beginning of the group, but by the end of the project the time went too quickly, which might have reflected the anxiety participants experienced at the start of the group compared with their more engaged experience later, so we were unsure if changing the length of session based on this alone would be advisable. Arranging for participants to come directly to the studio could reduce the anxiety of waiting on the gallery's ground floor. There might be a way of getting a better completion rate of outcome measures if these were completed immediately after the final session, and some of the outcome measures, while very useful in other contexts, may have been too long for this project. We might get more usable data if we had fewer and simpler outcome measures such as the Rosenberg Self-Esteem Scale (Rosenberg 1965).

One aspect of the group work was to try to identify further support young people might access in CYPS, the community, or both, after the end of the group. A future version of the BALTIC project could offer the opportunity to make links with other activities and projects for young people at BALTIC after the project finished, for instance by offering the option of joining one of the art activity groups run by BALTIC. Overall, while encountering some challenges, this type of collaborative project can be done with potential benefits for both the participants and the organisations involved.

Most importantly, we are grateful to the service users, their parents and carers who took part. What we have learned from the experience and from their feedback has been invaluable in helping plan further collaborations with BALTIC.

Acknowledgements

With thanks to Lesley-Anne Rose, Sarah Bradbury and the staff at BALTIC; our management at Northumberland, Tyne and Wear NHS Trust; James Blacklock, higher assistant psychologist; Simon Critchley and Mandy McCoull from NTW CYPS, who helped with planning; NTW Library and Knowledge Services and Research and Development; Val Huet and the staff at the British Association of Art Therapists. Photograph of BALTIC © Graeme Peacock.

References

Anderson, R. and Darlington, A. (1998) 'Introduction.' In R. Anderson and A. Darlington (eds) *Facing It Out*. London: Gerald Duckworth and Co.

BALTIC Centre for Contemporary Art (2015) *Fiona Tan: DEPOT: Interpretation Guide.*

BALTIC Centre for Contemporary Art (2018) *Learning and Civic Engagement Framework.*

Beck, A.T., Beck, J.S., Jolly, J. and Steer, R. (2001) *Beck Youth Inventories™ – Second Edition for Children and Adolescents Combination Booklet (BYI-II).* Harcourt Assessment (Current version by Pearson).

Chorpita, B., Yim, L., Moffitt, C., Umemoto, L. and Francis, S. (2000) Revised Children's Anxiety and Depression Scale (RCADS). Accessed on 13/6/2019 at www.childfirst.ucla.edu/resources.

Cole, A., Jenefsky, N., Ben-David, S. and Munson, M. (2018) 'Feeling connected and understood: The role of creative arts in engaging young adults in their mental health services.' *Social Work with Groups 41,* 1/ 2, 6–20.

Coles, A. and Harrison, F. (2018) 'Tapping into museums for art psychotherapy: An evaluation of a pilot group for young adults.' *International Journal of Art Therapy 23,* 3, 115–124.

Congreave, E., Kernohan, K., Dorris, L. and Broome, H. (2017) 'The clinical utility of an art psychotherapy group for young people with epilepsy and cognitive comorbidities.' *Developmental Medicine and Child Neurology 59,* 13.

Fry, C.E., Langley, K. and Shelton, K.H. (2017) 'A systematic review of cognitive functioning among young people who have experienced homelessness, foster care or poverty.' *Child Neuropsychology 23,* 8, 907–934.

Greenwood, H. and Layton, G. (1987) 'An out-patient art therapy group.' *Inscape Journal of Art Therapy,* Summer, 12–19.

Havsteen-Franklin, D. (2014) 'Consensus for using an arts-based response in art therapy.' *International Journal of Art Therapy 19,* 3, 107–113.

Higenbottam, W. (2004) 'In her image: A study in art therapy with adolescent females.' *Canadian Art Therapy Association Journal 17,* 1, 10–16.

Huet, V. (2011) 'Art therapy based organisational consultancy: A session at Tate Britain.' *International Journal of Art Therapy 16,* 1, 3–13.

Isserow, J. (2008) 'Looking together: Joint attention in art therapy.' *International Journal of Art Therapy 13,* 1, 34–42.

Jang, H. and Choi, S. (2012) 'Increasing ego-resilience using clay with low SES (Social Economic Status) adolescents in group art therapy.' *The Arts in Psychotherapy 39,* 4, 245–250.

Kaufman, R., Rinehardt, E., Hine, H., Wilkinson, B. *et al.* (2014) 'The effects of a museum art program on the self-concept of children.' *Art Therapy 31,* 3, 118–125.

Linesch, D. (1988) *Adolescent Art Therapy.* New York, NY: Brunner/Mazel Inc.

Linesch, D. (2004) 'Art therapy at the museum of tolerance: Responses to the life and work of Friedl Dicker-Brandeis.' *The Arts in Psychotherapy 31,* 2, 57–66.

Malone, E. (2017) 'The cold truth: Art as fulcrum for recovery in participants and for civic change.' *Journal of Social Work Practice 31,* 2, 227–236.

Marshall-Tierney, A. (2014) 'Making art with and without patients in acute settings.' *International Journal of Art Therapy 19,* 3, 96–106.

McNeilly, G. (1983) 'Directive and non-directive approaches in art therapy.' *The Arts in Psychotherapy 10,* 211–219.

Miller, G. (2012) 'Art Therapy with Adolescents.' In C. Malchiodi (ed.) *Hand Book of Art Therapy.* New York, NY: The Guilford Press.

Pepper Goldsmith, T. and Ben-Simon, N. (2012) 'The Creative Group Experience.' In J. Magagna (ed.) *The Silent Child: Communication Without Words.* London: Karnac Books.

Riley, S. (1999) *Contemporary Art Therapy with Adolescents.* London and Philadelphia, PA: Jessica Kingsley Publishers.

Rosenberg, M. (1965) *Rosenberg Self-Esteem Inventory, Society and the Adolescent Self-Image.* Princeton, NJ: Princeton University Press.

Salom, A. (2015) 'Weaving potential space and acculturation: Art therapy at the museum.' *Journal of Applied Arts and Health 6,* 1, 47–62.

Scaife, M. and Bruner, J. (1975) 'The capacity for joint visual attention in the infant.' *Nature 253,* 265–266.

Schleien, S., Mustonen, T. and Rynders, J. (1995) 'Participation of children with autism and nondisabled peers in a cooperatively structured, community art program.' *Journal of Autism and Developmental Disorders 25,* 397–413.

Silverman, L. (1989) '"Johnny show us the butterflies": The museum as a family therapy tool.' *Marriage and Family Review 13,* 3–4, 131–150.

Slayton, S. (2012) 'Building community as social action: An art therapy group with adolescent males.' *The Arts in Psychotherapy 39,* 3, 179–185.

Stiles, G. and Mermer-Welly, M. (1998) 'Children having children: Art therapy in a community-based early adolescent pregnancy program.' *Art Therapy: Journal of the American Art Therapy Association 15,* 3, 165–176.

Treadon, C., Rosal, M. and Thompson Wylder, V. (2006) 'Opening the doors of art museums for therapeutic purposes.' *The Arts in Psychotherapy 33,* 288–301.

Twigg, E., Barkham, M., Bewick, B.M., Mulhern, B., Connell, J. and Cooper, M. (2009) 'The Young Person's CORE: Development of a brief outcome measure for young people.' *Counselling and Psychotherapy Research: Linking Research with Practice 9,* 3, 160–168.

Waller, D. (1993) *Group Interactive Art Therapy.* London: Routledge.

PART 3

Wider Perspectives

CHAPTER 11

Further Conversations with Rembrandt in Space, Place and Time

How Rembrandt's Self-Portraits and the Gallery Setting Inform the Art Psychotherapy Review

Helen Jury

Introduction

The National Gallery in London represents a major international collection of renowned artworks through the centuries: 'All major traditions of Western European painting are represented, from the artists of late medieval and Renaissance Italy to the French Impressionists' (National Gallery n.d.). For art psychotherapists, it is an invaluable reserve for considering artist-based skills, together with the development of the artist identity (Health and Care Professions Council 2013 (Standards of Proficiency 13.17–13.23), 2016 (Standards of Conduct, Performance and Ethics 3.3)). As a significant collection, it is an important resource for creative thinking in our professional work with client populations, and to expand ideas around innovative clinical practice.

In this chapter, I look at the connection that can be made when viewing artwork in a gallery space and particular artworks on display, and how the possibilities and difficulties around this can inform our understanding of art psychotherapy practice. I consider the two self-portraits by Rembrandt displayed in the National Gallery and how these inform the therapeutic encounter in art psychotherapy in the context of space, place and time – both together and individually – as well as consideration of the art psychotherapy review.

Through visiting the two Rembrandt self-portraits over a long period of time, I developed an internal discourse and journal in response to Rembrandt as painter, and his paintings as an art form and technical construct. The two self-portraits became central to understanding an interpretation of inner self. *Something* caught my eye, held my attention and compelled me to keep returning to view them, to understand them better, and to converse with them. As Berger comments of Rembrandt's work, 'If the pictures convince, they do so because details, parts, emerge and come out to meet the eye' (Berger 2015, p.143). Central to my understanding is the challenge of holding in mind and keeping each portrait in vision internally, 'giving rise to thoughts concerning the temporal, mental and emotional space we experience and occupy when we hold in mind the sense of artwork created; whether our own, that of another artist, or that of the client' (Jury 2012).

Together with these thoughts – and essential to consider – was the challenge of the impossibility of viewing the two Rembrandt portraits together, as they were in different rooms within the National Gallery. This challenge is compared to the significance of referencing the diverse artworks of any and all types that are created during art psychotherapy by a client; art made in separate sessions as part of the exploratory, clinical representation and record of the client's sense of self. This, the art psychotherapist holds in mind both together and singly, as part of the total collective of the therapeutic artwork. The capacity to recall the visual significance of a piece of artwork alongside the non-verbal material generated through its making is unique to art psychotherapy in that the original, concrete object remains to prompt this process. All intervention with materials is considered confidential clinical material for the client to return to and to access at any point in the therapy, which aids this.

These factors inform the chapter, connecting with the distinct ages and stages of life when Rembrandt painted each portrait: 34 and 63. This is considered in relation to time, place and space and the relevance to the potential span of art psychotherapy sessions, alongside implications of any changes that might take place for the client circumstantially, environmentally, and as a result of therapeutic engagement, which in turn become part of the complete art psychotherapy experience.

The Rembrandt self-portraits

Rembrandt painted over 80 self-portraits. He was unafraid of self-reflection and self-examination, fascinated by depicting an inner self and inner state. Wieseman (2014) suggests of Rembrandt's later work that a demonstration of passion and extrovert nature in his early years gave way later to 'an intensive investigation of the inner life of his subjects' (p.42) and as a consequence his self-portraits:

> became more inwardly directed and subtly, profoundly expressive...he turned his experienced and intensely inquisitive eye, mind and hand to the consideration of his own ageing flesh, the emotional onslaughts of his tumultuous personal life...venturing bold experiments in presentation. (p.42)

Study the two Rembrandt portraits in the National Gallery for any length of time and it becomes apparent that although by the same artist, they are distinct in period, style, image and mood. Berger compares the divergent aspects of 'Rembrandt and Saskia in the Parable of the Prodigal Son' c.1635, and 'Rembrandt, Self-portrait at the age of 63', stating that 'all has gone except a sense of the question of existence, of existence as a question. And the painter in him who is both more and less than the old man, has found the means to express just that' (Berger 2015, p.142). The two self-portraits in the National Gallery are similarly intertwined: created by the same artist, the same man painting his own image in different eras. Twenty-nine years separate these self-representations, with intervening life experience and events. The person represented is the same, yet the mood and character depicted are different – they are 'states of mind apart' (Jury 2012). When working with clients in art psychotherapy, we notice this sense of increased self-reflection depicted in the artwork, as the therapeutic process becomes assimilated and psychological material is possible to explore in greater depth.

To see all of Rembrandt's self-portraits together would be a captivating prospect: 80-plus depictions of self together in one room, one gallery. A collective expression would be evident, as in a retrospective of any artist's work. But perhaps precisely because we *cannot* always see artworks together, we learn to consider the mood and mental and emotional state of the artist that leads to investment of self at any specific point in time and space in an artwork – in Rembrandt's case, in each self-portrait.

What visual conversation would be possible if we could see these two National Gallery self-portraits side by side? We can anticipate what we might learn from the visual contraction of the intervening years in which they were created; the consideration of the two self-portraits and all depicted life experience together, in one particular point in time. Arguably, this is what we perceive in the art psychotherapy review where personal expression in artwork made over a period of time comes together; a totality of experiences juxtaposed in one place, in one time frame. In my journal I wrote:

> I can either mirror, or alter the dimension I am exploring, by choosing to consider the portraits separately, or I can bring them together [through photography]. Bringing them together for joint viewing would alter one state of mind: that of the absence of physical comparison. If the two paintings are together, it temporarily reverses the tension that 'holding in mind' the two together might offer. The artwork, in the process of being made, creates its own impetus: the reference being the time and space in which it was created. The 'holding space' becomes the time between sessions and/or a potential review, a revisiting of the artwork. (Jury 2012, annotated)

The role of the portrait

The two paintings are of interest due to the context in which Rembrandt was painting, and how his approach to them and view of his own self was influenced. Berger remarks on Rembrandt's moral stance and comments that he showed an interest in the ethical frame, 'he was the first artist to take the tragic isolation of the individual as his recurring theme, just as he was the first great artist to experience a comparable alienation from his own society' (Berger 2015, p.139). Rembrandt appeals because we understand that the communication of empathy through his art depicts the state and living conditions of others, as well as his understanding of what it meant to be ostracised by society through personal life events. He can be said to reflect back to us what we are aware of in our own lives.

Portraits mirror the self and other, allowing the viewer to re/consider and question senses of identity and self. Carr and Hancock (2017) describe Wright's ideas on mirroring and attunement in portraiture and self-identities, stating that the painting's surface is 'derivative, or "analogue" of the mother's expressive face in infancy', acting as 'a responsive and mirroring extension of the self' or 'surrogate adaptive mother' (p.8). Mirroring and attunement as developed by Stern (1985) are important processes in the healthy maturation of the infant in communication and socialisation through learned responses that are first experienced between baby and caregiver. This becomes refined and developed through extended communication with the outside world, in to adulthood. The idea is demonstrated in Berger's exploration of sense of self as reflected back through self-portraiture:

> A painter can draw his left hand as if it belonged to somebody else. Using two mirrors he can draw his own profile as if observing a stranger. But when he looks straight into a mirror, he is caught in a trap: his reaction to the face he is seeing changes that face. Or, to put it in another way, that face can offer itself something it likes or loves. (Berger 2015, p.151)

Carr (2014) talks of co-creation of a client's portrait in art psychotherapy where 'the revisioning process and the manifestation of aspects of self-identity within externalised objects' allow for difficult feelings to be uncovered and explored 'so that they can be held, contained, moved, worked on and reflected upon' (p.18). The portrait is therefore a powerful medium of exploration of inner self and self-in-relation-to-other, at any point in time.

The review in art psychotherapy process

Each piece of artwork produced by the client in art psychotherapy is unique. Whether a copy of another artwork, diagrammatic image, or form to express mood or feeling, it communicates an internalised sense of self felt and conceived at a particular point in time, in a particular session, framed in the context of the overall therapeutic process. Art psychotherapists are trained to work with this expression and to prize the role of artwork in recovery. Arnheim suggests that 'art therapists must use *all* resources and information in an investigative manner such that the image is understood as more than just an amalgamation of parts' (cited in Curtis 2011, p.2). As such, the body of reviewed artwork possesses a distinct status and function, demonstrating a unique picture of the therapeutic work in hand. As Prokofiev (2013) states of the client's participation in the review, 'it allows the checking and cross referencing of memory and meaning' (p.4).

The review offers client and art psychotherapist an opportunity to work across a combined time and experience span that is created between the original making of the artwork and its re-evaluation in the review. It allows for significant reconsideration, plus possibility for new meaning-making. Curtis (2011) suggests that 'when clients make and view their art, it is an active and dynamic process that engages the whole person' (p.1) through 'visual perception as an active process involving the whole person who dynamically constructs meaning'. Here, the therapist focuses on the artwork, 'attending to and repeatedly returning to the art's sensory and formal qualities to look for meaning' (*ibid.*, pp.9–10). Drawing on Leclerc and Acosta, Curtis suggests that the experience goes beyond both the seen or interpreted and cannot be defined, but it implicates 'the observer's whole, personal self' (*ibid.*, p.10). The art psychotherapist is integral and contributory to sense-making in the review, a viewpoint endorsed by Prokofiev (2013), who states that it 'helps to isolate and foreground the narrative of the art making', describing Schaverien's analysis of the chronology of the reviewed work as an opportunity to 'explore meaning in a new context and observe where change occurs with the intention of comparing it to psychological change or improvements' (p.2).

The art psychotherapist holds distinct strands of client experience, response and history. Ellis (2008) recognises that this encompassing role allows for 'the socio-historical aspects of temporality' that 'can contribute to a richer and more complex understanding of an individual's experience' (p.156). The capacity of the art psychotherapist to co-construct a meaning around artworks with the client is a skill crucial for the integration of therapeutic benefit and allows the client's presentation and engagement up to this point to be held in mind. Coles (2014) reflects this view in her description of 'therapeutic presence as a spatial "ground" for what happens within therapy' which facilitates 'creating a rich, textural "felt" presence which is finely adjusted in response to the client' (p.80). How this is done is important; as Huss suggests, 'art therapists often naturally and unthinkingly do integrate different ways of seeing client art' but 'how this integration occurs, and what exactly is integrated, has yet to be articulated' (Huss cited in Curtis 2011, p.10). This is also explored through the counter-transference response described by Acosta as 'the knowledge one knows without knowing one knows it' (cited in Curtis 2011, p.10).

Clinical context

Reflecting on the circumstantial impossibility of viewing the two Rembrandt self-portraits together at the same time in the National Gallery helps us understand more about the sum of individual, including apparently unrelated, artworks created on different occasions in art psychotherapy. How artworks are seen together in the review provides opportunity for distinct and new understanding. Each separate artwork 'talks' to the others when spread out or 'galleried' around the room and the overall therapeutic journey is laid out for viewing through this visual lens of artwork. A sense of passage of time and experience in therapy can be contemplated and witnessed here, in the review.

Artwork might be created in one session, or it can be returned to and even developed over a period of time. It might be reconsidered, and the original spur for creating it revisited. It can depict a difficult period for the client, or be a visual representation of unarticulated thoughts and feelings. Artwork is sometimes discounted by the client as unimportant or irrelevant, or it is forgotten, and sometimes the content and its significance within therapy overall is a surprise in the review. Reassessment of the subject matter might be difficult, or there might be reconciliation and resolution of experiences, thoughts and feelings. However, there is also opportunity for integration with fresh thoughts and ideas about the original difficulty being revealed. Although artwork often retains challenging or evocative feelings, the review can offer a unique opportunity for exploration with the experiences of sessions leading up to that point helping to clarify greater understanding. Significant pieces of artwork are now accompanied, couched, embedded, and sometimes explained, through being grouped together when reviewed. The review can be consolidating and informative in function, and holds a particular place in the art psychotherapy process.

The implication of viewing all the artwork together, with its associated art-making and process in space, place and time, is present alongside the recollection of each piece made within that session. The viewer plays an important role too, as artist-art psychotherapist. Townsend (2013) suggests optimisation of psychological space generated by the artist is important in order to create artwork, and proposes that the viewer also needs ideal conditions to truly benefit from the artwork presented in order to be able 'to enter into a relationship with it' and thereby 'perhaps imbue the work with his or her own inner experience' (p.183). Acknowledging that not all artwork is viewed within a gallery setting, she continues 'wherever it is seen, if it is successful, the surroundings contribute to the experience, enabling the viewer to enter his or her own internal space' (*ibid.*, p.183). Baker (2009) supports this, citing Dufrenne who suggests that 'artwork and spectator not be considered as isolated entities, but as mutually invested in one another, so that to understand the work of art, it is necessary to study the aesthetic experience constituted by the intimate relationship between its subject and object' (p.18).

The right conditions in the review allow the client-viewer to assimilate the experience and nurture a capacity to creatively process what is witnessed. The context becomes 'a place set apart from everyday life', where the boundaries of art psychotherapy space take on significance in facilitating the review, and this 'in turn informs subsequent art-making, as well as [further] therapeutic interaction' (Jury 2012). Art psychotherapy involves close emotional and personal examination, allowing for new appraisal of the self together with an opportunity for psychological insight into processes that were not necessarily apparent or possible to consider prior to the review, thereby effecting advancement of self-discovery. In the review, previous clinical processes and artwork are brought together *en masse*. For clients, this experience can be both overawing and revelatory, according to 'Simone', a woman in her 40s in long-term art psychotherapy, who described the experience of the interim review as being as if the inner self was exposed, allowing recollection of issues explored, and where the safe environment of the therapeutic space became vitally important. The time for the interim review session drawing to a close, she found this stage difficult, and she was surprised at how emotional she felt. She paused, appearing uninclined to physically move and finish the sessions, affected by the experience and unexpectedly caught unawares.

Time, space and process

Time as process in art psychotherapy has different frames in relation to artwork and therapeutic intervention. First, there is the time *in* which the artwork is made – the external frame and circumstances of a client's life at a particular time that inspire particular artwork and use of materials. There is the time *at* which it is made – the conscious or unconscious point at which it occurs for the client in therapy, with all the reference it will contain of the client's revealed experience. Then there is *future* time, unexplored and unrevealed, that will be significant for the client. These time structures relating to artwork and process are intrinsically held in mind by therapist and client, including how this will feed back in to clinical work.

The *how* of artwork made by the client and retained in the mind of client and therapist, alongside what space and relevance it holds, is important in therapy. Why does one piece of artwork remain in mind rather than another? What determines the importance of one piece of artwork over another, for either client or therapist?

What is it that makes us notice a particular artwork in relation to clinical material expressed, rather than another? Similarly, what is it that draws us to view one artist's work in a gallery, rather than that of another artist? These are questions that are embedded in the practice of art psychotherapy and worked with through verbalised thoughts and feelings in conjunction with the client. There is also the more complex understanding of the mental space that the artwork occupies when seen anew at the review. At this point it is literally *re*viewed and has the potential to take on a different significance for the client, according to their perception of what particular meaning the whole body of artwork holds in this new context. This can involve the feelings it originally evoked on making, what inspired its creation, and what new thoughts or feelings are activated and initiated on *re*viewing it. It might be ignored, the previously potent feelings contained within it disallowed and disavowed, or these latter might reappear in future sessions.

When reviewing her artwork after a year of being in therapy, Simone found an exploration of the artwork all in one place at one time overpowering, with its experience of the levelling of temporal boundaries. The concentration of artwork collapsed time, place and feelings, condensed in one here-and-now moment, and this felt almost overwhelming to her. She sat quietly before considering what the exploration of the body of artwork meant to her. It appeared that each of the artworks became significant in three ways:

- What it had meant at the time of making, and frames of reference at that particular point in time.
- What it meant now in relation to a sense of progression/moving on/understanding where she had been, and the latent power and emotional content it still held.
- Its place among the rest of the artwork, in consideration of the body of work as a whole; what it reflected of the journey that she had been on or still felt herself to be on.

Simone found that the artwork as individual pieces, and as a collection, condensed time and space so that the images were not only a collection, but a mass, each separately and together representing states of mind, thoughts and emotions that were uncovered and then partially or wholly forgotten, or that were re-addressed and became subdued and less troubling. She was surprised, and initially overcome by her internal response and the reminder of feelings made tangible through the artwork. This subsequently allowed her to construct her previous experience in the context of the fresh view and structure of the review: at the same time both time-*less* and time-*laden*.

Reflecting on how artwork produced in art psychotherapy is kept in mind through space, time, and in relation to the emotional frame in which it was made (and how it might be recalled in particular sessions by the art psychotherapist who holds it in mind for the client in therapy), is integral to the overall frame of the therapy work taking place. How a piece of artwork is retained through time in the mind of the art psychotherapist, session by session, both when it was created and how, and what it represents of the feelings, thoughts and experiences as communicated by the client in the session – all these elements become fundamental to the construct and efficacy of art psychotherapy practice. While the entirety of the work is kept in mind by the art psychotherapist clinically, the visual, emotional and therapeutic impact of the *collective* view of the client's artwork witnessed in the review is experienced and worked with by *both* the art psychotherapist and the client together, at the same point in time. This subsequently informs future therapy.

It is important to consider what bringing together the entirety of the client's artwork in one space signifies, as well as the frequency of reviews and the implications of this. When reviewing her artwork, 'Ursula', a young woman in ongoing art psychotherapy, found in her initial review that it was unexpectedly powerful for various reasons:

- The concrete nature and *actuality* of the artwork displayed.
- The juxtaposed sense of timing inherent in all the pieces laid out together for viewing.
- The fact that material explored through the artwork in one particular session might not be explored verbally until some sessions later, or never referred to again.

For Ursula, in the review, memories and a recall of events merged and formed new realisations, propelling the therapeutic process into another psychological space on which to reflect. Time and unconscious material slipped and slid over one another causing areas of explored material to join up, sometimes to make greater and more impactful sense, and sometimes to allow new revelation of meaning. Experiences and memories took on different resonances, surging up in unexpected juxtaposition and connectedness to one another and consequently becoming even more powerful in affect.

The internal dialogic space

> [T]he spectator intercepts (overhears) dialogues between parts gone adrift, and these dialogues are so faithful to a corporeal experience that they speak to something everybody carries within them. Before his art, the spectator's body remembers its own inner experience. (Berger 2015, p.145)

When writing my journal, I asked, 'How can we hold the two frames of reference and the experience of viewing each artwork in the same space?' (Jury 2012). I travelled back and forth between the two Rembrandt self-portraits to hold in mind one, while trying to catch a living connection with the other. Each time, the influence of a refreshed review of the other interrupted my flow of thought and visual memory. This brings into question what happens when we hold in mind the client's artwork – exactly how do we hold each separate piece and its significance in mind? How does each individual piece of viewed artwork influence consideration of every subsequent piece of artwork made by the client? Furthermore, how does the client, involved as they are in the production of artwork on a regular basis in sessions, hold in mind each piece of artwork created over time, plus process the personal significance of each and the influence it might have on future artwork and therapy? Curtis (2011) describes how 'people construct meaning given different levels of experience with imagery', applying 'feelings' and 'intuition' among other skills to understand 'meaning as open to reinterpretation', that they 'continually return to the image to contemplate new meaning, synthesize ideas, and justify their hypotheses through visual evidence' (p.10). This is the objective, spectator-art-psychotherapist view, but there is also the subjective, personal element that inspires thinking and feeling, when the piece of artwork being studied by the client is artwork of the client's own creation.

Each of us maintains internal conversations and dialogues not only on a non-verbal level through the artwork we create, but through ongoing narrative via thoughts concerning the influence of life events, relationships, imagined fantasies. These dialogues relate to our worldview and our negotiation of the actual world around us. The therapeutic relationship depends on an awareness and preparedness by both therapist and client to reach across and within different understandings of internal conversations and world observations, to form a common dialogue with the client's internal worlds and constructs. This, in association with the processing and production of any artwork in art psychotherapy, allows for development of further thought and articulation of the client's sense of reality of self, and ultimately a sense-making of experience and events in the client's life.

As art psychotherapists, using visual and verbal journalling helps us maintain a fluid articulation of thought and feeling around engagement with art processes through contact with art materials and creation of our own artwork and in viewing and contemplating the artwork of others, both artists and clients. It allows us space to challenge ourselves in meaning-making about external events and circumstances and to interrogate previously accepted views of the world. It helps consideration of alternative viewpoints and ways of articulating and expressing ideas. With the client who tears the corrugation from the surface of the cardboard and uses it to print texturally, or who bleeds ink and oil together on paper to make an emulsive swirl, both these processes might challenge our previously accepted ways of thinking about art practices and the function of materials as the 'artist-art psychotherapist'. We might not notice these processes nor see them as significant if we have not broadened our own understanding of techniques that other artists employ in expression making, or viewed their work in galleries and museums. Viewing the work, techniques and practice of others expands our knowledge, skills and understanding of the potential of art practice, enlightening and informing us of clients' internal processes and unconscious thoughts. Museum and art gallery exhibits that challenge our ways of seeing and conceptualising art, and the use of materials as art, are important to enable us to appreciate versatility of mediums and form, and their usage. Destruction of work by a client, with the potential *absence-but-presence* of the artwork that is felt and at times acknowledged in the review (where although it cannot be seen, the absence is notable), can be an important reminder of the relevance of absent psychological material in therapy. This further informs us about the psychological space clients occupy and their functioning, explored in the next section via the Rembrandt portraits.

Absence: out of sight, out of mind?

During my conversations with Rembrandt, one of the self-portraits from the National Gallery went out on loan and was no longer possible to view. A brief note replaced the portrait, stating it had gone on tour and would return at some future date. I was indignant and felt acutely the sense of absence in relation to the corresponding self-portrait in the next room. Suddenly, there was the need to 'keep in mind' the missing portrait until it returned at some unknown date, along with the significance of absence, as well as any difficulty on my part in trying to recall the portrait meanwhile. I was struck that in a similar way, the client artwork remains out of sight but accessible to the client each session. The fact that the artwork is hypothetically available for viewing in any art psychotherapy session in a drawer, box, folder or similar, provides a parallel link in therapy, sustaining hope and constancy through a latent contract of future viewing. The stored artwork maintains a constant and concrete connection and positive reminder, an unformed sense of self, continually exploring and constructing, in therapy. It is a reminder of what has been explored in the safe environment of the therapeutic space, kept constant by the therapist and evidenced in the accessible artwork psychically present each session. How then, would the client feel if artwork went missing, was not available to view at any particular point, in the same way as the Rembrandt had gone walkabout? This could engender a sense of attack and insecurity regarding the therapeutic engagement. In this case, I was rationally aware that the National Gallery would eventually return the Rembrandt self-portrait to its location. But the attachment I had formed to it presumed an unquestioning expectation of its continued presence for me, whenever I might choose to view it.

Through the process of reviewing artwork in art psychotherapy there is unconscious awareness of the artwork as part of a larger sense of the client's trajectory in therapy: the linear process and narrative of whole life experience. In the journal, I noted:

> What do *I* bring to each Rembrandt self-portrait, and what do *I* take away? I am reminded of my own mortality. I am between the ages at which the paintings were made and can therefore be wise to a youthful Rembrandt, while mindful that I reject a certain knowledge of mortality I see in Rembrandt's later portrait, a *'he-knows-something-I-don't-and-I-don't-want-to-know'* that informs me he is aware of not only demise and death per se, but quite possibly his own. He died a year after it was painted. (Jury 2012)

Death as implicit in living is evident just as the ending is apparent at the beginning of therapy, and our conscious awareness of death and how we interact with the concept unconsciously dictates how we understand our relationship with time. Ellis (2008) emphasises the importance of this aspect of temporality through 'the importance of the fact of our death which is already inescapably present for us on the horizon of our lives' (p.177), and the significance of this in work with clients alongside consideration of endings in therapy. She goes on to explore age in relation to self-exploration, citing Reggiori who maintains that 'while aging unavoidably and invariably brings about a deterioration in some capacities, it may also enable increased playfulness and creativity' (*ibid.*, p.178). I felt this to be apparent in the Rembrandt portraits, mixed with reckoning and assimilated life experience, the older Rembrandt holding in mind the younger self depicted in the next room in the National Gallery.

Similarly, the artwork of the client represents the life story of the span of therapy, and has a beginning which we can see, and which is witnessed, and an end that can still only be supposed during interim reviews. The ending of the therapy work becomes implicitly present in the interim review and is a type of witnessing of death: a landmark pointer in the life of the therapy. Some clients manifest this when *re*viewing the artwork, becoming overwhelmed by what has gone before, and by implication, understanding the potential of what might be to come. While it is possible to recall how the artwork has come about through the sessions up to that point, there is no way of the client being able to anticipate what the final accumulation of artwork will represent in terms of psychological material, nor the events and life experience that will have happened by the next, or even final, review of the work.

The two Rembrandt self-portraits can be used to understand something further here. The later Rembrandt portrait in the National Gallery captures a sense of an afterlife of the picture that can only be surmised at this point. At this stage, Rembrandt did not have experience of the whole, or entirety, of his life, as it had not been completed. Perhaps we can assume he understood that the portraits he had painted would continue to have an individual presence through future existence when he, as the artist, did not. I feel he played with this idea in his portraiture: a concrete understanding of here-and-now representation within the unknown, potentiated future. Berger corroborates this idea when discussing Rembrandt's later works, saying that 'the late Rembrandt self-portraits contain or embody a paradox: they are clearly about old age, yet they address the future. They assume something coming towards them apart from Death' (Berger 2015, p.149).

Similarly, the artwork the client produces in sessions becomes a *memento mori*. By the tangible nature of its existence, it is a reminder of mortality – it exists, but could just as easily not. The artwork will continue in its 'here-and-now' state into the future, occupying present space in future and past contexts simultaneously, as long as it is kept and viewed anew. In the review, we are reminded of the hidden future capacity of psychological material, as yet unwitnessed and unexpressed in artwork form. Although not yet experienced, its future possibility is glimpsed in the context of the final review, spanning as it does all time frames including, implicitly, 'what is to come'. The client can have no knowledge of what is to come in terms of life and therapeutic experience, but there is portent in the review – the sense of linear time through creation of artwork also creates possibility of a future. When Simone reviewed her artwork, she also recognised possibility for fragmentation that she feared might come about if she explored too much through the art materials. She valued creativity very highly, but feared the sense of her creative self being overcome by the significance of what she created in the context of the art psychotherapy time span available. We were able to explore how she might cope in the context of the containing environment. This was an important discovery in her therapy of newfound capacity.

While there might be a glimpse of future self towards the end of therapy when the final review of artwork has happened, and the artwork has been collected up and removed from the therapy room, another knowledge of the psychological process also becomes possible: the cumulative effect of the whole. Here, art-making process, verbal exploration, and *re*viewing of the physical artwork begin to work together. The particular elements of the therapeutic experience sift down to validate the beneficial attributes. These are eventually internalised by the client and inform a sense of self in relation to psychological material and within an overview of their experience. In conversation about Berger's analysis of Rembrandt's works, Riach states:

> What Berger draws our attention to in the later Rembrandt self-portrait is a quality of human sympathy untainted by self-pity. It's one of the most difficult, but necessary things...a remembering accompanies the disintegration... And when we look at Rembrandt...what gives us authority and encouragement comes through, something essential, part of that recognition of what tragedy is. In Berger's phrase, that quality of inspiration is what all art delivers: the intimation of our own potential. (Riach and Moffat 2017)

The supervisory nature of reflective space

Regularly viewing the works of artists in galleries, museums, exhibitions and performances is an investment in both artist and art psychotherapist self, as explored previously. Coles refers to the need for the therapist to 'be in a state of heightened artistic sensitivity' (2014, p.80) to understand the different levels and degrees of expression of the client. Through reflection and exploration of works of artists and their handling of materials and ideas, we understand more not only the potential of materials, their scope and divergent uses, but also styles and symbolism. We come to understand a greater pictorial representation of a worldview, helping us acknowledge clients' states of mind. Reflection and contemplation of art psychotherapy practice through supervision are essential properties of clinical work, to benefit and maintain professional insight and sensitivity. Professional art psychotherapy supervision allows the supervisee to recall the artwork of the client through discussion to give space and opportunity for enriched reflective understanding, sometimes through reverie. During supervision, the supervisee can non-judgementally inhabit a contemplative and critical space where artwork and artwork process are jointly considered in relation to the client's presentation and presiding history. Here, the supervisee can work with specific artwork or refer to all artwork and psychological material, along with the time span they encompass, truncating time and gaining an overview. Unless otherwise consciously arranged, there is no other opportunity to overview, review, or work back and forth through all the artwork between sessions, apart from here, within supervision. However, this takes place for art psychotherapist and supervisor alone within the supervision space, holding a distinct function overall in the therapeutic context – the client is not physically present to respond or partake, but is recalled, conjured up, by the art psychotherapist.

The powerful and collective totality of viewing individual pieces of artwork in relation to one another, and/or as a whole body of work, is therefore not available to either client or therapist until a review. In the review, the experience is *clinically* reflective and is within the context of the art psychotherapy process, whereas in supervision, reviewing artwork is a professional consultation, an opportunity for the professional exploration of ideas by the therapist with an experienced colleague.

Conclusion

The art psychotherapy review is an opportunity for new connections and interconnections between thoughts, feelings, ideas and incidents previously hidden or unrealised to be uncovered. Had the artwork not been seen collectively as a whole, in its entirety and each artwork in relation to the other, these meanings might have remained hidden. New implications become apparent and re-examined as unconscious material is connected between work that was sometimes produced weeks or months apart, alongside the recalled process of making the art piece. The experience of the review can seem the equivalent of an exhibition's worth of artwork (corresponding to all the 80-plus Rembrandt self-portraits together, perhaps?) viewed in the boundaried construct and space of one art psychotherapy session. It can be the self, laid bare. It becomes the *in the moment* summation of thought and feelings; internalised and externalised experience brought together with all the here and now, in the present, transferential feelings and emotional responses that might occur within this experience. Time shortens and contracts, sometimes even appearing to stop when the entire scope of art psychotherapy sessions is laid out and made apparent through the artwork. Time telescopes and individual sessions lose longitudinal character with the artwork displayed in *one* space, at *one* time, and on *one* occasion – that of the review. The effect that it can have for the client, as they see their symbolic history displayed before them – feelings and thoughts, emotions and experience, all revealed – cannot be undone, and can lead to a sense of profound affect. As Ellis (2008) says, 'every moment produces a new moment for a different context of experience' (p.154).

And then I revisit the National Gallery to find that there has been a reorganisation. The gallery space has been repainted and the Rembrandts now appear together in one room. Among these, Rembrandt aged 63 appears to sympathetically consider his younger counterpart aged 34 across the gallery space; the younger version making sense, or not, of his future counterpart. I still cannot hold them both in view at the same time, even if I stand in the middle of the gallery and use peripheral vision, and so, tantalisingly, they cannot co-exist in the same span and moment. But the *awareness* of them being there together in that same space, provides a different viewpoint and a new consideration that is similar to a periodic review of clients' artwork, where the work is seen together and a new vision is created, but then returns to the folder/box/cupboard/storage. What remains is the knowledge of the work having been together collectively; the memory and the effect of each piece on the other and the subsequent, unseen mental process continuing work. The other Rembrandt works surrounding the self-portraits in the gallery and accompanying and informing them provide additional reference, context, information and knowledge – this is a new level discovered.

Acknowledgements

Fully informed consent has been given for all clinical work cited in this chapter for the purposes of research and publication. All contributions have been anonymised and any identifying factors removed. Sincere thanks and appreciation go to those who have contributed and advanced the thinking around the topics explored.

References

Baker, J. (2009) *The Tactile Eye: Touch and the Cinematic Experience*. London, Berkeley and Los Angeles: University of California Press.

Berger, J. (2015) *Portraits: John Berger on Artists*. London and New York, NY: Verso.

Carr, S. (2014) 'Revisioning self-identity: The role of portraits, neuroscience and the art of the therapist's "3rd hand".' *International Journal of Art Therapy 19*, 2, 54–70.

Carr, S. and Hancock, S. (2017) 'Healing the inner child through portrait therapy: Illness, identity and childhood trauma.' *International Journal of Art Therapy 22*, 1, 8–21.

Coles, A. (2014) '"Being Time": An exploration of personal experiences of time and implications for art psychotherapy practice.' *International Journal of Art Therapy 19*, 2, 71–81.

Curtis, E.K. (2011) 'Understanding client imagery in art therapy.' *Journal of Clinical Art Therapy 1*, 1, 9–15.

Ellis, M.L. (2008) *Time in Practice: Analytical Perspectives on the Times of Our Lives*. London: Karnac Books.

Health and Care Professions Council (HCPC) (2013) *Standards of Proficiency for Arts Therapists*. London: HCPC. Accessed on 31/10/18 at www.hcpc-uk.org/standards/standards-of-proficiency/arts-therapists.

Health and Care Professions Council (HCPC) (2016) *Standards of Conduct, Performance and Ethics*. London: HCPC. Accessed on 28/6/18 at www.hcpc-uk.org/aboutregistration/standards.

Jury, H. (2012 onwards) *Conversations with Rembrandt*. [Personal journal, unpublished].

Prokofiev, F. (2013) 'Allowing the artwork to speak: The use of a visual display as research method in a retrospective study of four years' artwork in art therapy with a four-year-old boy.' *ATOL: Art Therapy Online 4*, 1, 1–5.

Riach, A. and Moffat, A. (2017) 'In praise of John Berger Part Two: Scratching beneath the surface of art's canvas.' *The National Scot News* (24/2/17). Accessed on 24/2/17 at www.thenational.scot/news/15114086.in_praise_of_john_berger_part_two__scratching_beneath_the_surface_of_art___s_canvas.

Stern, D. (1985) *The Interpersonal World of the Infant*. New York, NY: Basic Books.

The National Gallery website (n.d) Accessed on 5/1/18 at www.nationalgallery.org.uk/paintings/collection-overview.

Townsend, P. (2013) 'Making Space.' In A. Kuhn (ed.) *Little Madnesses: Winnicott, Transitional Phenomena and Cultural Experience*. London and New York, NY: I.B. Tauris.

Wieseman, M.E. (2014) 'Rembrandt: The Late Self-Portraits.' In The National Gallery *Rembrandt: The Late Works*. Exhibition catalogue. London: The National Gallery.

CHAPTER 12

Temporary, Portable and Virtual

Making Galleries on the France–UK Border at Calais

Miriam Usiskin, Bobby Lloyd and Naomi Press

Introduction

This chapter proposes an innovative, even radical, approach to using arts-based psychosocial groups and curation as part of crisis support for refugees living in transit on the France–UK border at Calais and facing ongoing exposure to hostility and homelessness. It is delivered by a core team of art therapists from Art Refuge UK, and the potential spaces and art media used within this particular humanitarian setting become sites for intercultural and social connections, imagination and psychological survival. At times, they also become galleries – temporary, portable and virtual.

Refugees, volunteers, and workers from other organisations as well as ourselves as artists and art therapists make art alongside one another in diverse group settings which have included portacabins, tent studios, community centres, a day centre, a safe house, and a roadside distribution point. The work described here does not form part of clinical treatment as those we work with are neither patients nor clients. The settings are accessed by refugees on a drop-in basis, and people are free to join our groups for as long or short a time as they so wish.

Art installation, a box of postcards, a large map and the use of social media are discussed due to their particular relevance to the theme of this book. The photographs included were taken on our mobile phones by or alongside those we work with. We have chosen to curate this chapter thematically rather than in a linear way so as to reflect the complexity and richness of the work.

Context

Established in 2006, Art Refuge UK is a small, robust charity that offers specialist and imaginative art and art therapy spaces to people displaced due to war, persecution and poverty, including unaccompanied minors. Our work largely takes place through groups, and currently operates in London, Bristol and northern France. Art Refuge UK works in close partnership with local government and non-government organisations (NGOs) that provide infrastructure, local knowledge and mutual support, to ensure interventions are adapted and appropriate to each social, political and cultural context, and to enable sustainable working.

In September 2015, a small team of art therapists began offering psychological support on behalf of Art Refuge UK in the large makeshift refugee camp known as 'The Jungle' in Calais, northern France. To put numbers into context, around one million migrants and refugees arrived in Europe in 2015, while numbers at the border in Calais reached their height of around 10,000 people towards autumn 2016 (Stanton and Welander 2016). We worked with unaccompanied minors and adults, mostly fleeing war and persecution from North Africa and the Middle East, the majority risking their lives to get across the English Channel to claim asylum in the UK where many have family connections and/or a legal right to asylum.

In the camp, we delivered our work across two days each week in partnership with our French partners Médecins du Monde and Médecins Sans Frontières within their psychosocial programmes. Ours was one of the few services to offer a psychological space open to all, regardless of ethnicity, culture, age or gender. Following the camp population's eviction and its razing to the ground in October 2016, we have worked in various settings alongside the French associations Secours Catholique and Médecins du Monde, adapting our work to suit the changing context and needs.

Our team is made up of experienced UK Health and Care Professions Council registered art therapists who are also practising artists. Keeping the team small and focused allows us to remain steady in face of the significant challenges we encounter while working in this unique context. Team members work in rotation, never alone, with one core member acting as the cultural carrier from week to week, passing on knowledge, information and nuances from the previous week's work. Consistency of delivery is essential to allow for trust and knowledge accumulation to build, both within the work and with our partners. It also ensures effective, robust peer support. The latter is a crucial part of good practice and the editing and reforming of the social media posts we write at the end of each visit provide not just an online gallery, but also the structure for us to regularly check in with each other as to how, if, and by what means, we have been affected within the work. This peer supervision acts as a means of self-care for the team while working in the field, which is further supported by each member of the team's individual supervision back in the UK.

The extracts presented are adapted from Art Refuge UK's Facebook posts (2016–18) written each Friday by the team members on their way home from their shift in Calais. The varied and informal style captures something of the particular quality of experience from that week's work.

Temporary, portable and virtual

Our work began in various settings across the large camp: tents, a portacabin, a wooden shelter. From November 2016, it has taken place through outreach in the Calais area, in temporary housing, a safe house for unaccompanied teenagers, a day centre, and alongside a medical van at the main roadside distribution point. Art materials used in the various spaces range from focused, ordinary materials, to found objects, plasticine, postcards, filmmaking and animation, as well as cyanotypes, kite-making and large-scale mapping in the outdoor environments. Through witnessing, cataloguing, photographing and curating, and against the backdrop of widespread human rights abuses in the Calais area (Bochenek 2017; Welander and Gerlach 2018), the work draws on the team's knowledge and experience, the individual refugees' resilience and imaginative capacity, as well as the idiosyncrasies of the different physical spaces on offer (Andemicael 2011). All the work is supported by linking closely with our NGO partner organisations.

Our work is underpinned by the concept of Portable Studio (Kalmanowitz and Lloyd 2005, 2011, 2016), which offers an internal frame. Portable Studio emerged out of the work of Kalmanowitz and Lloyd in the former Yugoslavia in the mid 1990s and they described it as:

> based on the premise that the internal structure we carry as art therapists can allow for work to physically take place in a wide range of settings which, in the former Yugoslavia, extended from the refugee camp dining room and bedroom, to the hills surrounding the camp and, at one point, the local rubbish dump. This internal structure comprises a number of key elements which include an attitude both to the art and the individual making it. Central is a belief in the individual possessing internal resources rooted in experience, resilience and culture rather than being a powerless victim for whom the therapist alone holds the solutions. (Kalmanowitz and Lloyd 2005, p.108)

The notion of appreciating that people we encounter in our work carry with them their own inner resourcefulness is imperative in this context and helpful in informing the frame of our work. It is what the psychological aspect of this work hinges on and where we see time and again the way that the art-making, viewing, curating and exhibiting can both collaborate with and enhance personal resilience.

The work is responsive and nuanced, and as a team we have been through our own journey of doubt and hope and the need to re-inhabit our workspaces both psychologically and physically on each occasion. We make no assumptions and need to be congruent about our own cultural heritages and mindful about how these may be both received and seen.

In creating the galleries – both physical and virtual – we often need to literally inhabit spaces that have no walls. Interactions can be fleeting; the individuals we encounter often engage with little expectation other than a curiosity as to what we are doing and who we are. The ethos of the work is underpinned by core principles of art therapy practice, while as a team we acknowledge our need to adapt our models to respond to the psychological needs of the refugee population and keep a strong ethical frame (Hogan 2009). We are a specialist team of art therapists who view the work through a particular lens that is shaped by our extensive knowledge and active engagement in the here and now in this setting.

There is no avoidance of the complexities of this environment in which there are multiple, complicated, daily socio-political shifts, as we have explored in our article on 'virtual shelters' in this context (Lloyd, Press and Usiskin 2018a). Police, vigilante and mafia violence, and intimidation and destruction of property are all ongoing and all too familiar. We have to be honest about the limitations of the work, as well as the difficult grey areas (Kalmanowitz and Potash 2010) that need continual reflection and re-evaluation, and thoughtful and responsive interaction rather than a reactive response. 'An examination of motivations and intentions is essential to ethical practice. Unexamined attitudes and practices can perpetuate inequality in any cross-cultural situation' (Potash *et al.* 2017, p.75).

The team members are all visual artists who understand that each material or art medium has its own qualities and characteristics, alongside the need to be intentional when choosing materials for the widely disparate settings we encounter in Calais. Moon explores related ethical issues, stating, 'Ongoing, intentional consideration of the potential impact of materials on clients is an ethical responsibility of the art therapist' (Moon 2000 cited in Moon 2010, p.11). In addition, the team collectively carries a rich and diverse history of studying visual art; of gallery and museum visits worldwide; of making, exhibiting and involvement in art practices; of collecting books, postcards and other resources. As practitioners, we find that there is shared acknowledgement of the need to actively engage in contemporary art practice, researching appropriate images and references, and of keeping the work alive when not physically present in Calais.

A key element of the work is choosing context-specific materials, explored by Kalmanowitz and Lloyd (2016) when considering the use of kites in the makeshift Calais camp and the Idomeni camp on Greece's northern border with Macedonia in 2016:

> The making of kites honoured the tradition of the artist, art therapist and the kite makers. The therapists supported this physical engagement and creative problem-solving alongside the different psychological and social meanings. This work was tailored specifically to the people and context. (p.154)

Our work takes place in very particular locations influenced by their smells, physicality and sounds; the weather, the diversity of cultures we encounter; our perspective as a British team working in France; as well as the immediate social context, history and politics. Creating a space that is safe enough to make the work possible is imperative. With some individuals, we have seen an ability to relate to something outside themselves, perhaps as a means of alleviating feelings of being homesick. 'Homesick individuals have little interest in the new environment, which makes adaptation and settling virtually impossible' (Dieterich-Hartwell and Koch 2017, p.2).

This sense of homesickness is explored by Papadopoulos (2002), who proposes the idea of 'nostalgic disorientation' that sets off a yearning for a specific, tangible state of home and belonging. Much of the work we do involves holding this notion of homesickness in mind and trying to create some kind of space which can be temporarily inhabited – poignant in Calais, a border town and place of transit for so many who have not yet reached their hoped-for destination.

Art installation

Installation art has been a major strand of contemporary art practice since the 1960s. Often site specific, it might involve construction and assemblage and usually temporarily transforms a particular site into an active, and at times immersive, space that encourages an interactive experience (Bishop 2005; Gingko Press 2014). This idea helps us further enrich our understanding of the work, and was explored by Kalmanowitz and Lloyd (2011) to allow them to imaginatively re-vision their diverse studio spaces into viable working environments. We can also think about it in terms of the role of temporary galleries. Moon (2008) writes about installation as a site-specific artwork, the intention of which 'is to create a sense of place that is to be experienced rather than viewed' (p.82), which further helps us understand the context of the temporary gallery space, as below.

This first extract from our Facebook posts (Art Refuge UK 2016–18) comes from our work in a purpose-built psychosocial tent that we shared with Médecins du Monde over a number of months in 2016.

Extract one: 8–9 September, 2016

We returned to the Médecins du Monde space in the camp to prepare for the day. This involved laying out approximately 200 plasticine animals, objects and people made in the tent over the last few months so as to document, repair and re-present them back as a temporary art installation for those using the space [see Figure 12.1]. Several men recognised pieces they had made and new figures were added. As with yesterday, we felt acutely the harsh reality of distance, a sense of yearning; of the unbearableness of loss of family; of wanting familial attention with another person; of needing to tell aspects of the journey from home; of wanting to connect on an authentic level. Yesterday it was with us as mothers, today as fellow human beings – mothers, sisters, aunts.

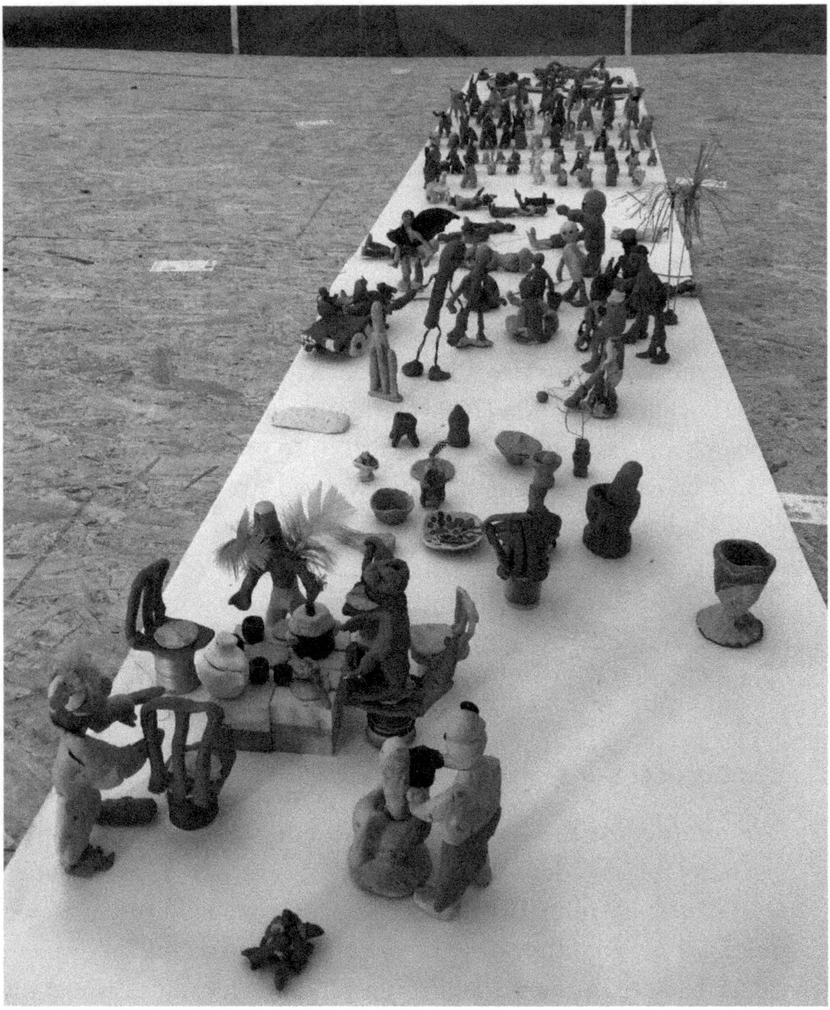

Figure 12.1 Plasticine installation

The plasticine objects transformed the tent into a space that individuals could inhabit. For this to happen we drew on our own identity as artists, and our experiences in transforming unlikely spaces into those for exhibition. Moon (2008) develops these ideas further:

> If we are to cultivate an artist identity in all aspects of our work, it makes sense that we use our artistic sensibilities to reconceptualize our workspaces. To consider our environments as works of art brings an intentional focus to the creation of therapeutic space

> and engages our artist identity in the process. Architecture, interior design, environmental sculpture, and installation art all have relevance for us when we begin to think of our physical spaces as works of art in and of themselves. (p.83)

The following extract is from our work at the Maria Skobtsova House in Calais. Maria Skobtsova (Smith 1967) was a Russian noblewoman, poet, nun, member of the French resistance and canonised martyr, who in 1930s Paris opened her house to refugees, the vulnerable, homeless and lonely. It also became a site for theological and intellectual discussion. The safe house in Calais works in this spirit to provide emergency accommodation and support for up to 22 vulnerable unaccompanied refugees of all faiths, while also acting as a house for prayer. At the time of writing, the house largely accommodates young men from Eritrea and Ethiopia. Since late 2016 we have offered three-hour sessions there on Friday afternoons around the dining room table, which then also becomes the site for installation.

> **Extract two: 6–7 April, 2017**
>
> The evening session was grounded by the presence at the table of the trusted safe house staff. Bringing a LEGO® boat, some ornamental model trees, rocks and concrete bricks onto the table allowed new landscapes to once again emerge, along with touching exchanges and periods of creative collaboration. An important historic Eritrean site was created by the same young man who had made a truck two weeks ago that represented the overcrowded vehicle he had been driven across the Sahara desert in on a frightening journey that most of these young men have experienced. After temporarily struggling with the bricks, he produced three towers in a landscape, pulling together a powerful scene, much as he had poignantly willed the making of the desert truck. In parallel, a second young man who had been director of lighting two weeks earlier now directed those around the table, inspired by the LEGO® boat to make his own plasticine sculpture of the boat he had travelled in from Libya to Italy. With humour and yet insistence that the forty or so tiny figures be made to

his specification, each wearing a life jacket, he also managed to create a powerful object embodying his experience. The two young men ended the afternoon stage-managing their artworks with backdrops, lighting and filters on their phones [Figure 12.2]. We were deeply moved that they had shared with us and the group such intimate experiences, and that the boat held meaning for all of them, as had the truck two weeks earlier.

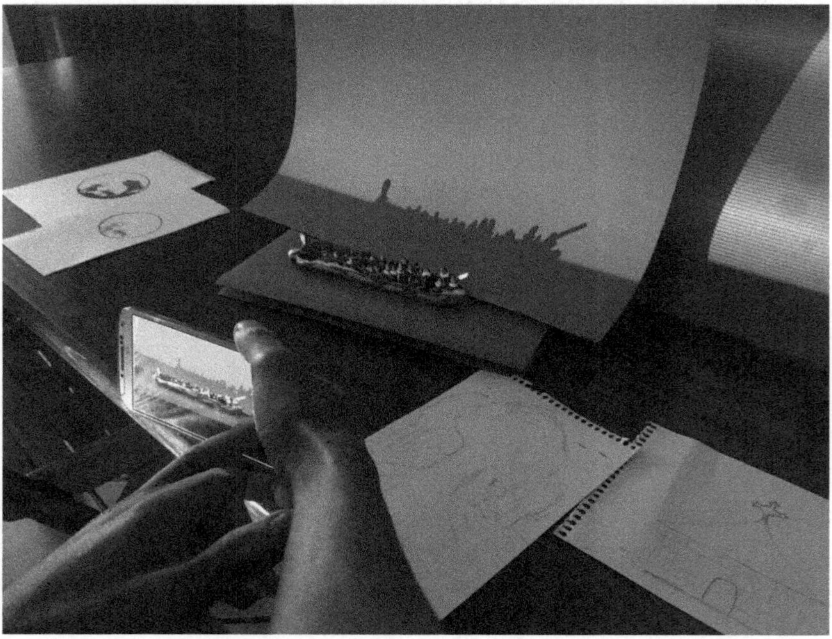

Figure 12.2 Stage-managing the boat

Box of postcards

We regularly use a collection of postcards in a small, map-lined cardboard suitcase. The small, portable size of the postcard has, by and large, remained uniform across time and cultures, hence their ability to stack neatly together in a box. This also makes them intimate. Our box of postcards referenced in the extracts below is carried, constantly re-formed and carefully curated, as an alive, collective, intercultural resource and acts in itself in the work like a mini portable gallery or museum containing meaningful contents.

The postcard has been a distinct artistic medium since the middle of the 20th century and this continues into contemporary art practice. The images in our eclectic collection range from landscapes to holiday destinations, reproductions of old masters to contemporary artists from around the world, and include images of artworks made by refugees within our work in Calais, which have been professionally printed up as postcards. Choosing an image from this wide collection allows for a subjective element and the potential connection with personal cultural narratives not imposed from the outside.

Postcards as a genre have particular resonance for our work with refugees. Phillips (2000) describes them as 'receptacles of memory, bearers of images and carriers of news' (p.16). Originating in the mid-19th century, they act as social tools and accessible forms for correspondence, communication, visual engagement, and advertising – of a place, idea, object, something perhaps longed for. Traditionally meant to be sent to another person as a form of communication, postcards are often sent across national borders. It is ironic that the images they hold can sometimes unwittingly cause religious or political offence, raising legal issues (Phillips 2000). As with those seeking asylum, the cards are also sometimes returned to the country of origin.

Berger (1974) talks about the intimacy of home noticeboards as another form of miniature museum or container for experience that are curated and displayed by individuals, and this again resonates with our work:

> [A]ll the images belong to the same language and all are more or less equal within it, because they have been chosen in a highly personal way to match and express the experience of the room's inhabitant. Logically, these boards should replace museums. (p.30)

A session we delivered in an apartment in Calais with a group of refugee friends from Sudan, Pakistan and Iran illustrates this well. We took our box of postcards and were moved by the poignant activity that followed between people, place, postcard and object, with an impromptu art exhibition resulting on the kitchen table.

Extract three: 5–6 October, 2017

The afternoon was spent with a familiar group of refugees in an apartment in Calais, the cosy domain of someone who has recently gained asylum in France. We sat sipping tea... We noticed the relocation of familiar clay and plasticine figures that had been made in previous groups at the hostel (where some of the men were currently living in temporary accommodation), which had then been physically moved by the group to the safer home of the apartment to be cared for and to bring comfort. The art objects brought identity into the space, making it personal, allowing it to become a home; being filled with friends both literally and figuratively. The friendship circle formed, the group sifted through postcards, choosing images and creating an impromptu exhibition [Figure 12.3]. The images held portraits from around the world, linking different people and cultures. The exhibition allowed those unable to use a shared verbal language to express themselves by sharing images.

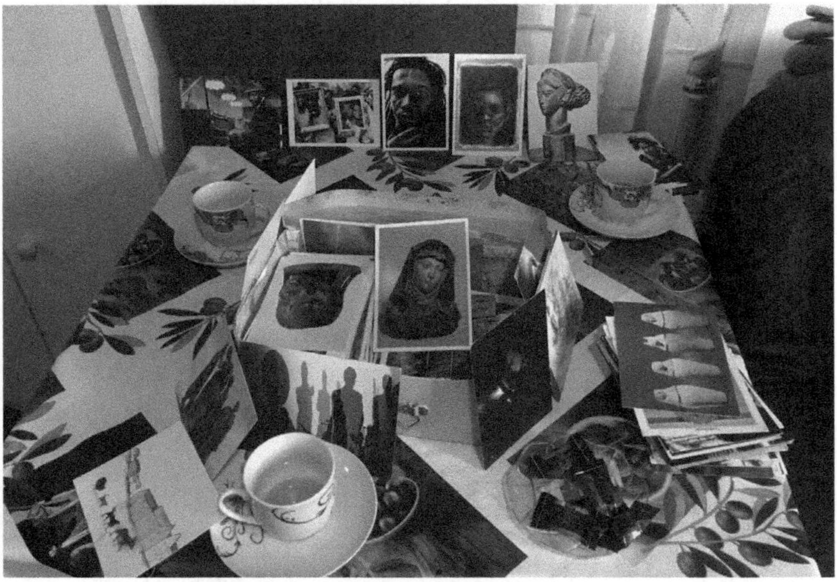

Figure 12.3 Postcard exhibition on the table

For the final few months of the Calais camp's life, a designated youth area was set up to support hundreds of unaccompanied minors living in the camp and who were considered of particular concern due to their vulnerability to traffickers, abuse and neglect. We offered weekly sessions from a shipping container with our partner Médecins Sans Frontières. The postcards as an art medium came into their own given their intimate size, helping to activate the space into one that felt emotionally contained and in which therapeutic work could take place.

Extract four: 8–9 September, 2016

Around 35 unaccompanied teenage boys joined us throughout the afternoon, both inside the container and on a table outside in the sun. One young man, when offered the box of postcards to look through, chose one that sparked his curiosity, leading him to embark on a watercolour. Others followed his lead. The postcards seemed to lend themselves to the size of the space and their inherent transience seemed to allow for both intimacy and familiarity for these boys so used to navigating small spaces [Figure 12.4]. There were extended periods of joint visual attention [Isserow 2013], the boys seeking close proximity with us and with each other. Several talked about hunger, lack of shoes, and fingerprints being taken forcefully in other countries in Europe. The area outside the container allowed for space around things, connection with other services, as well as freedom to come in and out of the art therapy space. A couple of hours into the afternoon, heavy tear gas (sprayed by the CRS police nearby) led several boys to join those already in the container, invited in by us and each other to find refuge in the space as if coming in from bad weather or a storm at sea. There was a sense of the space inside as safe in spite of the intrusion of the gas and the unlikely environment of a hot shipping container, as well as an atmosphere of camaraderie.

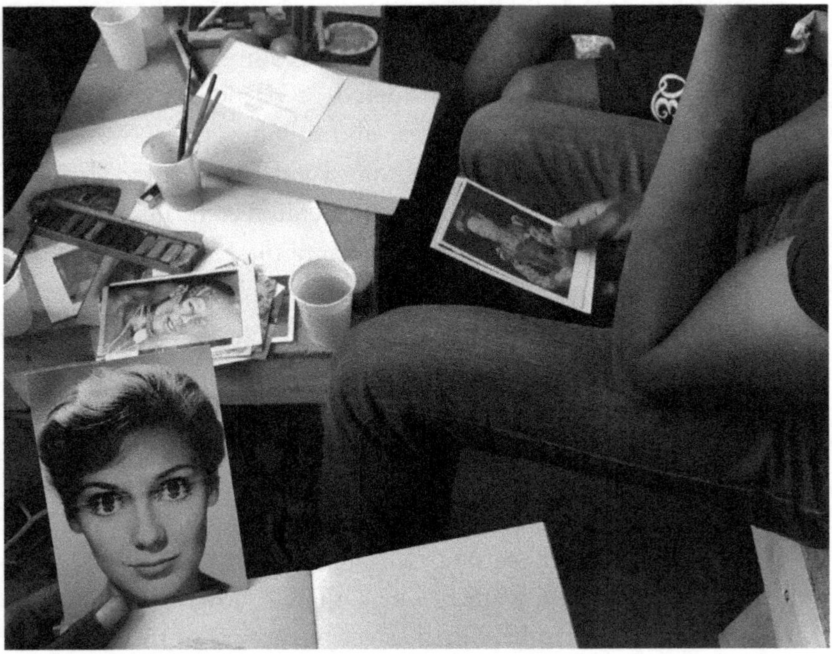

Figure 12.4 Drawing postcards in the shipping container

The collection of postcards inspires new drawings, watercolour paintings and visual translations which we often photograph and include in our weekly Facebook post (described below). These new reproductions cross borders digitally, carrying news or a narrative in much the same way a postcard might. This is in a context in which displacement, invisibility and lack of agency are commonly felt experiences.

Large map

The large map is an ongoing artwork exhibited in a range of settings. A first map covering Europe, Northern Africa and the Middle East began its journey taped to the outside of a wooden community space, later to the canvas walls within the Médecins du Monde tent, both in the southern half of the Calais camp (spring 2016). A second version was taped to the Médecins du Monde ambulance at the main distribution point (from autumn 2017) and has been used since, with a new world map added from May 2018. Individuals are invited to mark their routes from their country of origin to Calais.

A number of authors refer to a state of limbo as a liminal space in which the individual no longer feels at home (Dieterich-Hartwell and Koch 2017; Harris 2009). It is not a place in which a person can even begin to feel settled, since they have not reached their final destination. 'Liminality may be experienced with discomfort and uncertainty, yet this "in-between space" carries a significant potential for transformation and change' (Dieterich-Hartwell and Koch 2017, p.2). In our work in Calais over a number of years, this transitional space is always one of limbo which carries with it both pain and the potential for something to happen. The map here becomes a construct, a point of reference that is temporarily fixed in space. It is an object printed in vivid colour, deliberately chosen. It glows in the dark, on dull days and in all weathers. The map is robust (printed on a strong plastic material), and able to withstand the fierce Calais winds and driving rain. It is monumental; its scale and colour ensure it holds a strong presence as an artwork in its own right. It draws curiosity from refugees, volunteers, visitors and journalists alike. People come to the map to view it as they would a picture in a gallery, but the map is not fixed inside the four walls of a gallery space, it is taped to the side of a community space in a refugee camp, or the medical team's ambulance, or tied to the tall fence that cordons off one of the many spaces meant to deter refugees from setting up shelter.

The map is an interactive artwork installed in a specific place. The routes marked out are drawn over and over again by new visitors to the map. The map has become a snapshot of a particular time and place in history, with specific routes all leading to Calais. The map becomes not just a statement of the current situation on the France–UK border and a shared perspective, but a participatory art piece in situ. It draws attention to the environment in which it is shown, as much as it draws attention to itself and to those who view it or interact with it. In this sense, the map encourages the space around it to be occupied and activated, as in a site-specific art installation.

Extract five: 2–3 November, 2017

Several hundred people gathered at the distribution area across an afternoon with a clear blue sky and in strong autumnal sun. The Red Cross, Médecins du Monde's doctors, nurses and psychologist, and services providing food, clothing, toilets and youth support were all present. Groups gathered and football was played on the tarmac road. As usual, we placed the map on the outside of the ambulance, with two small tables that held postcards, plasticine and drawing materials. Around fifty or so individuals from Afghanistan, Sudan and Eritrea joined us, many in small groups, often with friends, drawn towards the large map. Many stayed for a while in conversation around the map and for art-making. As images or objects were made, a small, impromptu exhibition was created on the ambulance itself [Figure 12.5] next to the map.

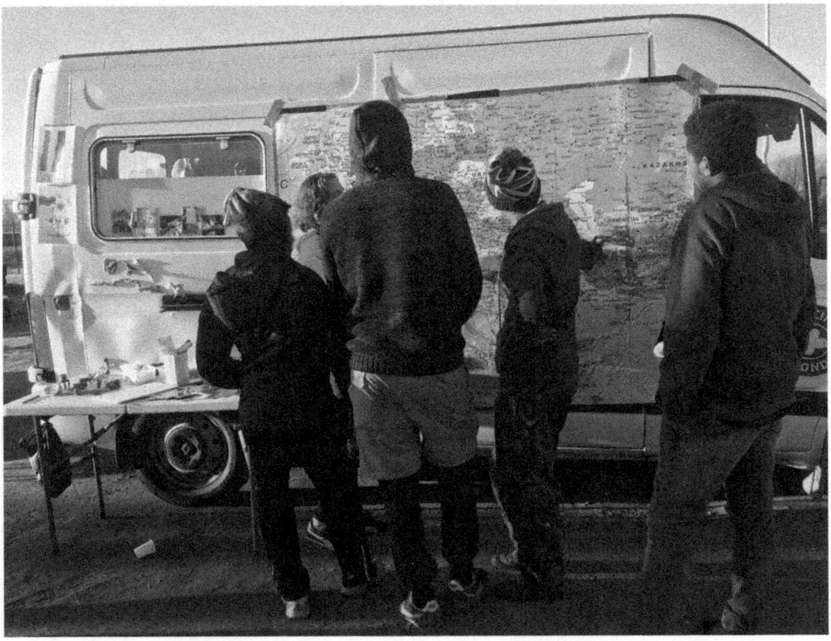

Figure 12.5 Viewing the map and exhibition

The routes described on the surface of the map may appear similar, yet all carry a unique narrative, a personal resonance. The lines are marked with different pens; gold and silver intermingle with black, red and green, the routes become iridescent and multidimensional; they seem to lift off the map's surface. Certain places are obscured as the traffic of pen marks becomes heavier. Each individual has left something behind but also made a mark on the changing face of Europe, lines and routes marked all over. Because of the 'pen traffic', Italy at certain sites becomes obliterated. The notion of being able to mark and contextualise where one was, where one is now, gives credence to the lines added; the marking becomes part of the map itself, adding to the marks already on the printed surface. There is curiosity about which country is where, a real sense of people looking together at the map. Borders are redrawn, and anticipated or hoped-for journeys are added. The map holds a collective narrative that can be viewed [Figure 12.6].

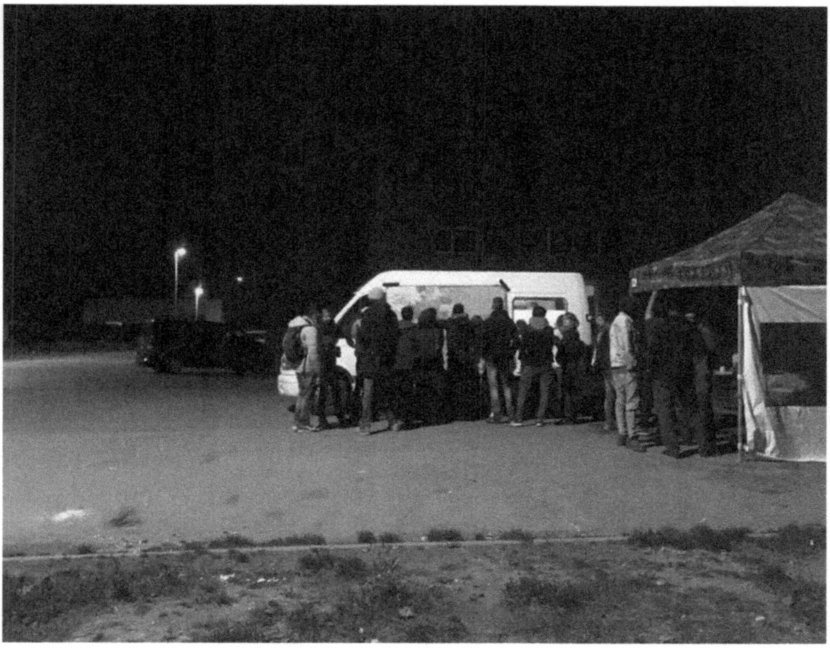

Figure 12.6 Viewing the map at night

In the final extract, the map and fence it is tied to are activated by its viewers to become a site for installation.

Extract six: 21–22 February, 2018

It was freezing cold with blue skies and temperatures dropping. There was a tense edge to the air with fewer refugees and isolated outbursts of aggressive, confrontational behaviour from some individuals towards others they did not know. With a table set up with bricks in the winter sunshine, it was only the map that offered useful diversion. We had first placed it on the ambulance out of the sun, only to move it to the border fence behind the van where it attracted small groups and acted as a catalyst for discussion. It also served as the focus for two men to talk independently of their plans to navigate different countries prior to finding the country they want to settle in. The cold appeared to make people draw upon internal resources, allowing their minds to wander. The security fence became an extended mapping area, with Canada, Iceland, South Africa and Australia marked out further on to the metal fence with imaginary lines.

Virtual galleries

Our active use of social media forms a key element of the work, acting as a platform from which this work can be shared and those participating in our groups can actively find voice and visibility. Each Friday evening, on our journey home from Calais to London via the Eurotunnel, we use the time to debrief about our work over the previous two days. We look through the images taken on our phones, reflect on the political context, weather, conversations and emerging themes. We choose a title. One of the team then sets about writing a Facebook post on their phone, read out to the team and re-edited before being shared online on the Art Refuge UK page by late Friday evening.

This editing and re-editing process is reminiscent of curating an exhibition or gallery space. It takes consultation by the team about what images might work and where and how words link to images. These are presented in the public domain and serve as a visual witness to the work of that particular week. The post is later adapted for Instagram and Twitter. The cumulative nature of the posts also means that we have a gallery archive and written narrative of the entire body of work from September 2015, which is recorded on the website as an ongoing blog and another form of viewing.

This work on the France–UK border takes place in a highly charged political context and often the nuanced experiences that we have each week on the ground in Calais can inform better than the voice of a visiting journalist. We document not just the violations taking place in this context, but also the psychological resilience, creativity and imaginative capacities of those we work with. The posts are regularly shared beyond our page. They also sit alongside an ongoing dialogue with the other NGOs working in Calais and with refugees across Europe, contributing to an online community of activists and aid organisations, and an alternative discourse to the dominant and dehumanising rhetoric of 'the refugee crisis' (The Guardian 2018) and all that follows in its wake.

Facebook is a contemporary medium, a virtual, participatory space. As a team, we try to have an informed understanding of the changing culture of social media and we think carefully about the potential pitfalls and ethical issues of posting images online. We monitor and debate these on an ongoing basis both among ourselves, with our trustees and partners and – where we can – with the participants themselves.

Artworks within our work increasingly take the form of temporary structures, installations or large-scale maps. They are photographed by us week by week, the photographs holding a visual record, and some participants take photos on their own mobile phones. We are careful to ask permission of individuals before taking images of their work, and often invite them to photograph their own artwork using our mobile phones. Where possible, we show the Facebook page to those participating in our groups alongside the potential context in which an image might be shared. We are scrupulous to ensure that no one can be identified through the posts, given the obvious sensitivity of the work.

Belkofer and McNutt (2011) suggest that social media offers an opportunity in many ways 'to revisit old models of storytelling' (p.160). They also explore ethical considerations for art therapists using social media, drawing on Martin (2008) and Rice (2009) and stating:

> It is evident that for many people, participation in digital media is providing a home base and a sense of control and certainty in a postmodern world where identity, community, and meaning are increasingly difficult to experience and define. (Belkofer and McNutt 2011, p.160)

There is an urgent, live debate in the art therapy profession about the role of social media in contemporary practice, demonstrated recently in Garner (2016) and Malchiodi (2018) who talk of harnessing the digital developments possible with social media while engaging with ethical issues. Malchiodi (2018) identifies the pitfalls and possibilities of using different social media platforms, such as Facebook, Instagram and Twitter, but also proposes that core ethical principles of practice can translate to these areas when consideration and respect for those we are working with are kept core to the work itself.

We have found social media to offer our work a powerful, contemporary tool that contributes to interpersonal learning and social participation. Ritual and routine allow for the work to feel responsibly held by the team; posting into the online community often feels cathartic for us as practitioners, but also allows it to enter a different zone where information sharing, advocacy, education and the influence of an online audience all become possible.

At the time of writing, Facebook is also the primary form of social media used by refugees for navigating routes, finding information and connecting with family and friends. As documented by Griswold (2018) who maps the journeys of Syria's diaspora artists, 'They are, at most, only half in France, Zeid explained. "Syria has moved to Facebook," she said. Salman added, "My home is the people, not the land"' (Griswold 2018).

From September 2015 to the time of writing this chapter, the posts are regularly looked at by the refugee artists and users of our spaces. These individuals have few possessions beyond the clothes they are wearing and, for many, their mobile phones. Knowing that we carefully select images to post online has provided reassurance for refugees who tell us that they can return to view them on their own mobiles, and discuss them with others, thus carrying on connections and a wider support network on which to draw.

When fire destroyed swathes of shelters in the large camp, one man from Kurdistan was relieved to know his artwork was not only physically in our safekeeping, but also digitally recorded. He asked if we could send him his portfolio via Messenger, so he could view his images, copy, and potentially download them when he reached his final destination. Another man from Sudan who joined our groups over a number of months in the Calais camp, his asylum claim now secure, sent us photos of himself standing in front of the 'Mona Lisa' and other famous images in the Louvre. He was finding a way through his museum visit and the common language of images, to safely and privately bridge the physical space between us.

Conclusion

The work in France is ongoing at the point of writing this chapter (2019), the team travelling from London to Calais on Thursday mornings and returning to the UK the following evening. The NGOs working in Calais are at capacity in providing for the basic needs of refugees: water, food, clothing, medical care. Until the closure of the large camp, this list included provision of shelter, largely not tolerated by the French state since the end of 2016. Psychological spaces continue to be scarce, even though the need for mental health support has been identified as urgent by our partners, other agencies and the refugees themselves (Einhorn Jardin 2015; Monk, Stanton and Welander 2017; Lloyd *et al.* 2018b), and evidenced by ongoing and constant numbers of people who continue to join our spaces.

The unique physical position on the border crossing of France and the UK creates an in-between space. Our practice has had to adapt to the continually changing political climate and local context in Calais, itself a tiny element in a much wider refugee situation that has developed across Europe since 2015.

Our response is interpersonal and improvisational. Through careful selection of art media, the work aims to actively connect with art historical and contemporary art practice references across cultures. The notion of creating site-specific installations and spaces in which postcards from across the world and large maps can be viewed both individually and collectively has become significant in a setting where the emergent themes are related to disorientation, dehumanisation and displacement.

In this context, shared activity of curating and viewing resonates with those we work with, as well as with the volunteers and workers. This underpins the key components of the work in which resilience is such a profound element. The viewer, the viewing and the viewed all have a place and role, the work taking place in groups, with others, in company, with witnesses and co-producers.

Acknowledgements

We would like to thank: our partners Médecins du Monde, Médecins Sans Frontières, Secours Catholique, Maria Skobtsova House; the wider Art Refuge UK team in France, including Anna Kälin, Jess Linton, Tony Gammidge, Sarah Robinson and Jayne McConkey; our dedicated board of trustees, funders (individual donors and family trusts); and our families for their ongoing support. Above all, we would like to acknowledge all those individuals who have participated in our work in northern France from whom we have learned so much about imagination, survival and what it is to be human.

References

Andemicael, A. (2011) *Positive Energy: A Review of the Role of Artistic Activities in Refugee Camps, Geneva.* UNHCR Policy Development and Evaluation Service, unpaginated. Accessed on 9/5/18 at www.unhcr.org/4def858a9.pdf.

Art Refuge UK (2016–18) Facebook posts. Accessed on 25/10/18 at www.facebook.com/artrefugeuk.

Belkofer, C.M. and McNutt, J.V. (2011) 'Understanding social media culture and its ethical challenges for art therapists.' *Art Therapy: Journal of the American Art Therapy Association 28,* 4, 159–164.

Berger, J. (1974) *Ways of Seeing.* Harmondsworth: Penguin Books.

Bishop, C. (2005) *Installation Art.* London: Tate Publishing.

Bochenek, M.G. (2017) *'Like Living in Hell': Police Abuses Against Child and Adult Migrants in Calais.* Human Rights Watch, unpaginated. Accessed on 22/10/18 at www.hrw.org/report/2017/07/26/living-hell/police-abuses-against-child-and-adult-migrants-calais.

Dieterich-Hartwell, R. and Koch, C. (2017) 'Creative arts therapies as temporary home for refugees: Insights from literature and practice.' *Behavioural Sciences Journal 7,* 4, 69–80.

Einhorn Jardin, L. (2015) *La Santé Mentale à Calais: Migrants, Intervenants, des Constats et des Préconisations d'Actions.* Médecins du Monde, unpaginated. Accessed on 9/5/18 at https://associationspp.files.wordpress.com/2018/01/mdm_rapport-de-mission-exploratoire-santc3a9-mentale_calais_2015.pdf.

Garner, R. (ed.) (2016) *Digital Art Therapy: Material, Methods and Applications*. London and Philadelphia, PA: Jessica Kingsley Publishers.

Ginkgo Press (2014) *Installation Art Now*. Berkeley, CA: Gingko Press.

Griswold, E. (2018) 'Mapping the journeys of Syria's artists; What happens when a culture disperses?' *The New Yorker*. Accessed on 20/6/18 at www.newyorker.com/culture/culture-desk/mapping-the-journeys-of-syrias-artists.

Guardian, The (2018) 'Five myths about the refugee crisis.' Accessed on 25/10/18 at www.theguardian.com/news/2018/jun/05/five-myths-about-the-refugee-crisis.

Harris, D.A. (2009) 'The paradox of expressing speechless terror: Ritual liminality in the creative arts therapies' treatment of posttraumatic distress.' *The Arts in Psychotherapy 36,* 94–104.

Hogan, S. (2009) 'The art therapy continuum: A useful tool for envisaging the diversity of practice in British art therapy.' *International Journal of Art Therapy 14,* 1, 29–37.

Isserow, J. (2013) 'Between water and words: Reflective self-awareness and symbol formation in art therapy.' *International Journal of Art Therapy 18,* 3, 122–131.

Kalmanowitz, D. and Lloyd, B. (eds) (2005) *Art Therapy and Political Violence: With Art, Without Illusion*. London and New York, NY: Routledge.

Kalmanowitz, D. and Lloyd, B. (2011) 'Inside Out Outside In: Portable Studio and Found Objects.' In E. Levine and S. Levine (eds) *Art in Action: Expressive Arts Therapy and Social Change*. London and Philadelphia, PA: Jessica Kingsley Publishers.

Kalmanowitz, D. and Lloyd, B. (2016) 'Art therapy at the border: Holding the line of the kite.' *Journal of Applied Arts & Health 7,* 2, 143–158.

Kalmanowitz, D. and Potash, J. (2010) 'Ethical considerations in the global teaching and promotion of art therapy to non-art therapists.' *The Arts in Psychotherapy 37*, 20–26.

Lloyd, B., Press, N. and Usiskin, M. (2018a) 'The Calais Winds took our plans away: Art therapy as shelter.' *Journal of Applied Arts & Health 9*, 2, 171–184.

Lloyd, B., Usiskin, M., Press, N. and Welander, M. (2018b) *Mental Health in Displacement – A Widespread Yet Largely Overlooked Crisis*. Accessed on 27/10/18 at www.law.ox.ac.uk/research-subject-groups/centre-criminology/centreborder-criminologies/blog/2018/10/mental-health.

Malchiodi, C. (ed.) (2018) *The Handbook of Art Therapy and Digital Technology*. London and Philadelphia, PA: Jessica Kingsley Publishers.

Martin, A. (2008) 'Digital Literacy and the "Digital Society".' In C. Lankshear and M. Knobel (eds) *Digital Literacies*. New York, NY: Peter Lang.

Monk, L., Stanton, N. and Welander, M. (2017) *Six Months On*. Refugee Rights Europe, unpaginated. Accessed on 23/5/18 at http://refugeerights.org.uk/wp-content/uploads/2017/04/RRDP_SixMonthsOn.pdf.

Moon, B. (2000) *Ethical Issues in Art Therapy*. Springfield, IL: Charles C. Thomas.

Moon, C. (2008) *Studio Art Therapy: Cultivating the Artist Identity in the Art Therapist*. London and Philadelphia, PA: Jessica Kingsley Publishers.

Moon C. (2010) *Materials and Media in Art Therapy: Critical Understandings of Diverse Artistic Vocabularies*. London and New York, NY: Routledge.

Papadopoulos, R. (ed.) (2002) *Therapeutic Care for Refugees: No Place Like Home*. London: Karnac Books.

Phillips, T. (2000) *The Postcard Century: 2000 Cards and Their Messages 1900–2000*. London: Hansjorg Mayer, Thames and Hudson.

Potash, J., Bardot, H., Moon, C., Napoli, M., Lyonsmith, A. and Hamilton, M. (2017) 'Ethical implications of cross-cultural international art therapy.' *The Arts in Psychotherapy 56*, 74–82.

Rice, J. (2009) *The Church of Facebook: How the Hyperconnected Are Redefining Community*. Colorado Springs, CO: David C. Cook.

Smith, S. (1967) *The Rebel Nun*. London: Pan Books.

Stanton, N. and Welander, M. (eds) (2016) *Still Here, Exploring Further Dynamics of the Calais Camp*. Refugee Rights Europe, unpaginated. Accessed on 25/10/18 at http://refugeerights.org.uk/wp-content/uploads/2018/08/RRE_StillHere.pdf.

Welander, M. and Gerlach, G. (2018) *A Brief Timeline of the Human Rights Situation in Calais*. Refugee Rights Europe. Accessed on 26/10/18 at http://refugeerights.org.uk/wp-content/uploads/2018/10/History-Of-Calais_Refugee-Rights-Europe.pdf.

CHAPTER 13

Art Therapy and Museums in the Colombian Context

Co-leading Collective Transformations

Andrée Salom

Introduction

The union between art therapy and museums is one that produces transformation in both fields. With the union, museums become spaces of therapeutic deed. Art therapy expands to highlight community and social actions. This chapter incorporates community art therapy perspectives and art therapists' ability to integrate different areas of knowledge as foundations for the art therapy/museum collaboration.

The first exhibition that I describe illustrates the transformation that occurs when different elements are mixed together. It serves as a metaphor for the transformations pertinent to this inquiry, which includes personal and cultural change. The other museum exhibitions and activities in the chapter show that the art scene in Colombia implements social themes related to a recent agreed-on peace treaty. The exhibitions have been unrelated to art therapy until now, when I contextualise them in therapeutic terms. I then portray potential art therapy directives related to four of the shows, to exemplify how art therapists can add to the intentional bond between art and wellbeing in the museum context. All of the museum endeavours presented are pertinent to our field as they evidence Colombians' readiness for art therapy/museum collaborations.

Transformation

I went to see artist Hicham Berrada mix reactive substances inside clear glass beakers filled with base solutions. He projected the microcosms created inside the beakers onto a big wall for everyone to see in the Sala de Proyectos El Garaje, at the Miguel Urrutia Art Museum (MUMA) in Bogotá. The title of the exhibition was *Reactive Landscapes* and the specific performance was titled *Pressage*. Writing on the wall described a reactive as 'a substance that produces a chemical reaction the moment it interacts with another substance. The result is a product of different characteristics and properties' (Subgerencia Cultural del Banco de la República 2017).

He sprinkled and poured ingredients, handled with surgeon's gloves, into one container at a time. Complementing or contrasting colour substances rose and fell. As they came into contact with one another, elements stretched, yielded, swirled and slid. Some were sandy, some cloudy, others glossy. As if breathing, the combinations produced tiny and large bubbles. Slowly, slowly, yet in retrospect relatively quickly, the elements interacted, creating suspensions, growth, tensions, expansions, collapses, resistance, support, and hide-and-seek dynamics. In relative speeds, transformation was visible: poetic transformation, scientific transformation, lifelike transformation.

I was attentive to Berrada and his choices, to the projection on the wall, to what its moving image impressed on me. I was curious about what the images caused in the other viewers, the children, the families. I wondered how the creative act would influence their dynamics after the show. I perceived everything and everyone as being transformed, at the very least influenced. Reactions arose.

Potential space (Winnicott 1971, 1989) refers to the phenomenon of transformation that happens when internal and external realities interact through play. Potential space is initiated in childhood and lasts throughout the lifespan by means of cultural venues (*ibid.*). It has been studied in relationship to museums (Froggett and Trustram 2014; Salom 2015). In part, the parallel is possible given that new museum paradigms and the postmodern view of art in general (Anderson 2004; Cameron 1971; Rancière 2009) promote interactions between the viewer of art and the art itself. Such interactions facilitate the ongoing construction and re-evaluation of interpretation, of the personal and subjective view attributed to external reality. The definition of the museum as a forum (Cameron 1971) opened doors for the socially responsible and inclusive functions of museums. Such an aperture enhances the transformation that can happen for a wide range of visitors of diverse backgrounds, as well as the meaning attributed to museums and the works they carry (Anderson 2004; Lavine and Karp 1991; Camic and Chatterjee 2013; Chatterjee and Noble 2013; De Montebello 2005; Silverman 2010). Regardless of being public, exhibitions transform us privately. In turn, we add to them; whether we say something or not, we interact with them, we infuse them with meaning (Froggett and Trustram 2014).

Colombian artist Carolina Rodriguez (personal communication 22 June 2017) said that the art scene benefits from exhibitions like *Pressage*, where illusion is present and the impact of the show persists long after the visit. Her words echo Silverstone (1992), who wrote that 'the meaning of an object [in an exhibit] continues in the imaginative work of the visitor who brings to it his or her own agenda, experiences and feelings' (p.35) and Rancière (2009), who defended viewers' subjective interpretation of art pieces (pp.14–17). Albeit not coming from psychoanalytic theory, they were referring to notions central to Winnicott's (1971) concept of potential space.

The Colombian political climate

At the time of writing (2018), after more than 50 years of violent confrontation, the Colombian population is currently traversing a collective social transformation, framed by the challenges of a peace process. The internal conflict in the country has many sources of influence. Tension between conservative and liberal parties starting in the 1940s led to a civil war, complicated by communist guerrilla groups that lost their ideals, violent paramilitary organisations that started out as counter-guerrilla armies, corruption, drug trafficking, and the war on drugs (Lobo-Guerrero 2013). There have been brutal confrontations between armed groups in rural areas for decades. This has forced more than seven million individuals (a third of whom are children and many of whom belong to a minority group) to move from their home areas and seek safety elsewhere within the country (ACNUR 2016).

A peace agreement was signed between the Colombian National Government and the armed guerrilla group FARC-EP in November 2016. The agreement aims to 'end...the enormous suffering that the conflict has caused' (Colombian National Government and FARC-EP 2016, p.6), and ensure 'that social conflicts can be resolved through [democratic] institutional channels' (p.6). The fifth point of the document is titled 'Agreements regarding the Victims of the Conflict: Comprehensive system of truth, justice, reparation and non recurrence, including special jurisdiction for peace; and commitment on human rights' (p.132). This chapter recognises victims as citizens who have experienced human rights violations and who are entitled to judicial and extrajudicial systems that can establish the truth of what occurred (p.131).

For the process of peacebuilding, the document emphasises participation and inclusion, not only through pluralistic political involvement, but also through social movements and organisations (p.35). It states that 'the participation of and dialogue between the various sectors of society contribute to a climate of trust and promote a culture of tolerance, respect, and coexistence' (p.7). The agreement specifies an 'equality-based and gender-based approach' (p.136) towards reparation, which considers the particularities of the victims, their territory, vulnerability, ethnicity and background.

Post-traumatic stress has been correlated with (although not limited to) victims and civilians living in situations of political violence (Summerfield in Lobo-Guerrero 2013, p.26). This correlation is pertinent to the Colombia population (p.1) as victims and civilians have undergone or witnessed massacres, tortures, disappearances of loved ones, kidnappings, the effects of anti-personnel mines, and many other atrocities related to the internal conflict. Although individual treatment can be useful, the Colombian problem is a social one, and thus merits social interventions (Ottemiller and Awais 2016). Individual psychotherapy is expensive and culturally alien for many Colombian groups. In addition, the Colombian population tends to process difficulty collectively (CNRR-GMH 2010), as is implied by the social emphasis of the peace agreement (Colombian National Government and FARC-EP 2016).

Arts and health at a collective level in Colombia

Colombia houses a cultural mix that includes tens of indigenous traditions, Afro-Colombian heritages, and European and Middle Eastern roots. This cultural amalgam comes with complex issues of privilege and power, reflected in the country's conflicts and artistic heritage. Imagery in Colombia has been used to influence social structures since before the Spanish conquest (Salom 2017); artistic elements such as golden masks and grand depictions of Spanish viceroys, and later of creole revolutionaries, have helped establish the ruling classes of the times (Londoño Vélez 2005).

Images have also been used to influence religious power. 'La Lechuga' (Figure 13.1) is the most famous Colombian monstrance, a liturgical object used in the Catholic ritual. It was finished in 1707 and is now exhibited at Museo La Casa de la Moneda del Banco de la República. 'La Lechuga' provides an example of the superimposition of symbols used to induce the conversion of indigenous people to Catholicism. The monstrance holds a consecrated host and a Christian cross in the traditional Catholic way. However, it was crafted using Colombian gold and 1485 emeralds found in the territory, and emphasises a detailed sun, a star revered by pre-Colombian ethnicities. The superimposition of symbols helps to establish the stories derived from images. To influence evangelisation, Londoño Vélez (in Salom 2017) explains that 'Catholic images were attributed with miraculous properties deriving from the spiritual traditions of Native and Afro-descendent population' (p.7).

The arts have also been used by the different ethnicities in Colombia to maintain and honour their cultural roots and identity, and to communicate with one another (CNRR-GMH 2010; Cobo 2013; Lobo-Guerrero 2013; Salom 2017). The different traditions in the territory have found means of expression and co-existence through carnivals, folk crafts, music, dance, and other cultural activities (*ibid.*). Many ritualistic, folkloric, academic and common uses of the arts are evident in Colombia for making sense of personal as well as social challenges (Salom 2017). As the themes of the Colombian art scene described below show, art has been applied to challenge established hierarchies, bond communities and promote citizen participation (*ibid.*, p.70).

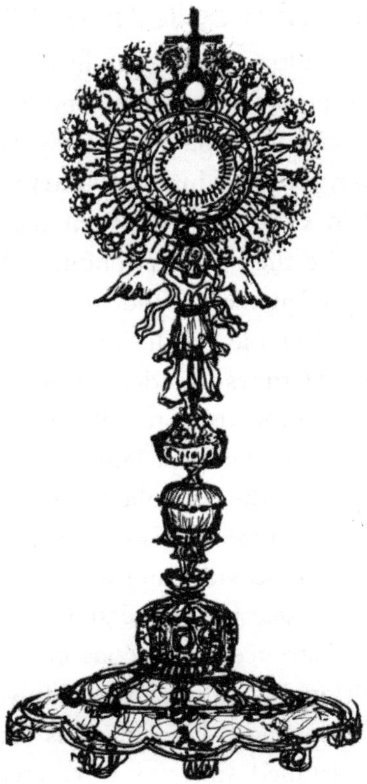

Figure 13.1 'La Lechuga' (drawing by author)

Among the unique themes that can be found in contemporary Colombian art, galleries, and art fairs, the role of memory stands out as a recurrent topic. Artists have documented historic events (many of them violent) with works which demand that public attention toward atrocity be paid and that it is not left unnoticed. Political and social themes related to power and privilege are being examined, as are ecological and geosocial topics, collective works, and initiatives that make analogies between art and education (*ibid.*).

Visual and performing arts have also been conventionally used in the country to process the particular atrocities of violence (CNRR-GMH 2010; Lobo-Guerrero 2013, p.30). Solutions to emotional needs produced by the socio-political conflict have drawn from this tradition, and thus community art initiatives are widespread (Lobo-Guerrero 2013). For instance, song writing and storytelling have been adapted to include themes related to hostility (p.30), and women have formed embroidery groups to process grief caused by human rights violations (p.31). The Director of Arts at the Ministry of Culture, Giomar Uribe, recognised the community and trust-building benefits that artistic programmes provide in the areas of the country that have been most affected by the war (Artera 2017). The prevalence of the arts as a tool for processing social injustice is fortunate, given that art can provide a means of bodily and environmental control that can be beneficial in the face of trauma (Herman 1997).

Professional art therapy initiatives in relationship to the post-conflict situation are slowly being initiated. For example, *Proyecto Chiva* is an art therapy process that art therapist Maria Reyes and I developed for displaced populations. Through it, individuals create a moving means of transportation (predominantly traditional Colombian buses) and fill it with those elements that they wish to take along with them throughout life. The elements may be objects, people, emotions, thoughts or values. The results from an initial pilot programme are being studied for publication.

Because the arts are innately used in Colombia 'to adapt and undergo cultural change' (Salom 2017, p.5) as well as to elaborate on conflict and pain (CNRR-GMH 2010; Lobo-Guerrero 2013), the establishment of art therapy in Colombia may take a prevalently social and community path. As such, art therapists in Colombia may form alliances with cultural institutions from early on.

Art therapy and museums

In museum visits, as in community art-making, emotional growth may be motivated even when the objectives of museum disciplines are far removed from the technical languages and frames of therapy (Salom 2008; Silverman 2010). However, in parallel to their natural emotional and educational influence, museums' explicit therapeutic potential is being developed and implemented by art therapists (Betts *et al.* 2015; Colbert *et al.* 2013; Coles and Harrison 2018; Deane, Carman and Fitch 2000; Kaufman *et al.* 2014; Pantagoutsou, Ioannides and Vaslamatzis 2017; Peacock 2012; Thaler *et al.* 2017; Treadon, Rosal and Thompson Wylder 2006; Salom 2011, 2015;

Shaer *et al.* 2008; Spraggins Rochford 2017). Art therapy programmes in museums have addressed issues of empathy, development, life stages, mental/physical health, trauma and disaster relief, among others. Collaborations between art therapists and museums have served a wide range of populations, including children, young adults and older adults, with psychological challenges (Coles and Harrison 2018; Pantagoutsou *et al.* 2017), eating disorders (Thaler *et al.* 2017), emotional and behavioural difficulties (Treadon *et al. 2006*) and a variety of health and social needs (Shaer *et al.* 2008). Through art therapy processes, the museum experience has gained therapeutic leverage.

A project developed by Coles and Harrison (2018) provided a clear example of art therapists' objectives when working in museums. Their programme ran 18 art therapy sessions for young adults with severe mental difficulties, at two museums in Gloucester. The aims established were 'to help participants to understand themselves better; to foster the ability to form and sustain positive relationships with others; to encourage social inclusion; and to inspire creativity' (*ibid.*, p.115). As the objectives illustrate, among the value that art therapy adds to the museum experience there is an emphasis on 'learning about ourselves through the content in [museums]' (Salom 2008, p.1) and on the emotional growth that happens from intentionally learning about others, from others and about the world (Peacock 2012; Salom 2008; Spraggins Rochford 2017). Art therapists aim to create safe spaces, where it is possible to handle difficult emotional subjects and interpersonal conflicts (Ottemiller and Awais 2016, p.145). The conscious and deliberate transformation of individuals' subjective interpretations marks the distinction from related practices (Marxen 2009; Salom 2015). These transformations can be associated to psychological, relational and social contexts (Kaplan 2007). The collective aspect of the art therapy/museum collaboration may be useful in Colombia, as social engagement may lessen the sense of isolation that is prevalent in many individuals who have undergone traumatic experiences (Herman 1997).

There are a variety of theoretical frameworks that have been applied in the art therapy/museum partnership, as Peacock (2012) and Spraggins Rochford (2017) have described in detail. The range in logistics, themes and frameworks corresponds to the wide scope of foci within the art therapy field (Bucciarelli 2016; Salom 2017). Some are closer to the psychotherapeutic end of the art therapy spectrum (Coles and Harrison 2018; Pantagoutsou *et al.* 2017). Some programmes focus on art processes as the primary therapeutic element. Other projects lean towards social action (Betts *et al.* 2015; Colbert *et al.* 2013; Deane *et al.* 2000; Kaufaman *et al.* 2014; Peacock 2012). All art therapy approaches in museums foster creativity and wellbeing and can be used in tandem with one another, depending on the population, the objectives and the therapists' training. They confront the definition, boundaries and application of both the art therapy and the museum fields and invite their evolution. With the collaboration, museums can offer deliberate therapeutic assistance, thus becoming institutions that can provide mental health services; simultaneously, art therapy can expand a museum's community and social action reach, as explained below.

Social action art therapy, community-based practices and the transdisciplinary view

Socially oriented art therapy/museum collaborations are suitable for communities seeking social reparation, peacebuilding, and citizen participation on a large scale. In the introduction to the book *Art Therapy and Social Action*, Frances Kaplan (2007) described art therapy starting out 'as a form of psychoanalysis that used visual imagery' (p.12). The field transformed to include group formats, diverse types of foci, and cultural sensitivity (*ibid.*, p.12). Introducing the rationale for social action art therapy, Kaplan (2007) proposed that cultural and social factors should be considered along with 'personal and relationship factors' (p.15). Similarly, Ottemiller and Awais (2016) advocated for the expansion of art therapy into 'community-based practices that embrace wellness and prevention' (p.144).

As we introduce art therapy into different cultures and contexts which process social factors in a collective manner, a transdisciplinary view may benefit the growth of the profession. The transdisciplinary art therapy model proposed by Bucciarelli (2016) includes five areas that interact and support one another according to the needs of the population. The areas are: art techniques and processes, psychological theories, biological understanding, sociocultural constructs, and educational models (*ibid.*, p.152). The areas do not compete, nor do they interact lightly. Rather, they are integrated into cohesive practices, with complex fusions unique to art therapy (*ibid.*). The model can embrace the different social, relational, systemic and social justice theories related to community-based art therapy practices (Ottemiller and Awais 2016, p.144).

The different areas within the profession enrich and foster the others through interaction (Salom 2017) and, like the reactive substances in Berrada's performance, respond to create entirely new dynamics reminiscent of potential space. Art therapists who can understand and speak several technical languages can establish relationships with professionals from various disciplines additional to psychologists, psychiatrists, social workers and occupational therapists. 'To further a culturally situated identity for the profession' (*ibid.*, p.72) attuned to community values, multidisciplinary collaborations may include experts on trauma, peace, social justice and museums as well as 'artisans, festival organizers, [and] community leaders' (*ibid.*, p.72). The range of training of art therapy professionals, which includes psychological and artistic proficiency among other skills related to human development, can provide cohesive collaborations with many groups of people (Bucciarelli 2016; Salom 2017). Our education and practice, which includes artistic, educational and sociocultural aspects, is akin to, and may facilitate the bond with, museums' undertakings.

Colombian museums and social action

Contemporary exhibitions and art initiatives inside Colombian museums indicate artists' and curators' roles in the building of a more just, dignified and peaceful society. Those described below reflect themes included in Chapter 5 of the 2016 peace agreement (Colombian National Government and FARC-EP 2016), even though some occurred before the current peace process was initiated. Premises and narratives related to social responsibility, symbolic restitution, reintegration and citizen participation are present throughout.

The War We Have Not Seen was an exhibition at MAMBO (Museo de Arte Moderno de Bogotá) in autumn 2009. The title marked the need to evidence the truth of events related to the armed conflict. It showed 90 paintings created by 80 individuals who had previously participated in armed guerrilla groups, paramilitary groups or the government's army. As the show's curator expressed (Tiscornia 2009), the exhibition thus challenged notions about the relationships between members of opposing sides in the war. Previous adversaries suspended judgement to paint, during a two-year span. Participants had no formal art instruction yet the works were detailed and expressive. They depicted personal memories, accounts and affidavits that defied the Colombian tendency towards the normalisation of violence, and disallowed forgetfulness of the war that occurred (*ibid.*). Artist Juan Manuel Echavarria created the event (*ibid.*).

An exhibition of Pedro Ruiz's work, *GOLD: Spirit and Nature of a Territory,* was also shown at MAMBO in 2009. The exhibition depicted canoes filled with rich icons of the cultural and geographic identity of internally displaced populations in Colombia. The icons included exuberant, blown-up images of fauna and flora. Internally displaced refugees in Colombia face extreme circumstances and acculturation challenges as they adapt to urban life, cultural differences, dispossession of belongings and the lack of even the most essential of basic needs. The delicacy of the images contrasted starkly with the broken identity and economic poverty of many displaced individuals. The work portrayed abundant and splendid heritages amidst the conflict, and delved into the concept of natural and cultural wealth (Ruiz 2009). Despite being the sole painter in the exhibition, Ruiz described this project as collective because it drew from the personal experiences of many (*ibid.*).

Diana Rico and Richard Décaillet, through Colectivo 4 Direcciones, presented *The Origin of the Night* at the Museo de Arte de la Universidad Nacional in 2016. A sound installation, looping the chants of spiritual leaders from six different ethnicities, it was intended to convert the 'art museum into a *maloca* igniting the spiritual healing of visitors' [emphasis added] (Rico and Décalliet 2016). A maloca is a community home, traditional to the indigenous people of the Amazons; 4 Direcciones brought the healing vibrations found inside malocas into the middle of the city, via the museum. Among the objectives, the exhibition intended to preserve, honour and carry forward the values and practices of indigenous peoples, as well as denounce the calamity that their cultures have faced in relation to Western paradigms and the internal conflict (*ibid.*). The exhibition destabilised the oppressive power dynamics, which rarely include indigenous expressions in the Colombian art scene. A tribute was made to heritage, multicultural collaboration and equality.

In a more metaphorical way, El Museo del Oro added to the collective notion of reparation through a temporary exhibition in 2018 called *Can this be Fixed: How and Why we Repair Things*. This show took place two years after the peace agreement was signed, showing a commitment to the ongoing and long-term process of change that is needed. The show presented techniques for repairing both precious and ordinary objects from different time periods. It included methods from pre-Hispanic times, such as hinges made from rolled out links of golden metal. Some techniques resemble the ones used to craft the pieces, while others are greatly different, combining the fundamental materials used in the original piece (such as clay) with another material (such as a cotton cord). Without directly mentioning the task of social reparation that the country is facing, the exhibit suggested reflections about brokenness, deterioration, use, value, ancestry and need. One of the exhibition labels addressed the issue succinctly: 'We fix things not only because it is possible to do so, but because it is personally, socially and culturally necessary' (Subgerencia Cultural del Banco de la República 2018).

Along with exhibitions, Colombian museums offer programmes to educate about peacemaking. The Museo Nacional, housing archaeological, ethnographic, historic and art collections, showed *The Past, Present and Future of Peace in Colombia* in 2018. The exhibition contained a series of iconographic posters that informed viewers about the peace agreements that have been signed in the country during the 20th and 21st centuries. The posters were freely distributed to libraries, museums and other institutions around the country (Museo Nacional de Colombia 2018).

The museums of the Banco de la República (Subgerencia Cultural del Banco de la República 2013a) have an initiative called *La Paz se Toma la Palabra* – a play on words which can be translated as *Peace Speaks Up*. The initiative generates and implements cultural dynamics for the construction of peace. For instance, the project called *Children Think About Peace* offered literary workshops for children around Colombia. It concluded with an illustrated book that presents children's written perspectives and requests related to the conflict (Gaviria and Naranjo Moreno 2015). The book includes directives for educators who want to replicate the workshops. *Facing an Other: Drawings in the Post Conflict* was initiated in 2013 (Subgerencia Cultural del Banco de la República 2013b) and was framed within an intervention to help 130 individuals reintegrate back into civilian life after leaving an armed group. Professional experts on reintegration worked alongside 12 graphic artists to lead drawing and comic-strip workshops. The resulting self-portraits generated discussion about identity and belonging.

Museums as art therapists' co-leaders

Animistic thought, found in the Colombian territory during pre-Hispanic times and still alive within many communities today, portrays objects and places as having autonomous intentions. Using animistic cosmology, it is viable to say that contemporary museums, exhibitions – and even individual art pieces – carry an active agency; each carries a certain theme and contains form, texture and colour configurations that influence visitors in particular ways. I worded this concept in the language of art therapy when I described the museum as an art therapy 'co-leader', and wrote that 'museums can confront or contain experiences, allow different pacing rhythms, and offer or restrain choices according to the population being served' (Salom 2011, p.82). Thinking about each museum as a 'co-leader' resonates with art therapists' training in metaphorical thought. This metaphor can be useful when planning what each museum and exhibition can provide in terms of content, history, atmosphere and logistics (*ibid.*).

For instance, the themes of the temporary exhibitions and projects described above responded to some of the collective needs of Colombian society and to the peacebuilding processes in various ways. Each exhibition, in a unique manner, documented the atrocities experienced by segments of the population, and did so in an aesthetic way that enhanced the life-affirming qualities of creativity. They leaned towards reparation by integrating the experiences, wisdom and knowing of different people, including marginalised and oppressed groups and adversaries. The exhibitions made problems visible. They modelled peaceful co-existence through art-making and addressed Colombian identity, inviting audiences to rethink it as resilient and culturally rich. The shows imparted historical information, promoting truth and memory. They produced reflections about transitions, change, tolerance, identity, equality, inclusion, participation and empowerment. They evidenced our need, desire and ability to repair and shift oppressive power dynamics. The museum exhibitions spoke to the process of social reconciliation through symbolic means and proposed restorative and socially participatory actions.

Art therapists can translate the objectives of exhibitions into therapeutic terms, as I have done above. However, we have a bigger influence to bring into action. First, art therapists' experience, training, supervision and ethical considerations can prevent many trial-and-error situations in the social arts initiatives that happen outside our discipline (Kalmanowitz and Potash 2010; Marxen 2009; Ottemiller and Awais 2016). As experts on processes of transformation kindled through metaphors, symbols, intrapersonal and interpersonal dynamics, we have a role to play in the evolution of the museum as an agent of social change.

Second, museums as 'co-leaders' point towards a socially and collectively inclined art therapy. As mentioned earlier, learning about ourselves includes learning about ourselves in a group and as part of society at large (Kaplan 2007; Ottemiller and Awais 2016). In museums, personal and relational themes can be explored as well as social, environmental and cultural ones (Kaplan 2007, p.15). We can design community-based art therapy directives (Betts *et al.* 2015; Spraggins Rochford 2017) to facilitate collective non-verbal dialogues between diverse populations (Ottemiller and Awais 2016; Peacock 2012). In further forging the transformation of art therapy and museums in socially based arenas, and as they react to each other's proximity, we can strive to ease personal as well as collective suffering.

The exhibitions described above stand out in my mind as transformative and socially restorative and, from an art therapist's perspective, visitors to the exhibitions can be involved therapeutically: emotionally, artistically and socially. Below, I discuss potential art therapy directives for visitors to four of the exhibitions.

Collective visual narratives

I envision visitors painting inside museums in response to the images shown in *The War We Have Not Seen*. Depending on the objectives established, art therapists could invite visitors to pictorially express their own memories, their own role in the unseen conflict, their empathy towards the actors in the war, and their grievances. Museum visitors could thus expand on the graphical documentation and processing of what has occurred. This would involve discussion with the artists, exhibition organisers and museum personnel about logistical considerations, and expectations, and informing visitors about the risks and benefits of participating (Ottemiller and Awais 2016; Salom 2011; Wadeson 2000). With agreement from participants, carefully chosen art responses could be delivered to the original artists, their families and their communities. With consent, reproductions of response art could travel along with reproductions of the original pieces to remote places in the country. Alternatively, the originals could be exhibited together with the responses at national museums and galleries. A public thread of collective visual narrative could emerge to elaborate events related to the war.

Personal totems

Like Pedro Ruiz's *GOLD*, *Proyecto Chiva* addresses identity, change and permanency. I propose for the two to be implemented in conjunction with one another. In my proposal, a work area overseen by an art therapist would be set behind the images of the golden canoes, providing durable three-dimensional art materials. *Proyecto Chiva* involves building a means of transportation and placing symbols of valuable resources inside it (Figure 13.2). I imagine visitors of all ages and backgrounds being inspired by *GOLD*, making and filling canoes with totems of their own fertile talents, their innate wild beauty and their creative capabilities. *Proyecto Chiva* includes a moment for sharing the sculptures and verbally elucidating the trajectories that they represent. This moment can happen at the work area or during scheduled workshops held by art therapists at museums. The constructed pieces can provoke extensive visual and verbal dialogues related to Colombians' collective resilience. The individual canoes can be taken home as reminders of personal esteem.

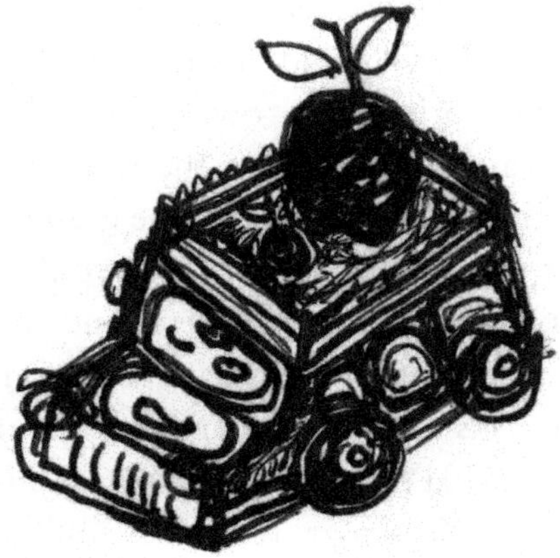

Figure 13.2 A personal chiva (drawing by author)

Shift in leadership

The Origin of the Night ignited in me a desire for a collective performance in which every participant adds a personal piece to the whole: an in situ woven mural of contrasting materials inspired by the chants, for instance. However, when collaborating with indigenous populations who have unbroken lineages related to the use of ritual and who have been underserved by cultural institutions, I believe the art therapist's first role is to ask questions and learn from the cultural traditions. Therefore, the initial art therapy action in relationship to this exhibition would include a dialogue with the presenters, the curators and the public. The dialogue could include verbal and art-based responses to the following questions: What occurred in each one of us as we listened to the deep voices being reproduced? Would it be culturally attuned to propose an additional collective action? Would the six indigenous groups be interested in leading such creation? Can it be safe for participants to transgress the boundaries between cosmologies and engage in collective work? Cultural sensitivity, awareness of power structures and use of systems perspectives can add to how art therapy approaches community dynamics (Ottemiler and Awais 2016).

Citizen participation

After seeing *Can this be Fixed*, I fancied the city filled with repair carts, loaded with tools for fixing all kinds of objects. In my proposed action, crafts people, technicians and volunteers lead the travelling workshops, assessing damaged items and providing strategies for restoration. For some individuals, the repair of their precious objects might be enough. For others, conversations about reparation could be taken into the personal, relational and social arenas, guided and structured by art therapists. Such conversations could happen as objects are being repaired, or later at an organised forum led by art therapists. Social participation steered by art therapists and museums can include extended groups of the population, both inside and beyond the walls of the museum.

Conclusion

Art therapy interventions in museums can adopt various unconventional formats. They can happen in large groups, or art therapists can be available for individual visitors wishing to gain personal insight through exhibitions. Whether made in a group, or in an individual session, visitors' artwork can be itinerant, taken home, curated or exhibited collectively in different cultural sites. The work can form part of printed booklets, formal books or video productions. Large-scale initiatives can help identify social problems and bring about dialogues regarding solutions (Kaplan 2007). Response art made by visitors at museums can provide further dynamism in the collective construction of meaning.

The theoretical frames, therapeutic boundaries and ethical considerations of collective work may stem from traditional group and individual art therapy approaches and from the emphasis that art therapists place on safe space. However, it is yet to be seen how these elements undergo a transformation and adapt to the needs of large-scale arrangements. A focus on clear expectations, limitations and goals can differentiate between community and clinical processes (Ottemiller and Awais 2016; Wadeson 2000). Clear theoretical frames and significant therapeutic relationships can demarcate the boundaries between art therapy and related practices (Arrington 2001; Marxen 2009).

I informally asked a few visitors for their responses to the *Pressage* performance. A woman told me she disliked the music because it induced emotion. One girl saw a castle projected on the wall. Another saw an alien and told me a whole story that developed from there on. A physicist explained minerals, the beginning of life on earth and bacterial mouth plaque. A mother showed me a video that she took of her son's silhouette moving in relation to a projection on the wall: an exploding flower, a boy reaching for it. People played, projected their intimacies and saw according to their training, life stories and circumstances. The elements in the beakers were transformed, as well as the viewers.

The art therapy/museum junction is kindling a change in both disciplines involved. In turn, their interaction can be generative for museum visitors, their view of the world and their subjective experiences. By stabilising our bond with museum educators to provide ongoing art therapy services, we can play an important role, not only for the benefit of marginalised groups but also for the wellbeing of the public at large. Our cultural beliefs around social conflict, psychological suffering, collective identity and creativity can be modified through transdisciplinary initiatives. As cultural institutions continue to provide transformative experiences for citizen participation and reparation, novel dynamics and social justice will be part of the art therapy/museum agenda.

References

Alto Comisionado de las Naciones Unidas para los Refugiados (ACNUR) (2016) *Tendencias Globales Sobre Refugiados y Otras Personas de Interés del ACNUR*. www.acnur.org/recursos/estadisticas.

Anderson, G. (ed.) (2004) *Reinventing the Museum: Historical and Contemporary Perspective on the Paradigm Shift*. Walnut Creek, CA: Altamira.

Arrington, D. (2001) 'Why do we make art? A reflective paper.' *Art Therapy: Journal of the American Art Therapy Association 18*, 2, 105–108.

Artera, C. (June 22, 2017) '¿Y si el arte y la cultura fueran las claves de la reconciliación en Colombia?' *Revista Semana*. Accessed on 15/8/2018 at www.semana.com/nacion/articulo/el-arte-y-la-cultura-como-agentes-de-transformacion-y-reconciliacion-en-colombia/529466.

Betts, D.J., Potash, J.S., Luke, J.J. and Kelso, M. (2015) 'An art therapy study of visitor reactions to the United States Holocaust Memorial Museum.' *Museum Management and Curatorship 30*, 1, 21–43.

Bucciarelli, A. (2016) 'Art therapy: A transdisciplinary approach.' *Art Therapy: Journal of the American Art Therapy Association 33*, 155–158.

Cameron, D.F. (1971) 'The museum, a temple or the forum.' *Curator: The Museum Journal 14*, 1, 11–24.

Camic, P.M. and Chatterjee, H.J. (2013) 'Museums and art galleries as partners for public health interventions.' *Perspectives in Public Health 133*, 1, 66–71.

Chatterjee, H.J. and Noble, G. (2013) *Museums, Health and Well-Being*. Farnham: Ashgate.

Cobo, M. (2013) *The Voice of Colombian Art Therapists: Cultural Considerations for Art Therapists in the Colombian Territory*. (Master's thesis). Lesley University.

Colbert, S., Cooke, A., Camic, P.M. and Springham, N. (2013) 'The art-gallery as a resource for recovery for people who have experienced psychosis.' *The Arts in Psychotherapy 40*, 2, 250–56.

Coles, A. and Harrison, F. (2018) 'Tapping into museums for art psychotherapy: An evaluation of a pilot group for young adults.' *International Journal of Art Therapy 23*, 3, 115–124.

Colombian National Government and FARC-EP (2016) *Final Agreement to End the Armed Conflict and Build a Stable and Lasting Peace*. Accessed on 13/7/2019 at http://especiales.presidencia.gov.co/Documents/20170620-dejacion-armas/acuerdos/acuerdo-final-ingles.pdf

Comisión Nacional de Reparación y Reconciliación-Grupo de Memoria Histórica (CNRR-GMH) (2010) *Bojayá, la Guerra sin Límites*. Bogotá: Ediciones Semana.

Deane, K., Carman, M. and Fitch, M. (2000) 'The cancer journey: Bridging art therapy and museum education.' *Canadian Oncology Nursing Journal 10*, 4, 140–42.

De Montebello, P. (2005) 'Museums: Why should we care?' *Leisure and Arts*, editorial page. Accessed on 10/3/2006 at www.opinionjournal.com/la/?id=110006760.

Froggett, L. and Trustram, M. (2014) 'Object relations in the museum: A psychosocial perspective.' *Museum Management and Curatorship 29*, 5, 1–16.

Gaviria, P. and Naranjo Moreno, J. (2015) *Los Niños Piensan la Paz*. Bogotá: Banco de la República.

Herman, J. (1997) *Trauma and Recovery: The Aftermath of Violence – from Domestic Abuse to Political Terror*. New York, NY: Basic Books.

Kalmanowitz, D. and Potash, J. S. (2010) 'Ethical considerations in the global teaching and promotion of art therapy to non-art therapists.' *The Arts in Psychotherapy 37*, 1, 20–26.

Kaplan, F.F. (ed.) (2007) *Art Therapy and Social Action*. London and Philadelphia, PA: Jessica Kingsley Publishers.

Kaufman, R., Rinehardt, E., Hine, H., Wilkinson, B. *et al.* (2014) 'The effects of a museum art programme on the self-concept of children.' *Art Therapy: Journal of the American Art Therapy Association 31*, 3, 118–125.

Lavine, S. and Karp, I. (1991) *Exhibiting Cultures: The Poetics and Politics of Museum Display*. Washington DC: Smithsonian Institution Press.

Lobo-Guerrero, N. (2013) 'Art Therapy to Reduce PTSD Symptoms of Displaced Women in Colombia.' (Unpublished master's thesis). Pratt Institute.

Londoño Vélez, S. (2005) *Breve Historia de la Pintura en Colombia*. Bogotá: Fondo de Cultura Económica.

Marxen, E. (2009) 'Therapeutic thinking in contemporary art: Or psychotherapy in the arts.' *The Arts in Psychotherapy 36*, 131–139.

Museo Nacional de Colombia (2018) *Presente, Pasado y Futuro de la Paz en Colombia* (*Present, Past and Future of Peace in Colombia*). Accessed on 15/8/2018 at www.museonacional.gov.co/exposiciones/carteles/paz/Paginas/Paz%20en%20Colombia.aspx.

Ottemiller, D. and Awais, Y.J. (2016) 'A model for art therapists in community-based practice.' *Art Therapy: Journal of the American Art Therapy Association 33*, 3, 144–150.

Pantagoutsou, A., Ioannides, E. and Vaslamatzis, G. (2017) 'Exploring the museum's images – Exploring my image (Exploration des images du musée, exploration de mon image).' *Canadian Art Therapy Association Journal 30*, 2, 69–77.

Peacock, K. (2012) 'Museum education and art therapy: Exploring an innovative partnership.' *Art Therapy: Journal of the American Art Therapy Association 29*, 3, 133–137.

Rancière, J. (2009) *The Emancipated Spectator*. London: Verso.

Rico, D. and Décalliet, R. (2016) *El Origen de la Noche* (*The Origin of the Night*). Accessed on 15/8/2018 at www.4direcciones.tv/el-origen-de-la-noche.

Ruiz, P. (2009) *ORO: Espíritu y Naturaleza de un Territorio* (*GOLD: Spirit and Nature of a Territory*). Accessed on 15/8/2018 at www.pedroruiz.co/past-works.

Salom, A. (2008) 'The therapeutic potentials of a museum visit.' *International Journal of Transpersonal Studies 27*, 1, 98–103.

Salom, A. (2011) 'Reinventing the setting: Art therapy in museums.' *The Arts in Psychotherapy 38*, 2, 81–85.

Salom, A. (2015) 'Weaving potential space and acculturation: Art therapy at the museum.' *Journal of Applied Arts & Health 6*, 1, 47–62.

Salom, A. (2017) 'Claiming the polarity of art therapy: Lessons from the field in Colombia.' *Art Therapy: Journal of the American Art Therapy Association 34*, 2, 68–74.

Shaer, D., Beaven, K., Springham, N., Pillinger, S. *et al.* (2008) 'The role of art therapy in a pilot for art-based information prescriptions at Tate Britain.' *International Journal of Art Therapy 13,* 1, 25–33.
Silverman, L.H. (2010) *The Social Work of Museums.* London: Routledge.
Silverstone, R. (1992) 'The Medium is the Museum: On Objects and Logics in Times and Spaces.' In J. Durant (ed.) *Museums and the Public Understanding of Science.* London: NMSI Trading.
Spraggins Rochford, J. (2017) 'Art therapy and art museum education: A visitor-focused collaboration.' *Art Therapy: Journal of the American Art Therapy Association 34,* 4, 209–214.
Subgerencia Cultural del Banco de la República (2013a) *Proyecto de Paz: Frente al Otro* (*Peace Project: Facing Another*). Accessed on 15/8/2018 at www.banrepcultural.org/proyecto-paz/frente-al-otro.
Subgerencia Cultural del Banco de la República (2013b) *Proyecto de Paz los Niños Piensan la Paz* (*Peace Project Children Think about Peace*). Accessed on 15/8/2018 at www.banrepcultural.org/proyecto-paz/los-ninos-piensan-la-paz/que-es-el-proyecto-los-ninos-piensan-la-paz.
Subgerencia Cultural del Banco de la República (2017) *Paisajes Reactivas* (*Reactive Landscapes*). Accessed on 15/8/2018 at www.arteinformado.com/agenda/f/hicham-berrada-paisajes-reactivos-141155.
Subgerencia Cultural del Banco de la República (2018) *Esto Tiene Arreglo* (*Can this be Fixed*). Accessed on 15/8/2018 at www.banrepcultural.org/bogota/contenido/esto-tiene-arreglo.
Thaler, L., Drapeau, C.E., Leclerc, J., Lajeunesse, M. *et al.* (2017) 'An adjunctive, museum-based art therapy experience in the treatment of women with severe eating disorders.' *The Arts in Psychotherapy 56,* 1–6. http://dx.doi.org/doi:10.1016/j.aip.2017.08.002.
Tiscornia, A. (2009) *The War We Have Not Seen* (*La Guerra que no Hemos Visto*). Accessed on 15/8/2018 at www.laguerraquenohemosvisto.com/english/ensayo_tiscornia.html.
Treadon, C.B., Rosal, M. and Thompson Wylder, V.D.T. (2006) 'Opening the doors of art museums for therapeutic processes.' *The Arts in Psychotherapy 33,* 4, 288–301.
Wadeson, H. (2000) *Art Therapy Practice: Innovative Approaches with Diverse Populations.* New York, NY: John Wiley and Sons.
Winnicott, D.W. (1971) *Playing and Reality.* New York, NY: Basic Books.
Winnicott, D.W. (1989) 'The Fate of the Transitional Object.' In C. Winnicott, R. Shepherd, and M. Davis (eds) *Psycho-Analytic Explorations.* Cambridge, MA: Harvard University Press.

Biographies

Mary Chamberlain has worked for over twenty years as a creative practitioner with marginalised people. Her experience includes work within the NHS, Modern Art Oxford, Support a Survivor of Torture and the Helen Bamber Foundation. She is also a professional artist, trained art therapist and has served as a trustee of Arts and Health South West.

Ali Coles has master's degrees in art psychotherapy and in museum and gallery management. She is an art psychotherapist for Gloucestershire Health and Care NHS Foundation Trust in England and lectures in art psychotherapy at the University of South Wales.

Michael Fischer has worked as an art therapist in child and adolescent mental health services for 17 years. He is also a practising sculptor focusing on woodcarving and ceramics.

Fiona Fitzpatrick is an art psychotherapist and founder and Director of the community interest company Arts Psychotherapies UK, working with a wide range of groups and individual clients.

Louise Giroux, BA, BFA, has worked in museum education for more than 20 years and is Programme Officer for Well-Being at the Montreal Museum of Fine Arts. She is committed to the principle and practice that art brings people together in their shared humanity.

Sheila Grandison is an art psychotherapist (Goldsmiths) and group-analytic supervisor (IGA). She is currently Training & Development Lead for Arts Therapies, East London NHS Foundation Trust, and Visiting Lecturer, School of Health Sciences, City, University of London.

Simon Hackett, PhD, is Principal Arts Psychotherapist at Northumberland, Tyne and Wear NHS Foundation Trust and Honorary Senior Clinical Lecturer at the Institute of Health and Society, Newcastle University. Simon is a clinical-academic art psychotherapist.

Emma Hollamby is Art and Dementia Programme Manager at Ben Uri Gallery and Museum. Broadening access to visual art and understanding its benefit, particularly for older people, has led Emma to both facilitation and research.

Sue Holttum, PhD, AFBPsS, CPsychol, works as a senior lecturer at the Salomons Institute for Applied Psychology, Canterbury Christ Church University, England, and as a part-time research officer for the British Association of Art Therapists.

Elaine Homer is a UK HCPC registered art psychotherapist working in schools and with adults in the community. With a background in media education, she also offers professional development for teachers.

Helen Jury established the MA in Art Psychotherapy at the University of South Wales, then moved to doctoral research at University College London. Art psychotherapist experience in the NHS, CAMHS, institutional, and supervisory work informs her current practice in student psychological services and independent practice.

Marilyn Lajeunesse, BA, BEd, MEd, has worked in museum education for over 25 years. She has created programmes, educational texts and audio guides. She initiated and continues to coordinate the ongoing Montreal Museum of Fine Arts *Sharing the Museum* inclusion programme.

Jane Landes is a UK HCPC registered art therapist with a background in adult mental health, private practice and art therapy education. Her focus is now on her own visual art practice.

Stephen Legari, MA, MSc(A), ATPQ, ATR, CFT, is an art therapist, couple and family therapist, and art therapy supervisor based in Montreal, Quebec. He is the Programme Officer for Art Therapy at the Montreal Museum of Fine Arts.

Bobby Lloyd is a visual artist, HCPC registered art therapist, supervisor and educator working in the UK and internationally. As Chief Executive Officer of Art Refuge UK, she leads its programme in northern France.

Karen Lund is an art therapist who facilitates groups with poor mental health, multiple sclerosis and brain damage in private practice and organisations, and with groups at risk of social exclusion, in the Bilbao Fine Arts Museum.

Ruth McGovern, PhD, is a lecturer in public health research and National Institute for Health Research Postdoctoral Research Fellow at the Institute of Health and Society, Newcastle University. Ruth's research aims to reduce lifestyle risk to help improve health and social outcomes.

Jordan Potash, PhD, ATR-BC, REAT, LCAT, LPCAT is a US registered, board certified, and licensed art therapist, a registered expressive arts therapist, and Associate Professor, Art Therapy Graduate Program, The George Washington University.

Naomi Press is an HCPC registered art therapist, supervisor, educator and visual artist based in France and working internationally. She is a core member of the Art Refuge UK team working in northern France.

Andrée Salom, MPS, ATR, is Academic Director of the Creative Arts Program at Universidad de los Andes and Co-founder of the Colombian Art Therapy Association. She is a children's book author and runs an art therapy practice in Bogotá.

Whittaker Scott has worked in the NHS as an art psychotherapist in England with children and young people since 1996. He also has an interest in landscape photography and landscape painting.

Miriam Usiskin is an HCPC registered art therapist, educator and supervisor. Working in the UK and internationally, she is senior lecturer at the University of Hertfordshire and a core Art Refuge UK team member in northern France.

Nana Zhvitiashvili MA is a UK HCPC registered art psychotherapist, group therapy practitioner and art historian. She worked as a museum curator, developing art therapy programmes. She works in paediatric and adult oncology.

Subject Index

accessibility
in art therapy 57
in museums 57–8
alcohol misuse
and *Creative Dialogues* project 133–54
'Associate Artists' scheme (Modern Art Oxford) 65, 66–7
adults with eating disorders
research on art therapy 33–4
adults with mental health issues
research on art therapy 31–3
adults without identified health difficulties
research on art therapy 34
Aivazovsky, Ivan 90, 91
art galleries
environment of 72
focus on visual in 96
Art Hive (Montreal Museum of Fine Arts) 173–4
art psychotherapy
absence of portraits 257–60
clinical context 250–2
and gallery artworks 244–5
internal dialogic space in 255–7
process of 249–50
reflective space for 260–1
and Rembrandt self-portraits 245–8, 250, 258–9, 262–3, 247
review in 246–257, 259, 261–265
role of the portrait in 247–8
time, space and process in 252–5
Art Refuge UK 265, 266, 267, 282
art therapy
accessibility and inclusivity in 57
and emotional attachment to museums 47–8
ideas of containment in 49–50
research on 28–34
research on in museums 159–60, 170, 171–3
and social action 297–8
therapeutic benefits of 27
therapeutic factors in museums and galleries 35–6
art therapy courses 170–1
Art Therapy and Social Action (Kaplan) 297
arts activities
access to 181, 182–3
benefits of 26–7
asylum seekers
and *Making Space Safe* group 63–79
BALTIC Centre for Contemporary Art
artist in art therapy group 231–3
attendance at project 231
background to project in 224–5
discussions with local NHS 229–30
exhibition from project 234–6
initial networking 229
outcomes from project 236–40
parent/carer involvement 231
recruitment for project 230–1
space and equipment for project 233–4
Beck Youth Inventories 237
Ben Uri Gallery and Museum *see Starting with Art* project
Berrada, Hicham 290
Berson, Lazar 109
Beveridge, Philippa 11–12
Bilbao Fine Arts Museum (BFAM) *see Let's Include the Museum* programme
Blacklock, James 231
Body Satisfaction Scale 172

Calais transit camps
art installation 271–4
box of postcards 274–8
context of 266–7

Calais transit camps *cont.*
description of project 265–6
map in artwork 278–82
nature of work 267–70
virtual galleries in 282–5
cancer
research on art therapy 28
Colombian museums
collective arts in 293–5
Hicham Berrada installation 290
museums as art therapy co-leaders in 301–5
political background to 291–2
social action in 298–301
cost-effectiveness of art therapy 38–9
Creative Dialogues project
art therapist's role in 144–5
background to 133–6
exhibition from 146–51
group agreement 139
museum visits 137–42
results of 151–4
themes of 136–7
Culture on Demand (DCMS) 189
curatorial staff
and art therapy 97–102
skill sharing 96–7
staff education 96–7

Décaillet, Richard 299
dementia
and the arts 109
in *Starting with Art* project 108–30
statistics on 109
drug misuse
and *Creative Dialogues* project 133–54

East London NHS Foundation Trust *see* ELFT/Tate partnership
eating disorders
research on art therapy 33–4
ELFT/Tate partnership
art therapy context for 183–8
description of 182
group dialogue in 194–9
phases of 190
policy context for 188–93
working model for 193–4
Ellis, Liz 189
Equality, Diversity and the Creative Case (Arts Council England) 181
ethnic minorities
attitude to museums 48–9
evaluation
of art therapy in museums 94
Let's Include the Museum programme 211–12
at Montreal Museum of Fine Arts 162, 172
research on 31–2, 36–7
Starting with Art project 126–8
Evans, Laura 172

Fischer, Michael 231, 238
Fitzpatrick, Fiona 134
Fuirer, Michèle 189
future approaches for research 36–9

Glasser, David 110

Hackett, Simon 134
Hall, Rose 190
Hands, Stephanie 190
Helen Bamber Foundation (HBF) 64
Heller, Vera 171–2

inclusion
in art therapy 57
in museums 57–8
integration
encouragement of 94–5

Korzinski, Michael 64

Lajeunesse, Marilyn 175
Lambert, Jacinthe 173
Lamy, Yvon 163
Leading Change, Adding Value: A Framework for Nursing, Midwifery and Care Staff (NHS England) 192
Lees, Diane 183
Legari, Stephen 160
Let's Include the Museum programme
creative responses to 213–14
evaluation of 211–12
experiences of 214–20
formation of group 212–13
objectives of 204–5
structure of activities 208–11
setting up 203–4
Lingard, Rebecca 190
'Lost and Found' (Beveridge) 11–12

MacDougall, Sarah 117
Making Space Safe group (Modern Art Oxford)
and 'Associate Artists' scheme 65, 66–7
background to group 64
basement usage 75–8
description of group 67–9
name for 63–4, 71
physical setting for 65–6, 72–8
in Project Space 72–5
referral process for 69–70
setting of Modern Art Oxford 70–1
Manifesto for a Humanist Fine Arts Museum 158–9
McGovern, Ruth 134
meaning making 100–1

Médecins du Monde 266–7, 270, 277, 278, 280
mental health carers
research on art therapy 29–30
mental health issues
and ELFT/Tate partnership 181–200
at BALTIC Centre for Contemporary Art 223–41
research on art therapy 31–3
mental health staff
research on art therapy 30
military veterans
research on art therapy 33
Modern Art Oxford *see* *Making Space Safe* group
Montreal Museum of Fine Arts (MMFA)
Art Hive 173–4
art therapy at 160–2
art therapy courses at 170–1
co-creation in 161
description of 157–8
early collaborations at 163–7
evaluation at 162, 172
exhibitions of participants 162
humanist approach in 158–9
later collaborations at 167–9
philanthropy in 176–7
roles in 161–2
sharing best practice 174–6
museum collections
multiple interpretations of 92–3
narratives through 99–100
museums
accessibility in 57–8
as co-leaders in art therapy 301–5
as custodians of heritage 49–53
differing interpretations in 102
as educational space 53–6
and ethnic minorities 48–9
ideas about 44–5
inclusion in 57–8
interactions in 101–2, 290–1
meaning making in 100–1
negative attitudes about 48
as places of play 56
positive attitudes about 46–8
purpose of 45–6
research on art therapy in 159–60, 170, 171–3, 227–8, 295–7
skill sharing 96–7
staff education 96–7
threats to 58–9

National Gallery, London 21, 246–249, 252, 260–261, 265
National Portrait Gallery 44
Neale, Aimee 190

older people
research on art therapy 30–1
in *Starting with Art* project 108–30

partnerships
importance of 92
Philippa Beveridge 11–12
Platonova, Olga 87
Profile of Mood States (POMS-BI) 172
Project Space (Modern Art Oxford) 72–5
Psychological Outcome Profiles (PSYCHLOPS) 31–2, 37
Public Perceptions of – and Attitudes to – the Purposes of Museums in Society (BritainThinks) 45–6

Quirion, Rémi 171

reflective practice
development of 93
refugees
and Calais transit camps project 265–86
and *Making Space Safe* group 63–79
research on art therapy
adults with eating disorders 33–4
adults with mental health difficulties 31–3
adults without identified health difficulties 34
cancer diagnosis 28
cost-effectiveness of 38–9
evaluation in 31–2, 36–7
future approaches 36–9
mental health carers 29–30
mental health staff 30
military veterans 33
in museums 159–60, 170, 171–3, 227–8, 295–7
older people 30–1
therapeutic factors 35–6
wellbeing 37–8
young people 28–9, 226–8
Revised Children's Anxiety and Depression Scale 237
Reyes, Maria 295
Riach 260
Rice, Barbara 189–90
Rico, Diana 299
Rose, Lesley-Anne 231, 238
Rosenberg Self-Esteem Scale 31, 37, 237, 240
Ruiz, Pedro 299

Russia
development of museum-based art therapy 82–6
working with young people with learning difficulties 88–91

safe spaces
importance of 77–8
Sandford, Stephen 190
Scott, Whittaker 229, 231, 238
Seeds of Hope: An arts-based approach to raising awareness about suicide and fostering resiliency project 171–2
Sharing the Museum (Le Musée en partage) program (Montreal Museum of Fine Art–MMFA) 175–6
Silverman, Yehudit 171
skill sharing in museums 96–7, 174–6
Smallwood, Ellen 173
social action
and art therapy 297–8
and Colombian museums 298–301
social prescribing 98–9
Somerset House 117
staff education 96–7
Standards of Proficiency for Arts Therapists (HCPC) 125, 244
Starting with Art project (Ben Uri Gallery and Museum)
art-making in 124–5
artworks used 118–21
clinical placement in 112–13
day centre for 114
description of museum 109–10
evaluation of 126–8
group for chosen 115–16
identity as theme 123–4
migration as theme 121–3
museum visits 116–17
reasons for using art therapy 112
results of 128–30
start of project 110–12
Stone, Emily 189
Strengths and Difficulties Questionnaire (SDQ) 37
substance misuse
and *Creative Dialogues* project 133–54

Tan, Fiona 234
Tate Encounters: Britishness and Visual Culture (Dewdney, Dibosa and Walsh) 194
Tate Modern see ELFT/Tate partnership
Taylor, Aimée 111
Through Different Eyes exhibition (State Russian Museum) 84–6
Timm-Bottos, Janis 170–1, 173

Universal Declaration of Human Rights (United Nations 1948) 181
University College London (UCL) Museum Wellbeing Measure 31, 32, 37–8, 126, 127

Vestergaard, Claire 190

Warwick-Edinburgh Mental Wellbeing Scale 37
wellbeing
research on 37–8
Williams, Jamie 190

young people
at BALTIC Centre for Contemporary Art 223–41
research on art therapy 28–9, 226–8
young people with learning difficulties
Russian case study 88–91
Young Person's CORE 237

Author Index

ACNUR 291
Age and Opportunity 30
Age UK Policy and Research Department 128
Aletraris, L. 136
All-Party Parliamentary Group on Arts, Health and Wellbeing (APPGAHW) 26, 27, 31, 35, 36, 37, 38, 76, 160, 199
Allen, P.B. 174
Alter-Muri, S. 159, 214
Alzheimer's Society 109
Andemicael, A. 268
Ander, F. 48, 58
Anderson, R. 226, 290, 291
Arrington, D. 306
Art Refuge UK 271
Artera, C. 296
Arts Council England 181, 182, 183, 194
Ashworth, M. 31, 37
Aston-Mansfield 184
Awais, Y.J. 292, 296, 298, 302, 303, 305, 306

Babock, J.L. 170
Bachelard, G. 75
Baddeley, G. 33, 165, 172, 173
Baker, J. 251
BALTIC Centre for Contemporary Art 224, 234, 236
Barrett, S.H. 82
Beard, R.I. 112, 126
Beck, A.T. 237
Bedford, L. 54, 152
Belkofer, C.M. 283, 284
Ben-Simon, N. 226
Ben Uri 110, 128
Bennington, R. 159
Berger, J. 101, 245, 246, 247–8, 255, 259, 275
Betts, D.J. 34, 295, 297, 302
Bilbao Fine Arts Museum (BFAM) 214
Bion, W. 50, 101
Bishop, C. 271
Bochenek, M.G. 268
Bockler, J. 39
Bollas, C. 44, 60
Bolwerk, A. 27, 31
Bondil, N. 158
Bourdieu, P. 137, 154
Borghol, N. 27
Bottorff, J.L. 173
Bourriaud, N. 97
Bowlby, J. 47
Boyko, A. 102
Braun, V. 30, 38
BritainThinks 45, 46, 47, 48, 49, 52, 53, 58, 60
British Association of Art Therapists 49, 116, 122
British Association of Art Therapists – Museums and Galleries Special Interest Group (MagSIG) 113
Brooker, J. 140
Bruner, J. 235
Bucciarelli, A. 297, 298
Bull, S. 87
Burnham, J. 194
Burns, M. 171
Byers, A. 124
Bygren, I.O. 26, 27, 98

Callaghan, K. 78
Cameron, D.F. 290, 291
Camic, P.M. 27, 47, 168, 291
Canas, F. 159
Carman, M. 28, 159, 295
Carr, D. 50, 54
Carr, S. 248
Case, C. 50, 205, 206
Casement, P. 211
Cavendish, C. 190
Chaney, D. 96
Chatterjee, H.J. 31, 38, 47, 126, 152, 168, 291
Choi, S. 227
Chorpita, B. 237
Clarke, V. 30, 38
Cloud, W. 136, 153, 154
Clow, A. 27
CNRR-GMH 292, 293, 294, 295
Cobo, M. 293
Colbert, S. 31, 36, 159, 295, 297
Cole, A. 226
Coles, A. 31, 32, 33, 36, 47, 48, 50, 51, 52, 53, 54, 56, 58, 99, 127, 159, 228, 260, 295, 296, 297
Collie, K. 173
Colombian National Government and FARC-EP 292, 298
Concordia University 171
Congreave, E. 226
Cozolino, L. 27

Crawford, M.J. 186
Creative Dialogues 133, 141, 146, 150, 152
Critchley, S. 87
Curtis, E.K. 249, 250, 255

Dalley, T. 50, 203, 204, 205, 206, 210
Darlington, A. 226
De Botton, A. 72
De Montebello, P. 291
Deane, K. 28, 29, 32, 36, 159, 173, 174, 295, 297
Décaillet, R. 299
Deco, S. 174
Deeny, K. 192
Delaney, H. 185
Deliss, C. 71
Delucia, J.M. 32, 33, 36
Department for Culture, Media and Sport 189
Department for Digital, Culture, Media and Sport 49
Derry, C. 56
Desmarais, S. 152
Dewdney, A. 194
Dibosa, D. 194
Dieterich-Hartwell, R. 270, 279
Dodd, J. 85
Doering, Z. 57
Dumison, K. 113

Edlin, G. 120
Edson, G. 54
Edwards, D. 50, 144
Ehresman, C. 109, 112
Einhorn Jardin, L. 285
Ellis, M.L. 250, 262

Falk, A. 123
Fancourt, D. 27
Federov, N. 85
Firm, K. 171
Fisher, S. 172
Fitch, M. 28, 159, 295
Flatt, J.D. 30
Fleming, D. 55
Foucault, M. 84
Francis, R. 190
Fredhoi, C. 27
Freud, S. 99
Froggett, L. 50, 53, 54, 55, 99, 101, 290, 291
Fry, C.E. 227

Gabel, A. 27, 32, 35, 36, 38
Gantt, L. 52
Garner, R. 284
Gaviria, P. 301
Gerlach, G. 268
Gilroy, A. 97, 209, 213
Gingko Press 271
Giroux, Louise 176
Glasser, D. 110
Goldschmidt, M. 120
Goodman, A. 37
Goodman, R. 37
Granfield, R. 137, 153, 154
Greater London Authority 182
Greenblatt, S. 99
Greenwood, H. 232
Griswold, E. 284
Guardian, The 283

Hackett, S. 136
Hamblin, K. 30
Hamil, S. 113, 159, 170
Hancock, S. 248
Harper, S. 30
Harris, D.A. 279
Harrison, F. 31, 32, 33, 36, 47, 52, 54, 56, 58, 99, 127, 159, 228, 295, 296, 297
Havlena, J. 173
Havsteen-Franklin, D. 233
Hawley Reagan, L. 97, 98, 102
Heal, S. 54
Health and Care Professions Council (HCPC) 57, 125
Health Education England 190
Hennessy, E.A. 136
Herman, J.I. 69, 295, 296
Heynen, E. 54
Higenbottam, W. 226
Ho, R.T.H. 34
Hogan, S. 269
Holden, H. 39
Holttum, S. 38
Horsburgh, M. 30
Hosea, H. 174
Housen, A. 96
Huet, V. 30, 35, 38, 99, 235

International Council of Museums Documentation Committee 51
INVOLVE 38
Ioannides, E. 34, 35, 50, 54–5, 57, 99, 111, 159, 295
Isserow, J. 93, 235

James, I. 114
Janes, R.R. 55
Jang, H. 227
Jensen, S.M. 112
Jones, C. 85
Jordanova, L. 100
Jury, H. 35, 113, 159, 245, 246, 252, 255, 258

Kalmanowitz, D. 136, 268, 269, 270, 271, 302
Kaplan, F. 57, 297, 302, 305
Karp, I. 291
Kaufman, R. 227, 295, 297
Keller, M. 160
Killick, K. 101, 102
King, I. 170
Kislev, E. 207
Klein, D.L. 170, 214
Koch, C. 270, 279
Krezinski, A.J. 173
Kurimanzutto 142

Lackoi, K. 138
Lambert, J. 173
Landes, J. 35, 113, 159

Langley, K. 227
Laub, J.H. 154
Lavine, S. 291
Layton, G. 232
Leavy, P. 38
Leggett, J.A. 30
Liebmann, M. 210
Linesch, D. 28, 29, 31, 36, 226, 227
Lloyd, B. 136, 268, 269, 270, 271
Lobban, J. 33
Lobo-Guerrero, N. 291, 292, 293, 294, 295
London, I. 138
London Arts in Health Forum 109
Londoño Vélez, S. 293
Long, B.C. 173
Longabaugh, R. 154
López Martínez, M.D. 214
Lorr, M. 172

MacDougall, S. 117, 123, 124
Maclagan, D. 209
Macpherson of Cluny, W. 187
MagSIG 113
Mahony, J. 209
Malchiodi, C. 174, 284
Malone, E. 228
Marin, A. 159
Marshall-Tierney, A. 233
Martin, A. 283
Marxen, E. 97, 296, 302, 306
McGuigan, K.A. 30
McLaughlin, K.A. 29
McNair, D.M. 172
McNeilly, G. 232
McNiff, S. 35, 146
McNutt, J.V. 283, 284
Memphis Brooks Museum of Art 160
Mermer-Welly, M.J. 159, 228
Miller, G. 227
Moffat, A. 260
Monk, L. 285
Montreal Museum of Fine Arts (MMFA) 163, 168
Moon, B. 269, 271, 272–3
Moreau, A. 170
Murphy, D. 33
Museums Association 45–6, 47, 57, 58
Museo Nacional de Colombia 300
Mustonen, T. 228

Naranjo Moreno, J. 301
Nathoo, S.S. 47
National Collaborating Centre for Mental Health (NCCMH) 185
National Gallery of Art 13
National Health Service (NHS) 127
National Institute for Arts in Health 160
National Institute for Health and Care Excellence 109, 185
Nekrasova-Karateeva, O. 92
NHS England 192
Noble, G. 291

O'Brien, F. 141–2, 149
O'Doherty, B. 76–7
O'Farrell, K. 87
O'Neill, M. 98–9
Osorina, M. 92
Ottemiller, D. 292, 296, 298, 302, 303, 305, 306

Pantagoutsou, A. 34, 35, 295, 296, 297
Papadopoulos, R.K. 64, 270
Parashak, S.T. 159, 174
Patterson, S. 186
Peacock, K. 99, 113, 295, 296, 297, 302
Pearce, S.M. 52
Pepper Goldsmith, T. 226
Phillips, T. 275
Pink, S. 38
Pisani, R. 186
Platonova, O. 92
Point of Care Foundation 38
Potash, J. 269, 302
Press, N. 269
Prokofiev, F. 249
Putnam, R. 137

Radermacher, H. 63, 69, 78
Ramos i Portas, C. 207
Rancière, J. 290, 291
Ranger, D. 173
Rasanen, M. 88–9
Rasmuson, S. 26
Rayner, E. 125
Rees, M. 87
Reilly, R.C. 174
Riach, A. 260
Rice, J. 283
Rico, D. 299
Riley, S. 226
Robb, M. 27, 32, 35, 36, 38
Roberts, S. 27, 29
Rochford, J.S. 174
Rodriguez, C. 291
Rogers, C. 158
Ronnestad, M.H. 113
Rosal, M. 29, 85, 174, 227, 295
Rosen, M. 182–3
Rosenberg, M. 31, 37, 237, 240
Rothwell, K. 136
Royal College of Psychiatrists 185
Ruiz, P. 299
Rusted, L. 129
Rynders, J. 228

Sainsbury Centre for Mental Health 188
Salom, A. 30, 35, 37, 47, 53, 54, 228, 290, 293, 295, 296, 297, 298, 301, 303
Sampson, R.J. 154
Sandell, R. 55, 57

Sandler, I. 29
Scaife, M. 235
Schaverien, J. 50, 104, 118, 136, 138
Schleien, S. 228
Schubert, K. 97
Shaer, D. 29, 30, 58, 100, 159, 202, 215, 296
Sheldon Memory Lab 173
Shelton, K.H. 227
Sheppard, L. 129
Silverman, I.H. 295
Silverman, L. 50, 60, 227
Silverman, Y. 171
Silverstone, R. 291
Simon, N. 195
Simpson, M.G. 83
Skovholt, T.M. 113
Slade, P.D. 172
Slayton, S. 226
Sloan, L. 170
Smallwood, E. 173
Smith, A. 120
Smith, F. 171
Smith, S. 273
Solway, R. 100
Spooner, H. 160
Spraggins Rochford, J. 159, 296, 302
Springham, N. 27
Stafstrom, C.E. 173
Stanton, N. 266, 285
Stern, D. 248
Stevens, J. 36, 38
Stewart-Brown, S. 37
Stiles, G.J. 159, 228
Subgerencia Cultural del Banco de la República 290, 300, 301

Tanizaki, J. 77
Tapia, J.M. 82
Taylor, P. 109
Thaler, I. 33, 34, 38, 159, 165, 166, 167, 172, 295, 296
Thompson, G. 29, 159
Thompson Wylder, V.D. 29, 85, 174, 227, 295
Thomson, I.J. 37, 126, 160
Thumin, N. 100
Thyme, K.F. 173
Times of Israel 121
Timm-Bottos, J. 174
Tinnin, L.W. 52
Tiscornia, A. 299
Tissier, D. 49
Todd, S. 33, 47
Townsend, P. 251
Treadon, C.B. 29, 85, 170, 174, 227, 295
Trustrum, M. 44–5, 49, 50, 53, 54, 55, 59, 60, 99, 101, 290, 291
Twigg, E. 237

United Nations 181
Usiskin, M. 269

Van Butsele, G. 12
Van der Kolk, B. 52, 68, 77
Van Lith, T. 160
Vaslamatzis, G. 34, 295
Victoria and Albert Museum 55
Visnola, D. 27

Wacquant, L. 137, 154
Wadeson, H. 174, 303, 306
Wald, J. 124
Waller, D. 96, 109, 114, 126, 129, 207, 210, 226
Walsh, V. 194
Welander, M. 266, 268, 285
Wertheim-Cahen, T. 69
Whelan, G. 39
White, W. 137
Willig, C. 37
Winnicott, D.W. 49, 56, 99, 101, 148, 219, 290, 291
Wieseman, M.E. 246
Wood, C. 29

Yalom, I. 30, 31, 35, 53, 118
Yenawine, P. 96
Yin, R. 37
Yukhnevich, M. 83

Zhvitiashvili, N. 92
Zinchenko, V. 96